ROBUSTNESS IN IDENTIFICATION AND CONTROL

APPLIED INFORMATION TECHNOLOGY

INDUSTRIAL ARTIFICIAL INTELLIGENCE SYSTEMS
Lucas Pun

KNOWLEDGE BASED SYSTEM DIAGNOSIS, SUPERVISION, AND CONTROL
Edited by Spyros G. Tzafestas

PARALLEL PROCESSING TECHNIQUES FOR SIMULATION
Edited by M. G. Singh, A. Y. Allidina, and B. K. Daniels

ROBUSTNESS IN IDENTIFICATION AND CONTROL
Edited by M. Milanese, R. Tempo, and A. Vicino

ROBUSTNESS IN IDENTIFICATION AND CONTROL

Edited by

M. Milanese and R. Tempo

Turin Polytechnic
Turin, Italy

and

A. Vicino

University of Florence
Florence, Italy

PLENUM PRESS • NEW YORK AND LONDON

Library of Congress Cataloging in Publication Data

International Workshop on Robustness in Identification and Control (1988: Turin, Italy)
Robustness in identification and control / edited by M. Milanese and R. Tempo and A. Vicino.
p. cm.—(Applied information technology)
Includes bibliographical references and index.
ISBN-13: 978-1-4615-9554-0 e-ISBN-13: 978-1-4615-9552-6
DOI: 10.1007/978-1-4615-9552-6
1. System identification—Congresses. 2. Control theory—Congresses. I. Milanese, M. II. Tempo, R. III. Vicino, A. IV. Title. V. Series.
QA402.I585 1988 89-16081
004.2'1—dc20 CIP

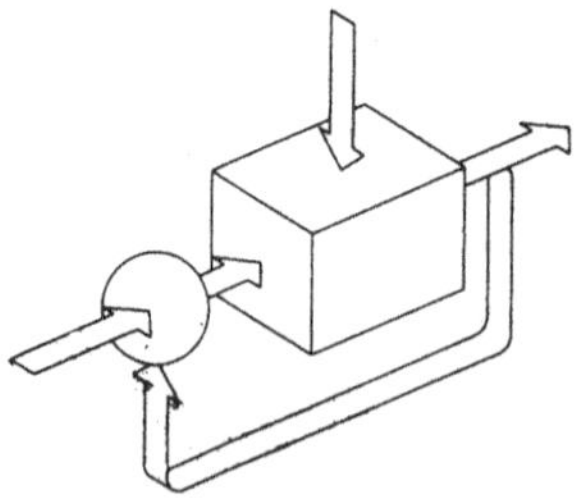

Proceedings of an International Workshop on Robustness in Identification and Control, held June 10–12, 1988, in Turin, Italy

Softcover reprint of the hardcover 1st edition 1989

A Division of Plenum Publishing Corporation
233 Spring Street, New York, N.Y. 10013

FOREWORD

This volume collects most of the papers presented at the *International Workshop on Robustness in Identification and Control*, held in Torino (Italy) in 1988. The main focal point of the workshop was *Unknown But Bounded* uncertainty and associated robustness issues in identification and control.

Recent years have seen a growing interest in studying models which include unknown but bounded uncertainty. The motivation for dealing with such models is derived from robustness considerations. In many applications, some performance specification must be met for all admissible variations of the uncertain parameters. A second motivation for models with this type of uncertainty stems from the fact that the statistical description of uncertain variables may not be well known or even not suitable. For example, in some cases, only a small number of measurements is available and the resulting errors are due to analog-digital conversion, modelling approximation or round-off, so that a statistical description may actually be unreliable.

The interest in unknown but bounded setting is certainly not new. In fact, engineering practice demands for appropriate algorithms in dealing with finite sample properties, finite parameter variations, tolerance analysis, etc. Despite the natural need for such methods, the lack of sufficiently well assessed theoretical results and algorithms prevented a systematic use of these procedures until recent years. However, in the last few years, important advances have been made both in estimation theory and in stability analysis.

The aim of the workshop was to bring together leading researchers in these areas, in order to assess the current state of the art and to discuss future trends and new promising research directions. Researchers from different fields, including mathematics, information-based complexity, circuit theory, modelling, identification and control, attended the workshop looking for sinergy of approaches developed and used in different research areas.

The workshop was held under the auspices of Ministero della Ricerca Scientifica e Tecnologica, Regione Piemonte, Cittá di Torino and Politecnico di Torino. We are pleased to thank the financial contribution of Assessorato della Cultura della Regione Piemonte, Assessorati al Lavoro e al Turismo della Cittá di Torino, Camera di Commercio di Torino and FIAT. We would like to acknowledge the support of Dipartimento di Automatica e Informatica (Politecnico di Torino) and of Centro di Elaborazione Numerale dei Segnali (Consiglio Nazionale delle Ricerche).

Finally, we are indebted to B. Ross Barmish (University of Wisconsin-Madison), Gustavo Belforte and Basilio Bona (Politecnico di Torino) who acted, together with the editors of this volume, as Scientific and Organizing Committee.

M. Milanese, R. Tempo and A. Vicino

Torino, February 1989

CONTENTS

1. Robust Identification and Complexity

2. Robust Stability and Control

1. ROBUST IDENTIFICATION AND COMPLEXITY

ESTIMATION AND PREDICTION IN THE PRESENCE OF UNKNOWN BUT BOUNDED UNCERTAINTY: A SURVEY

M.Milanese
Dipartimento di Automatica e Informatica
Politecnico di Torino
Corso Duca degli Abruzzi 24
10129 Torino- Italy
e-mail MILANESE@ITOPOLI.BITNET

INTRODUCTION

Many different problems such as linear and nonlinear regressions, parameter and state estimation of dynamic systems, state space and time series prediction, interpolation,smoothing, function approximation have a common general structure that here is referred to as *generalized estimation problem.* In all these problems one has to evaluate some unknown variable using available data (often obtained by measurements on a real process). Available data are always associated with some uncertainty and it is necessary to evaluate how this uncertainty affects the estimated variables.

Obviously the solution of the problem depends on the type of assumptions that are made on the uncertainty. The cases most investigated so far are unquestionably related to the assumption that uncertainty is given by an additive random noise with (partially) known probabilty density function (pdf). Within this context, the most important and widely used results are related to the theory of Maximum Likelihood Estimators (MLE). However, the application of the theory to real word problems may be not appropriate, due to many drawbacks such as the ones briefly recalled in the following.

MLE are asymptotically efficient, but it is difficult to evaluate if the available data are sufficient to be "near" to efficiency, that is to the Cramer-Rao lower bound of the estimates covariance matrix. For small number of data it should be useful to have an upper bound of the estimates covariance matrix as well. However tight upper bounds are difficult to evaluate. In this condition the evaluation of the Cramer-Rao lower bound may be critical. As a result, the indications on the estimates uncertainty may be by no means reliable. It is difficult to evaluate the effect of not exact verification of assumed statistical hypotheses (form of the pdf, correlations,etc).

Moreover in many situations the very random nature of uncertainty may be questionable. For example the real process generating the actual data may be very complex (large scale, nonlinear, time varying) so that only simplified models can be practically used in the estimation process. Then the residuals of the estimated model have a component due to deterministic structural errors, and treating them as purely random variables may lead to very disappointing results.

An interesting alternative approach, referred to as *set membership or Unknown But Bounded (UBB)* error description, has been pioneered by the work of Witsenhusen and Schweppe in the late 60's ([1,2,3]). In this approach uncertainty is described by an additive noise which is known only to have given upper and lower bounds. Motivation for this approach is the fact that in many practical cases the UBB error description is more realistic and less demanding than the statistical one. However despite the appeal of its features, the UBB approach has not yet reached a wide diffusion. An important reason for this is certainly the fact that until the first 80's reasonable results and algorithms had been obtained only for uncertainty bounds of integral type (mainly l_2), while in practical applications pointwise bounds (l_∞) are mainly of interest.

Real advances have been obtained in the last few years for the pointwise bounds case, leading to theoretical results and algorithms which can be properly applied to practical problems where the use of statistical techniques is questionable.

The purpose of this paper is to review these results and to present them in a unified framework in order to contribute to a better understanding of the present state of the art in the field and to stimulate further basic and applied researches.

Of course, a survey of a field by an author working actively on the subject is certainly biased by the author's opinion and experience. This survey is no exception.

PROBLEM FORMULATION AND MAIN CONCEPTS

This section provides main definitions and notation used in the paper. We formulate a general framework allowing the main results in the literature to be presented in a unifying view. Such formulation can be sketched as follows ([4,5]).

We have a problem element λ (for example a dynamic system or a time function) and we are interested in evaluating some function $S(\lambda)$ of this problem element (for example some parameter of the dynamic system or particular value of the time function). We suppose not to know exactly λ, but to have only some information on it. In particular we assume that it is an element of a set K of possible problem elements and that some function $F(\lambda)$ is measured. Moreover we suppose that exact measurements are not available and actual measurements y are corrupted by some error ρ.

The estimation problem consists in finding an estimator ϕ providing an approximation $\phi(y) \approx S(\lambda)$ using the available data y and evaluating some measure of such approximation. A geometric sketch is shown in Fig.1.

To be more precise let us now proceed to formal definitions.

Spaces and operators

Let Λ be linear normed n-dimensional space over the real field. Consider a given operator S, called a *solution operator*, which maps Λ into Z

$$S : \Lambda \rightarrow Z \tag{1}$$

where Z is a linear normed l-dimensional space over the real field. Our aim is to estimate an element $S(\lambda)$ of the space Z, knowing approximate information about

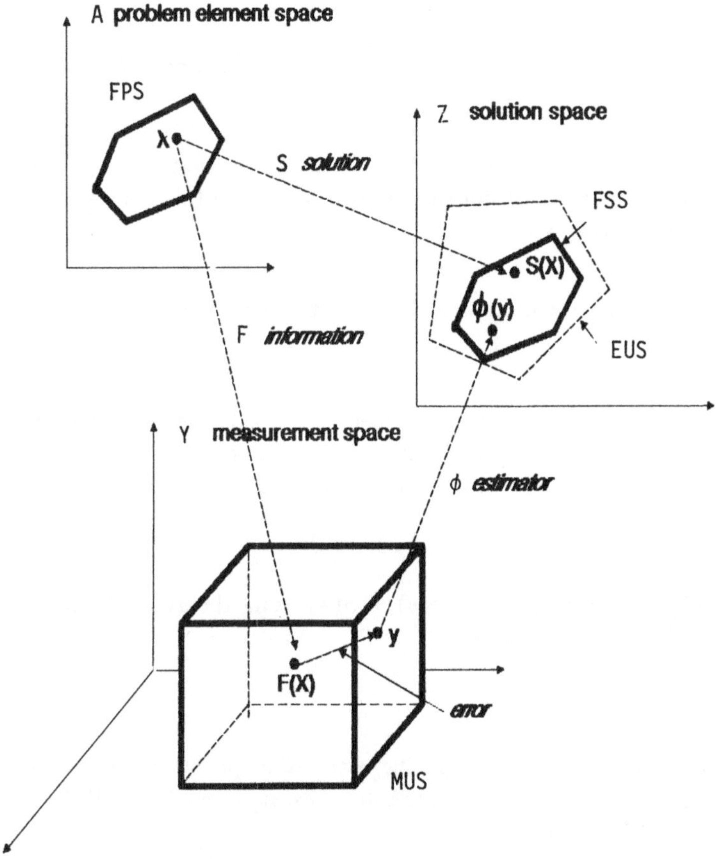

Fig.1 Generalized Estimation Problem

the element λ. We suppose that two kinds of information may be available. The first one (often referred to as a priori information) is expressed by assuming that $\lambda \in K$, where K is a subset of Λ. In most cases K is given as:

$$K = \{\lambda \in \Lambda; ||P(\lambda - \lambda_0)|| \leq 1\} \tag{2}$$

where P is a linear operator and λ_0 is a known problem element. The second kind of information is usually provided by the knowledge of some function $F(\lambda)$, where F, called *information operator*, maps Λ into a linear normed m-dimensional space Y

$$F : \Lambda \to Y. \tag{3}$$

Spaces Λ, Z, Y are called respectively *problem element*, *solution* and *measurement* spaces. In the following, unless otherwise specified, we assume that Λ and Z are equipped with l_∞ norms and Y is equipped with an l_∞^w norm[1].

In general, due to the presence of noise, exact information $F(\lambda)$ about λ is not available and only perturbed information y is given. In this context, uncertainty is assumed to be additive, i.e.

$$y = F(\lambda) + \rho \tag{4}$$

where the error term ρ is unknown but bounded some given positive number ϵ

$$||y - F(\lambda)|| \leq \epsilon \tag{5}$$

Note that if an l_∞^w norm in measurement space Y is used,pointwise bounds with different values on every measurement can be treated.

An *algorithm* ϕ is an operator (in general nonlinear) from Y into Z

$$\phi : Y \to Z \tag{6}$$

i.e., it provides an approximation $\phi(y)$ of $S(\lambda)$ using the available data y. Such an algorithm is also called *estimator*.

Example

As a simple example of how a specific estimation problem fits into this general framework, consider a problem of parameter estimation of an ARMA model. Let us consider the ARMA model

$$y_k = \sum_{i=1}^{p} \nu_i y_{k-i} + \sum_{i=1}^{q} \theta_i \rho_{k-i} + \rho_k \tag{7}$$

where ρ_k is an unknown but bounded sequence

$$|\rho_k| \leq \epsilon_k, \quad \forall k \tag{8}$$

To keep notation as simple as possible, consider the case $p = q$.

[1]The l_∞^w norm is defined as

$$||y||_\infty^w = \max_i w_i |y_i|, \quad w_i > 0$$

Suppose that m values $[y_1, ..., y_m]$ are known and the aim is to estimate parameters $[\nu_i, \theta_i]$.

Λ can be defined as the $2p+m-1$-dimensional space with elements

$$\lambda = [\nu_1, ..., \nu_p, \theta_1, ..., \theta_p, \rho_1, ..., \rho_{m-1}]^T \tag{9}$$

being K defined by (8). Z is the $2p$-dimensional space with elements

$$z = [\nu_1, ..., \nu_p, \theta_1, ..., \theta_p]^T . \tag{10}$$

$S(\lambda)$ is linear and is given by

$$S(\lambda) = [I_{2p} \mid \emptyset]\lambda \tag{11}$$

where I_{2p} is the identity matrix of dimension $(2p, 2p)$ and $\emptyset$ is the null matrix of dimension $(2p, m-1)$.

Y is an $m-p$ dimensional space with elements $y = [y_{p+1}, ...y_m]^T$.

$F(\lambda)$ is given by

$$\begin{bmatrix} F_1(\lambda) \\ ... \\ F_{m-p}(\lambda) \end{bmatrix} = \begin{bmatrix} \nu_1 y_p + & \cdots & +\nu_p y_1 + \theta_1 \rho_p + & \cdots & +\theta_p \rho_1 \\ ... & ... & ... & ... & ... \\ \nu_1 y_{m-1} + & \cdots & +\nu_p y_{m-p} + \theta_1 \rho_{m-1} + & \cdots & \theta_p \rho_{m-p} \end{bmatrix} \tag{12}$$

Relevant sets

Now we introduce the following sets which play key roles in defining the main concepts and results.

- MUS_y:*Measurement Uncertainty Set*

$$MUS_y = \{\tilde{y} \in Y : ||\tilde{y} - y||_\infty^w \leq \epsilon\} \tag{13}$$

- EUS_ϕ: *Estimates Uncertainty Set* (for a given estimator ϕ)

$$EUS_\phi = \phi(MUS_y) \tag{14}$$

- FPS_y: *Feasible Problems Set*

$$FPS_y = \{\lambda \in K : ||y - F(\lambda)||_\infty^w \leq \epsilon\} \tag{15}$$

- FSS_y: *Feasible Solutions Set*

$$FSS_y = S(FPS_y) \tag{16}$$

Note the difference between EUS_ϕ and FSS_y. The former depends on the particular estimator ϕ used and gives all possible estimated values that could be obtained for all possible measurements consistent with the actual measurement y and the given error bounds. The latter depends only on the data of the problem and gives all possible values which are consistent with the available information on the problem. In the literature FSS_y has been given also different names such as membership-set estimate and likelihood set. We assume that FSS_y is nonempty, i.e., that the model structure is able to represent the data y . We also assume that FSS_y is bounded; otherwise, information $F(\lambda)$ is too poor to solve the problem with finite error, i.e.there are identifiability problems.

An exact description of FSS_y or EUS_ϕ is in general not simple. Then approximate descriptions are often looked for, using simply shaped sets like boxes or ellipsoids containing *(outer bounding)* or contained in *(inner bounding)* the set of interest (see Fig.2). In particular Minimum volume Outer Box (MOB) or Ellipsoid (MOE) and Maximum volume Inner Box (MIB) or Ellipsoid (MIE) are clearly of interest. Information of great practical interest is also provided by the Values Uncertainty Intervals (VUI) and Estimates Uncertainty Intervals (EUI), giving the maximum range of possible variations of, respectively, the feasible values and the estimated ones. The VUI's are defined as

$$VUI_i = [z_i^m, z_i^M] \quad i = 1, \ldots, l\,. \tag{17}$$

where

$$\begin{aligned} z_i^m &= \inf_{z \in FSS_y} z_i \quad i = 1, \ldots, l \\ z_i^M &= \sup_{z \in FSS_y} z_i \quad i = 1, \ldots, l \end{aligned} \tag{18}$$

Note that the VUI's are the sizes (along coordinate axis) of the MOB_{FSS} (MOB containing FSS_y), so that these two problems are equivalent.

The EUI's are defined in the same way substituting EUS_ϕ for FSS_y.

Errors and optimality concepts

Algorithm approximation will be measured according to the following errors:

- *Y-local* error $E_y^\epsilon(\phi)$

$$E_y^\epsilon(\phi) = \sup_{\lambda \in FPS_y} \|S(\lambda) - \phi(y)\| \tag{19}$$

- *Λ-local* error $E_\lambda^\epsilon(\phi)$

$$E_\lambda^\epsilon(\phi) = \sup_{y \in MUS_{F(\lambda)}} \|S(\lambda) - \phi(\ y)\| \tag{20}$$

- *global* error $E^\epsilon(\phi)$

$$E^\epsilon(\phi) = \sup_{y \in Y} E_y^\epsilon(\phi) \tag{21}$$

Dependence on ϵ will be dropped out in subsequent notation, except when necessary.

Algorithms minimizing these types of errors will be indicated respectively as $Y-$ *locally*, $\Lambda -$ *locally* and *globally* optimal.

It is worthwhile to observe that local optimality is a stronger property than global optimality. In fact, for example, a Y-locally optimal algorithm minimizes the local error $E_y(\phi)$ for all data y, while a globally optimal algorithm minimizes the global error $E(\phi)$ only for the worst data. In other words, a Y-locally optimal algorithm is also globally optimal, while the converse is not necessarily true.

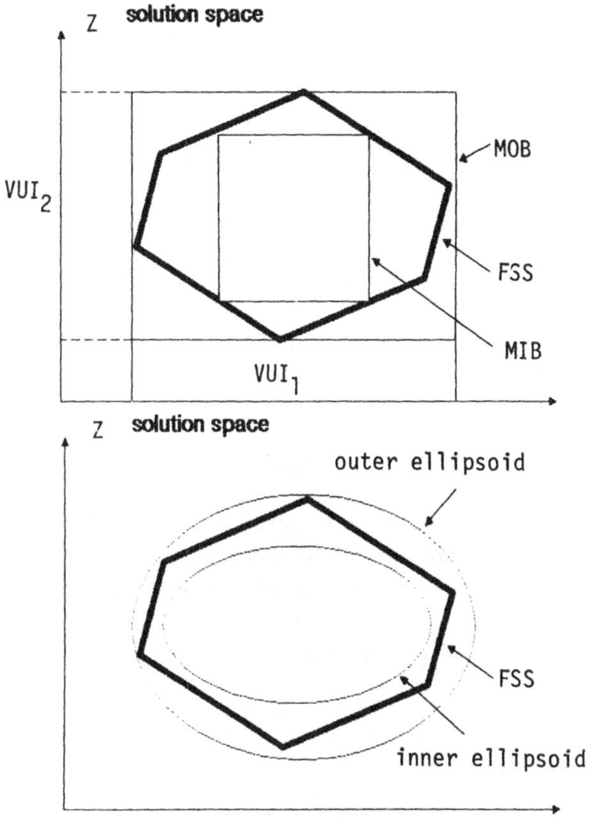

Fig.2 Box and ellipsoid bounding

We notice that Y−local optimality is of particular interest in system identification problems, in which a set of measurements y is available and one wants to determine the best achievable estimate $S(\lambda)$ for each possible y using an algorithm $\phi(y)$. Also Λ-local optimality is a particularly meaningful property in estimation problems, since it ensures the minimum uncertainty of the estimates for the worst measurement y, for any (unknown) element $\lambda \in K$.

Classes of estimators

Now we introduce some class of estimators whose properties have been investigated in the literature.

The first one is related to the idea of taking as estimate of $S(\lambda)$ the Chebicheff center of FSS_y. The center of FSS_y, $c(FSS_y) \in Z$, and the corresponding radius, $rad(FSS_y)$, are defined by

$$\sup_{z \in FSS_y} \|c(FSS_y) - z\| = \inf_{\tilde{z} \in Z} \sup_{z \in FSS_y} \|\tilde{z} - z\| = rad(FSS_y) \tag{22}$$

A *central estimator* ϕ^c is defined as

$$\phi^c(y) = c(FSS_y) \tag{23}$$

The second class is the analogous of unbiased estimators in statistical theory, which give exact values if applied to exact data.

An estimator ϕ is *correct* if

$$\phi(F(\lambda)) = S(\lambda) \quad \forall \lambda \in \Lambda \tag{24}$$

Clearly such class is meaningful when $l < m$, that is when there are more measurements then variables to estimate, as it happens in most practical cases. This class contains most of the commonly used estimators, such as for example projection estimators.

A *projection estimator* ϕ^p is defined as

$$\phi^p(y) = S(\lambda_y) \tag{25}$$

where $\lambda_y \in \Lambda$ is such that

$$\|y - S(\lambda_y)\| = \inf_{\lambda \in \Lambda} \|y - S(\lambda)\| \tag{26}$$

The most widely investigated and used estimators in this class are Least Square estimators (ϕ^{LS}), which are projection estimators when Hilbert (l_2) norm in used in space Y. Also l_1 and l_∞ projection estimators have been often considered.

In the next sections we will review the results available in the literature regarding the following aspects:

- existence and characterization of estimators, optimal with respect to some of the above defined optimality concepts.
- actual computation of the derived optimal estimator
- evaluation of the errors of such estimators
- description of FSS_y and EUS_ϕ.

Whenever possible, a statistical counterpart of the presented results will be indicated, based on the analogy: Y-local optimality$\Longleftrightarrow$minimum variance optimality, $EUS_\phi$$\Longleftrightarrow$estimate's pdf, EUI's $\Longleftrightarrow$ estimate's confidence intervals.

NON LINEAR PROBLEMS

A first important result is related to the existence of a Y-locally optimal estimator. It is worthnoting that no general results are available for Λ-locally optimal estimators.

Result 1 ([4,6])

- A central estimator ϕ^c is $Y-$locally optimal

$$E_y(\phi^c) \leq E_y(\phi) \quad \forall y \in Y, \, \forall \phi \tag{27}$$

- Its Y-local error is

$$E_y(\phi^c) = rad(FSS_y) \tag{28}$$

□

This result is the counterpart of the conditional mean theorem in statistics. As it happens for conditional mean estimators, central estimators are in general difficult to be actually computed. In fact the computation of ϕ^c involves the knowlwdge of FSS_y, which may be a very complex set (not convex, not simply connected), and difficult to computationally describe.

Several approaches have been proposed to describe FSS_y, mainly in papers related to dynamic systems parameter estimation. In [7] a random sample of parameters is generated by a Monte Carlo technique, and their belonging to FSS_y is verified directly through use of (4) and (5).

In [8] and [9] global optimization methods based on random search are used to construct the boundary of FSS_y. In [8] projections of FSS_y onto coordinate one-dimensional or two-dimensional subspaces are looked for. In [9] intersections of the boundary of FSS_y with bundles of straight lines centered at points inside FSS_y are searched. In particular, these numerical methods can generate a sequence of boxes contained in the MOB_{FSS} and converging to it with probability one (or, in other words, a sequence of approximate uncertainty intervals contained in the true VUI's and converging to them with probability one). However, this convergence property is not very useful in practice, because *no estimate is given of the distance of the achieved solution from the global solution.* Moreover all these approaches suffer the curse of dimensionality. These reasons motivate the interest in looking for less detailed but more easily computable information on FSS_y.

A first important result in this direction is that the computation of ϕ^c and of its Y-local error do not require the exact knowledge of FSS_y, but only of the MOB_{FSS}.

Result 2 ([5])

- The center $c(FSS_y)$ can be computed as

$$c_i(FSS_y) = (z_i^M + z_i^m)/2 \quad i = 1,\dots,l \tag{29}$$

- The radius $rad(FSS_y)$ can be computed as

$$rad(FSS_y) = \max_i (z_i^M - z_i^m)/2 \tag{30}$$

where z_i^m and z_i^M are given by (18).

□

Result 2 implies that the computation of central algorithm,of VUI'S and of MOB_{FSS} are equivalent problems. Their solution requires the solution of only $2l$ optimizations problems of the type (18), which however are in general not convex, exhibiting local extrema.

Any of the methods available in the literature, ranging from random global searches used in the previously cited papers to techniques of successive linearizations ([10]), give only approximate solutions and, more seriously, they do not provide any assesment on how far the approximate solution is from the correct one.

Exact solutions have been derived for two interesting classes of problems. The first one is related to the case in which (4) represents output-error equations and the sign of the unknown parameters is known.

Result 3 ([11])

- Let

$$y_k = \tilde{y}_k + \rho_k \quad k = 1,\dots,m \tag{31}$$

$$\tilde{y}_k = \sum_{i=1}^{p} \nu_i \tilde{y}_{k-i} + \sum_{i=1}^{q} \theta_i u_{k-i} \tag{32}$$

where u_k is a known sequence and ρ_k is an unknown but bounded sequence

$$|\rho_k| \leq \epsilon_k, \quad \forall k \tag{33}$$

- The set of all feasible unknown parameters $[\theta_i, \nu_i]$ is described by the following set of inequalities for k=1,...,m

$$\sum_{i=1}^{p} \nu_i[-y_{k-i} - sign(\nu_i)\epsilon_{k-i}] + \sum_{i=1}^{q} \theta_i u_{k-i} \leq y_k + \epsilon_k \tag{34}$$

$$\sum_{i=1}^{p} \nu_i[-y_{k-i} + sign(\nu_i)\epsilon_{k-i}] + \sum_{i=1}^{q} \theta_i u_{k-i} \geq y_k - \epsilon_k \tag{35}$$

□

If $sign(\nu_i), i = 1, \ldots, p$ is known, (34) and (35) are linear inequalities defining the feasible parameter set, which is a polytope. Then its center, its inner and outer bounding boxes or ellipsoids and the parameter uncertainty intervals can be computed by the methods exposed in the next section.

The second (more general) class of problems, for which exact solutions to computation of ϕ^c, of MOB_{FSS} and of VUI's can be found, is the one for which $S(\lambda)$ and $F(\lambda)$ are polynomial functions.

Result 4 ([12])

- If $S(\lambda)$ and $F(\lambda)$ are polynomial and $\lambda \geq 0$, optimization problems (18) are signomial problems.

□

Signomial problems are in general not convex and may exhibit local extrema, but iterative algorithms can be designed, able to evaluate at each iteration lower and upper bounds of the global extremum. Moreover the sequences of *lower and upper bounds are guaranteed to converge monotonically to the global solution* ([13,12]).

The hypothesis of Result 4 covers large classes of problems of practical interest. In fact in ([12]) it is shown for example that *parameter estimation and prediction of multiexponential, ARMA, and state space discrete models lead to $S(\lambda)$ and $F(\lambda)$ polynomial.* Moreover the condition that all parameters are positive ($\lambda \geq 0$) is not a serious restriction. In fact, if a rough knowlewdge of the order of magnitude of the parameter range is available, it is possible to bring the set FSS_y in the positive orthant of Λ by means of a suitable translation of the origin of the problem element space. From these considerations and Result 2 it can be concluded that *an optimal estimator and its error can be exactly computed for several nonlinear problems of practical interest. No analogous result is available in the statistical context.*

It must be remarked that most of the papers in the literature focus on studying FSS_y, while very few results are available on EUS_ϕ. We now report a result showing that, for any correct estimator, FSS_y is an inner bounding set of EUS_ϕ.

Result 5 ([14])

- If ϕ is correct then

$$FSS_y \subseteq EUS_\phi \quad \forall y \in Y \tag{36}$$

□

Then it also results that, for correct estimators, the VUI's are lower bounds of the EUI's, that is

$$VUI_i \subseteq EUI_i \quad i = 1, \ldots, l \tag{37}$$

Computation of the EUI's is a difficult task, and in general only methods giving lower bounds of the EUI's are known (see for example [10] for an efficient method in the case of least square estimators).

The same difficulties occur in the statistical context, where only the Cramer-Rao lower bound of the estimates covariance matrix can be computed and it is not possible to estimate how bigger the actual covariance matrix is (unless Monte Carlo simulation is used). A difference is that in the UBB context, according to Result 4, the VUI's can be computed exactly for many nonlinear problems of practical interest. On the contrary the Cramer-Rao lower bound can only be approximately evaluated.

Now we consider the properties of projection estimators. In general they are not optimal with respect to any of the three considered type of errors ([15]). However they are "almost" Y-locally optimal (within a factor 2) as shown by the following result.

__Result 6__ ([15])

- For a projection operator ϕ^p it results

$$E_y(\phi^p) \leq 2\ \mathrm{rad}(FSS_y) \leq 2E_y(\phi) \quad \forall y \in Y,\ \forall \phi \tag{38}$$

□

Projection estimators have interesting properties of robustness with respect to inexact knowledge of uncertainty bound ϵ. Central estimators are not robust in such a sense: a central algorithm computed supposing that $\epsilon = \epsilon_0$ may be not optimal if the actual ϵ is different. A central estimates $\phi^c(y)$ may not even belong to the actual FSS_y and its Y-local error $E_y(\phi^c)$ may be greater than 2 rad(FSS_y).

On the contrary projection estimators preserve their almost Y-locally optimality properties in presence of bounded uncertainty on ϵ as shown by the next result.

__Result 7__ ([16])

- Let ϕ^p the projection estimator computed with $\epsilon = \epsilon_0$. Then

$$E_y^\epsilon(\phi^p) \leq 2\ \mathrm{rad}(FSS_y) \leq 2E_y^\epsilon(\phi) \quad \forall y \in Y,\ \forall \phi,\ \forall \epsilon \leq \epsilon_0 \tag{39}$$

□

Result 7 can be rephrased saying that *projection estimators are robustly almost Y-locally optimal.*

Note that projection estimators have nice properties also in a statistical context. For example l_2-projection estimator is the MLE if noise ρ is supposed gaussian, l_1-projection estimator is the MLE if noise is supposed to have Laplace pdf, l_∞-projection estimator is a MLE if noise is uniformly distributed. l_∞-projection estimators has also interesting robustness properties with respect to uncertainty in the pdf's knowledge ([17,18]).

LINEAR PROBLEMS

In this section we consider the case in which $S(\lambda)$ and $F(\lambda)$ are linear. In this case equation (4) is written as

$$y = \mathcal{A}\lambda + \rho \tag{40}$$

where $\mathcal{A}$ is a matrix of dimension (m, n).

These assumptions are restrictive, but include cases of practical interest such as parameter estimation of linear regressions, of AR models with polynomial trends and harmonic components ([14,5,19]), state estimation of dynamic systems ([20]), time series forecasting ([21]). Moreover if uncertainty bounds are not too large, linear theory can be used for a first approximate analysis using some linearization techniques.

Example

As an example of linear problem, let us consider state estimation of the following discrete, linear, time invariant dynamic system

$$\begin{cases} x(i+1) & = Ax(i) + Bu(i) \\ y(i) & = Cx(i) + \rho(i) \end{cases} \tag{41}$$

where $x(i)$, $y(i)$, $u(i)$ and $\rho(i)$ are, respectively, the state, observation, process noise and observation noise vectors; A, B and C are given matrices. For the sake of notation simplicity we suppose that x is l-dimensional and y, u, ρ are 1-dimensional.

We assume that the process and observation noise samples are unknown but bounded

$$|u(i)| \leq U_i, \quad \forall i \tag{42}$$

$$|\rho(i)| \leq \epsilon_i, \quad \forall i \tag{43}$$

Suppose that m values $[y(1), \ldots, y(m)]$ are known and the aim is to estimate $x(m)$.

Λ can be defined as the $l+m-1$-dimensional space with elements

$$\lambda = [x(1), u(1), \ldots, u(m-1)]^T \tag{44}$$

being K defined by (42).

Z is the l-dimensional space with elements

$$z = x(m) \tag{45}$$

Y is the $m-$dimensional space with elements

$$y = [y(1), \ldots, y(m)] \tag{46}$$

Solution and information operator are linear and are given by

$$S(\lambda) = [A^{m-1}, A^{m-2}B, \ldots, AB, B]\lambda \tag{47}$$

$$F(\lambda) = \begin{pmatrix} C & 0 & \ldots & 0 & 0 \\ CA & CB & \ldots & 0 & 0 \\ CA^2 & CAB & \ldots & 0 & 0 \\ \vdots & \vdots & \ddots & \vdots & \vdots \\ CA^{m-2} & CA^{m-3}B & \ldots & CB & 0 \\ CA^{m-1} & CA^{m-2}B & \ldots & CAB & CB \end{pmatrix} \lambda \tag{48}$$

□

From Result 1 we know that in general a central estimator is Y-locally and globally optimal. Next result shows that it is also correct and Λ-locally optimal in the class os correct estimators.

<u>**Result 8**</u> ([22])

- ϕ^c is correct
- ϕ^c is Y-locally optimal

$$E_y(\phi^c) \leq E_y(\phi) \quad \forall \phi \tag{49}$$

- ϕ^c is Λ-locally optimal (among correct estimators)

$$E_\lambda(\phi^c) \leq E_\lambda(\phi) \quad \forall \lambda \in K, \ \forall \phi \text{ correct} \tag{50}$$

□

In ([15]) Result 8 is shown to hold for any norm in Y.

Note that under the present assumptions FSS_y and FPS_y are polytopes. Then from Result 2 it follows that ϕ^c and its Y-local error $E_y(\phi^c)$ can be obtained by solving the $2l$ linear programming problems (18).

Next result shows that a linear estimator can be computed, which is correct, globally optimal, and Λ-locally optimal within the class of correct estimators, representing the counterpart of the Gauss-Markov theory in statistical estimation.

<u>**Result 9**</u> ([14,5])

Let $K = \Lambda$ and $m \geq n$. Then there exists a linear estimator H^* such that

- H^* is correct
- H^* is globally optimal

$$E(H^*) \leq E(\phi) \quad \forall \phi \tag{51}$$

- H^* is Λ-locally optimal (among correct estimators)

$$E_\lambda(H^*) \leq E_\lambda(\phi) \quad \forall \lambda \in \Lambda, \ \forall \phi \text{ correct} \tag{52}$$

- Its errors are

$$E(H^*) = E_\lambda(H^*) = E_{A\lambda}(H^*) = \text{rad}(FSS_{A\lambda}) \quad \forall \lambda \in \Lambda \tag{53}$$

□

Estimator H^* can be computed from the knowledge of the active constraints of the linear programming problems (18) with $y = 0$ ([14,5]).

In case that an l_2 norm is used in Y, H^* can be be computed by least square. In fact, under this assumption, least square estimator is linear and correct, robustly Y-locally optimal and Λ-locally optimal within the class of correct estimators, as shown by the following result.

Result 10 ([15,16])

Let $K = \Lambda$, $m \geq n$ and Y be a Hilbert space. Let ϕ^{LS} be the projection (Least Square) estimator computed with $\epsilon = \epsilon_0$. Then

- ϕ^{LS} is central
- ϕ^{LS} is linear and correct
- ϕ^{LS} is robustly Y-locally optimal

$$E_y^\epsilon(\phi^{LS}) \leq E_y^\epsilon(\phi) \quad \forall y \in Y,\ \forall \phi,\ \forall \epsilon \leq \epsilon_0 \tag{54}$$

- ϕ^{LS} is Λ-locally optimal (among correct estimators)

$$E_\lambda(\phi^{LS}) \leq E_\lambda(\phi) \quad \forall \lambda \in \Lambda,\ \forall \phi \text{ correct} \tag{55}$$

□

Sets FPS_y, FSS_y and EUS_ϕ,(for linear ϕ), are polytopes defined by sets of linear inequalities. This is not the simplest way to describe them (for example many linear inequalities may not concur to defining the polytope) and simpler descriptions could be of interest. Perhaps the simplest way to characterize a polytope P is through its vertices. Algorithms exist able to compute recursively the vertices of a polytope P_k, defined by the first k measurements, from the knowledge of P_{k-1} and the k-th measurement ([23,24,25]). It is interesting to note that the number of vertices is usually much smaller than $2l^m$ (theorical maximum). For example Monte Carlo simulations on ARMAX models parameter estimation ([25]), have shown that the mean number of vertices of FSS_y is approximately constant for $m > 50$. For $l = 4$ and $l = 5$, for example, they are around 5 and 15 respectively.

Polytopes can be represented alternatively by describing their faces. In ([26]) this representation is used to derive a recursive algorithm. This approach seems more involved than the previous one, but it allows also the recursive computation of an outer bounding polytope with a fixed number of faces, leading to an approximate description of the polytope of interest by means of a polytope of prescribed complexity.

The most investigated approaches to approximate description of polytopes are through ellipsoid and box bounding. A recursive algorithm for outer bounding ellipsoid computation has been proposed in ([27]), for the case of parameter estimation, where the polytope of interest is the feasible parameter set. The underlying idea is as follows.

Let OE_{k-1} be the outer ellipsoid bounding P_{k-1}. Let R_k be the feasible parameter set corresponding only to the k-th measurement

$$R_k = \{\lambda \in \Lambda : y_k - \epsilon_k \leq a_k^T \lambda \leq y_k + \epsilon_k\} \tag{56}$$

where a_k^T is the k-th row of $\mathcal{A}$.

Clearly $P_k \subseteq OE_{k-1} \cap R_k$. OE_k is computed as the minimal volume ellipsoid containing $OE_{k-1} \cap R_k$, and then containing P_k also.

If ellipsoids OE_k are defined by their centers λ_k^c and positive definite matrix Σ_k according to

$$OE_k = \{\lambda \in \Lambda : (\lambda - \lambda_k^c)^T \Sigma_k^{-1} (\lambda - \lambda_k^c) \leq 1\} \tag{57}$$

the following recursive algorithm results, very similar to recursive least squares algorithm (Kalman filter).

<u>**Result 11**</u> ([27])

- OE_k can be computed by the recursion

$$\lambda_k^c = \lambda_{k-1}^c + \frac{\sigma_k V_k a_k \nu_k}{\epsilon_k^2} \tag{58}$$

$$\Sigma_k = (1 + \sigma_k - \frac{\sigma_k \nu_k^2}{\epsilon_k^2 + \sigma_k \mu_k}) V_k \tag{59}$$

where

$$V_k = \Sigma_{k-1} - \frac{\sigma_k \Sigma_{k-1} a_k a_k^T \Sigma_{k-1}}{\epsilon_k^2 + \sigma_k \mu_k} \tag{60}$$

$$\nu_k = y_k - a_k^T \lambda_{k-1} \tag{61}$$

$$\mu_k = a_k^T \Sigma_{k-1} a_k \tag{62}$$

and σ_k is the positive solution of the equation

$$(l-1)\mu_k^2 \sigma_k^2 + [(2l-1)\epsilon_k^2 - \mu_k + \nu_k^2]\mu_k \sigma_k + \epsilon_k^2 [l(\epsilon_k^2 - \nu_k^2) - \mu_k] = 0 \tag{63}$$

□

A similar approach can be used for the recursive computation of inner bounding ellipsoids ([19]). Let IE_{k-1} the inner bounding ellipsoid contained in P_{k-1}. Then IE_k is chosen as the maximal volume ellipsoid such that

$$IE_k \subseteq IE_{k-1} \cap R_k \subseteq P_k \tag{64}$$

The resulting recursive algorithm is much as for the outer bounding ellipsoid and is not reported here.

The main drawback of these recursive algorithms is that *they do not give the minimal and maximal volume ellipsoids bounding the feasible parameter set* ([28,19]). Since IE_k has an unfortunate tendency to shrink rapidly and soon vanish, it turns out that the inclusion $IE_k \subset P_k \subset OE_k$ in practice may not give any reasonable information on how loose bound OE_k is.

On the contrary extremal volume inner and outer boxes can be exactly computed.

MOB_{FSS} can be computed using linear programming directly from (18) or using the vertices of FSS_y (if known). With the first method one has to solve $2l$ linear programming problems with n variables and $2m$ inequalities constraints.

Methods to compute the maximal volume box contained in FSS_y (MIB_{FSS}) are at present not known, unless the shape of the box is given. We assume that the box looked for belongs to a family of boxes $B^c_v(\delta)$ of fixed shape and centered at some point λ^c

$$B^c_v(\delta) = \{\lambda \in \Lambda : \|\lambda - \lambda^c\|^v_\infty \leq \delta\}, \quad \delta \geq 0, \quad v_1, \ldots, v_n \geq 0 \tag{65}$$

where $v_1, \ldots, v_n$ are given weights which determine the shape of the box.

The following result shows that the MIB_{FSS} of given shape can be computed by solving one linear programming problem with $n+1$ variables and $2m+1$ inequalities constraints.

Result 12 ([29])

- The MIB_{FSS} of the form (65) has size $\bar{\delta}$ and center $\bar{\lambda^c}$ solution of

$$\sup_{\delta,\lambda^c:\left\{\begin{array}{c}\delta > 0\\ y^- + \delta|\mathcal{A}|v \leq \mathcal{A}\lambda^c \leq y^+ - \delta|\mathcal{A}|v\end{array}\right.} \delta \tag{66}$$

where

$$\begin{aligned}
|\mathcal{A}| &= \{|a_{ij}|\} && (67)\\
v &= [v_1, \ldots, v_n]^T && (68)\\
y^+ &= [y_1 + \epsilon w_1, \ldots, y_m + \epsilon w_m]^T && (69)\\
y^- &= [y_1 - \epsilon w_1, \ldots, y_m - \epsilon w_m]^T && (70)
\end{aligned}$$

□

OTHER TYPE OF RESULTS

In this section we briefly recall papers on topics related to estimation theory such as experiment design, estimation with reduced order models, uncertainty in the information operator. Almost all these papers consider linear problems.

Experiment design

In the previous sections information operator $\mathcal{A}$ is supposed given. In some practical application it is possible to choose among different information operators $\mathcal{A}$. For example it may be possible to choose the sampling times at which measurements are taken of the input and the output of a dynamic system to be identified. Then a natural choice is the one minimizing the error $E_\lambda(\phi^c)$ (*optimal information problem*). In ([30]) some results are given for the case in which information is provided by sampling. In ([22]) similar results are derived for more general classes of information. It is also shown that the optimal sampling times can be chosen a priori, and no improvements can be obtained by means of more sophisticated sampling schemes.

Another criterion is to minimize the volume of FSS_y. In ([19]) a recursive selection procedure is given, based on heuristics which avoids poor choices without guaranteeing the best. In ([31]), a characterization is given of the minimum number of sampling times assuring minimum volume $FSS_{A\lambda}$.

Reduced order models

In the previous sections it is supposed that the structure of the problem is given, for example the number of autoregressive and moving average terms for an ARMA model. In many cases, however, the structure of the problem and in particular the dimension of space Λ is not known and must be evaluated from the available information (*order determination problems*). In ([32]) some methods are discussed. Some of them are analogous to methods widely used for order determination in statistical contexts, such as the principal component analysys and singular value decomposition. A method is also proposed, based on the expected behaviour of FSS_y for overparametrized and underparametrized structures. A discussion on order determination problems can also be found in ([33]).

A second important problem is how estimation algorithms can take into account that approximated structures are used. The usual approach in statistical contexts is to ignore the deterministic nature of modeling errors, and eventually discard badly approximated structures with residuals evidently not satisfying the assumed statistical hypotheses. In the UBB approach modeling errors can be taken into account in a more natural way, since it is possible to evaluate bounds on such modeling errors ([34]). A deeper analysis is carried out in ([35]), where it is considered explicitely that using approximated structures corresponds to restrict the analysys to a subset $K \subset \Lambda$ *not containing the "true" problem element* λ. The concept of conditionally central estimator is introduced as an extension of central estimator, and it is shown that it is Y−locally optimal. In the same paper it is also shown that there are two possible ways of extending least squares estimators. The first one (indicated as RLSE, Reduced Least Squares Estimator), corresponds to what is usuallly done (more or less explicitly) when dealing with reduced order models. RLSE, however, does not preserve any of the interesting optimality properties of least squares estimators. A second type of extension is introduced (indicated as CLSE, Conditional Least Squares Estimator), which is shown to have interesting Λ−locally and Y−locally optimality properties.

Uncertain information operator

In some papers the case in which information matrix $\mathcal{A}$ is not exactly known, is studied. In particular perturbation of the type $\mathcal{A} = \mathcal{A}_o + \Delta\mathcal{A}$ have been considered, where $\mathcal{A}_o$ is given and $\Delta\mathcal{A}$ is not known but bounded. In ([36]) a modification of the recursive algorithm for outer ellipsoid bounding reported in Result 11 is proposed. In ([37]) and ([33]) two different extensions of FPS_y are considered. In ([37]) FPS_y is defined by considering that (15) holds for all $\Delta\mathcal{A}$ and is described by a set of $m2^{n+1}$ linear inequalities. In ([33]) FPS_y is defined by considering that (15) holds for some $\Delta\mathcal{A}$, and the problem of finding the corresponding MOB by means of suitable linear programming problems is also discussed.

APPLICATIONS

The UBB approach is now beginning to be applied to various application fields. Without pretending to give an exhaustive list of references, we cite some papers reporting applications to real word problems arising in biology ([14,38,39]), pharmacokinetics ([40]), time series prediction ([21]), economy ([41]), chemistry ([42]), image processing ([43]), ecology ([44,45]), measurement ([8,33,46]), tracking([47]).

ACKNOWLEDGMENTS

This work was partially supported by Ministero della Pubblica Amministrazione and Camera di Commercio di Torino.

References

[1] H.S. Witsenhausen, Sets of possible states of linear systems given perturbed observations. *IEEE Trans. Autom. Control,* vol. AC-13, pp.556-558, 1968.

[2] F.C. Schweppe, Recursive state estimation: unknown but bounded errors and system inputs. *IEEE Trans. Autom. Control,* vol. AC-13, pp.22-28, 1968.

[3] F.C. Schweppe, *Uncertain Dynamic Systems.* Prentice Halls ,Englewood Cliffs N.J., 1973.

[4] J.F. Traub and H. Woźniakowski, *A General Theory of Optimal Algorithms.* Academic Press, New York, 1980.

[5] M. Milanese and R. Tempo, Optimal algorithms theory for robust estimation and prediction. *IEEE Trans. Automat. Contr.*, vol. AC-30, pp. 730-738, 1985.

[6] C. A. Micchelli and T. J. Rivlin, A survey of optimal recovery, in: C. A. Micchelli and T. J. Rivlin, Eds. *Optimal Estimation in Approximation Theory,* pp. 1-54, Plenum, New York, 1977.

[7] K. Keesman,G.van Straten, Embedding of random scanning and principal component analysis in set-theoretic approach to parameter estimation. *Proc.12th IMACS World Congress,* Paris, 1988.

[8] M. K. Smit, A novel approach to the solution of indirect measurement problems with minimal error propagation. *Measurement,* vol. 1, pp. 181-190, 1983.

[9] E. Walter, H. Piet-Lahanier, Robust nonlinear parameter estimation in the bounded noise case. *Proc. 25th Conf. on Decision and Control,* Athens, 1986.

[10] G. Belforte, M. Milanese , Uncertainty intervals evaluation in presence of unknown but bounded errors. Nonlinear families of models. *Proc. 1st IASTED Symp. Modelling, Identification and Control,* Davos, 1981.

[11] T. Clement, Estimation d'incertitude parametrique dans un contexte de bruit inconnue mais borne. These de Doctorat, Institute National Polytechnique de Grenoble, 1987.

[12] M. Milanese, A. Vicino, Robust estimation and exact uncertainty intervals evaluation for nonlinear models. *Proc. of IMACS SMS88,* Cetraro, 1988.

[13] J.G. Ecker, Geometric programming: methods, computations and applications. *SIAM Review* , vol.1, n.3,pp. 339-362, 1980.

[14] M. Milanese, G. Belforte, Estimation theory and uncertainty intervals evaluation in presence of unknown but bounded errors. Linear families of models and estimators. *IEEE Trans. Autom. Control,* vol. AC-27, pp. 408-414, 1982.

[15] B.Z. Kacewicz, M. Milanese, R. Tempo and A. Vicino, Optimality of central and projection algorithms for bounded uncertainty, *Systems and Control Letters*, vol. 8, pp. 161-171, 1986.

[16] R. Tempo and G. Wasilkowski, Maximum likelihood estimators and worst case optimal algorithms for system identification. *Systems on Control Letters*, vol.10, pp.265-270, 1988.

[17] R.L. Launer and G.N. Wilkinson Eds. *Robustness in Statistics*. Academic Press, 1979.

[18] B.T. Poljak and J.Z. Tsypkin,Robust identification. *Automatica*, vol. 16, pp 53-63, 1980.

[19] J.P. Norton, Identification and application of bounded- parameter models. *Automatica*, vol. 23, pp. 497-507, 1987.

[20] R. Tempo, Robust estimation and filtering in the presence of bounded noise. *IEEE Trans. Automat. Contr.*, vol. AC-33, pp. 864-867, 1988.

[21] A. Vicino, R. Tempo, R. Genesio and M. Milanese,Optimal error and GMDH predictors: a comparison with some statistical techniques. *The Int. J. of Forecasting*, vol. 2, pp. 313-328, 1987.

[22] M. Milanese, R. Tempo and A. Vicino, Strongly optimal algorithms and optimal information in estimation problems. *J. Complexity*, vol. 2, pp. 78-94, 1986.

[23] V.V. Kapitonenko, Minmax identification in the case of uncertain original information. *Autom. and Remote Control,* pp. 166-169, 1982.

[24] H. Piet-Lahanier,E. Walter, Practical implementation of an exact and recursive algorithm for characterizing likelihood sets. *Proc.12th IMACS World Congress,* Paris, 1988.

[25] S.H. Mo,J.P. Norton, Recursive parameter-bounding algorithms which compute polytope bounds. *Proc.12th IMACS World Congress,* Paris, 1988.

[26] V.Broman, M.J. Shensa, A compact algorithm for the intersection and approximation of n-dimensional polytopes. *Proc.12th IMACS World Congress,* Paris, 1988.

[27] E. Fogel and F. Huang, On the value of information in system identification-Bounded noise case. *Automatica*, vol. 18, pp. 140-142, 1982.

[28] Belforte, G., B. Bona, An improved parameter identification algorithm for signals with unknown but bounded errors. *7th IFAC Symp. on Identification and System parameter Estimation*, York, 1985.

[29] G. Belforte, R. Tempo, A. Vicino, Robust parameter estimation for linear models with set-membership uncertainty. *Proc. of 8th IFAC Symposium on Identification and Parameter Estimation*, Beijing, 1988.

[30] G. Belforte, B. Bona and S. Frediani, Optimal sampling schedule for parameter estimation of linear models with unknown but bounded measurement errors. *IEEE Trans. on Automat. Contr.*, vol. AC-32, pp.179-182, 1987.

[31] L. Pronzato, E. Walter, Experiment design for membership set estimation: linear models with homogeneous and heterogeneous measurement errors. *Proc. First International Conference on Optimal Design and Analysis of Experiment,* Neuchâtel, 1988.

[32] J.P. Norton, Bounding techniques for model-structure selection, this volume.

[33] G. Belforte, B. Bona, V. Cerone, A bounded error approach to the tuning of a digital voltmeter. *Proc.12th IMACS World Congress,* Paris, 1988.

[34] R. Genesio, M. Milanese, A note on derivation and use of reduced order models. *IEEE Trans. on Automat. Contr.*, vol.AC-21, pp.118-122, 1976.

[35] B.Z. Kacewicz, M. Milanese and A. Vicino, Conditionally optimal algorithms and estimation of reduced order models. *Journal of Complexity*, vol.4, pp 73-85, 1988.

[36] T. Clement, S. Gentil, Recursive membership set estimation for ARMAX models: an output error approach. *Proc.12th IMACS World Congress,* Paris, 1988.

[37] R. Tempo, B.R. Barmish, J. Trujillo, Robust estimation and prediction using ARMA models: a nonstatistical approach. *Proc. of 8th IFAC Symposium on Identification and Parameter Estimation*, Beijing, 1988.

[38] G. Belforte, B. Bona, M. Milanese, Advanced modeling and identification techniques for metabolic processes. *CRC Journal Biomed. Eng.*, vol. 10, n. 4, pp. 275-316, 1983.

[39] J.P. Norton, Problems in identifying the dynamics of biological systems from very short records. *Proc.25th Conf. on Decision and Control,* Athens, 1986.

[40] R. Gomeni, H. Lahanier, E. Walter, Study of the pharmacokinetics of Betaxolol using set membership set estimation. *Proc. 3rd IMEKO Congress on Measurements in Clinical Medicine*, Edinbourg, 1986.

[41] M. Milanese, R. Tempo, A. Vicino, Optimal error predictor for economic models. *Int. J. Systems Sci.*, vol.19, n. 7, pp. 1189-1200, 1988.

[42] E. Walter, Y. Lecourtier, J. Happel, J.Y. Kao, Identifiabilty and distinguishability of fundamental parameters in catalytic methanation. *AIChE* , vol. 32, pp. 1360-1366, 1986.

[43] A. Venot, L. Pronzato, E. Walter, J.F. Lebruchec, A distribution-free criterion for robust identification with applications in system modelling and image processing. *Automatica,* vol. 22, n. 1, pp. 105-109, 1986.

[44] G. Van Straten, Analytical methods for parameter space delimitation and application to shallow-lake phytoplankton dynamics modeling. *Appl. Math. and Comp.*, vol. 17, pp. 459-482, 1985

[45] K.J. Keesman, G. Van Straten, Modified set theoretic identification of an ill defined water quality system from poor data. *Proc. of IAWPRC Symp. on System Analysis in Water Quality Management,* Pergamon Press, 1987.

[46] G. Belforte, B. Bona, E. Canuto, F. Donati, F. Ferraris, I. Gorini, S. Morei, M. Peisino, S. Sartori, Coordinate measuring machine and machine tools self calibration and error correction, *Annals CIRP*, vol. 36, n. 1, pp. 359-364, 1987.

[47] V.Broman, M.J. Shensa, Polytopes, a novel approach to tracking.*Proc.25th Conf. on Decision and Control,* Athens, 1986.

OPTIMAL SAMPLING DESIGN FOR PARAMETER ESTIMATION AND P-WIDTHS UNDER STOCHASTIC AND DETERMINISTIC NOISE

Charles A. Micchelli

Department of Mathematical Sciences
IBM Research Division
Thomas J. Watson Research Center
P.O. Box 218
Yorktown Heights, NY 10598

1. INTRODUCTION

We follow the interesting developments in the recent work of Milanese and Belforte [7], Belforte, Bona, and Frediani [1,2], and Milanese and Vicino [8] and address some questions suggested by these papers on the subject of parameter estimation in linear models subject to unknown additive and bounded noise. In addition, we treat the question of model selection for a given class of signals constrained to lie in some known set. We approach this latter question by presenting two formulations of p-widths subject to measurement errors and identify optimal linear models in some concrete cases. Both stochastic and deterministic p-widths are studied.

2. PARAMETER ESTIMATION

Let us begin with a general formulation of the problem which we will address. We are given a data vector $y \in \mathbb{R}^N$ which is supposed to represent $\Lambda\mu$ for some parameter vector $\mu \in \mathbb{R}^p$ where Λ is a given $N \times p$ matrix, $p \leq N$. Thus, under ideal circumstances there is some $\mu \in \mathbb{R}^p$ such that $y = \Lambda\mu$. However, in actual applications both measurement error and/or modeling errors are always present and so it is realistic to assume only that

$$y = \Lambda\mu + \varepsilon \tag{2.1}$$

where $\varepsilon \in \mathbb{R}^N$ is some unknown error vector. In the particular case of determining optimal sampling schedules, [1,2], a linear subspace of functions

$$\Lambda(t;\mu) = \sum_{j=1}^{p} \Lambda_j(t)\mu_j, \quad \mu = (\mu_1, \ldots, \mu_p) \tag{2.2}$$

defined over some set T are prescribed in advance. Observations $y = (y_1, \ldots, y_N)$ are available at some time parameters $\{t_1, \ldots, t_N\} \subseteq T$. Thus the parameter estimation problem becomes

$$y_i = \sum_{j=1}^{p} \Lambda_j(t_i)\mu_j + \varepsilon_i, \quad i = 1, \ldots, N$$

where it is desired to recover $\mu \in \mathbb{R}^p$ from this information.

Generally, the problem of parameter estimation requires finding a good choice for μ that best represents the data y in the model (2.1). The choice is always based on some information about the nature of the error vector which, as with the choice of Λ, are dependent on the application environment. Typically, ε is viewed as a random vector with a given covariance matrix. This leads to statistical estimation procedures for the selection of parameters. Alternatively, following [1,2,7,8] we consider parameter selection based on deterministic errors, which may take the form of simple linear inequalities on the error vector

$$|\varepsilon_i| \leq \delta_i, \quad i = 1, 2, \ldots, N. \tag{2.3}$$

Here $\delta_i > 0$ are known maximal error levels prescribed in advance. Equivalently, we may conveniently express these inequalities as $\|\varepsilon\|_\delta \leq 1$ by using the norm

$$\|\varepsilon\|_\delta := \max \{(\delta_i)^{-1} |\varepsilon_i| : 1 \leq i \leq N\}. \tag{2.4}$$

Any parameter selection strategy must be based on some measure of the size of the uncertainty set

$$U(y) := \{\mu : \|y - \Lambda\mu\| \leq 1\} \tag{2.5}$$

where here we allow for the choice of some other norm $\|\cdot\|$ on $\mathbb{R}^N$, besides $\|\cdot\|_\delta$ defined by (2.4). For instance, in the context of optimal sampling schedules the *Parameter Uncertainty Interval*

$$PUI_i := [\mu_i^m, \mu_i^M] \tag{2.6}$$

where

$$\begin{aligned} \mu_i^m &:= \min \{\mu_i : \mu \in U(y)\} \\ \mu_i^M &:= \max \{\mu_i : \mu \in U(y)\} \end{aligned}$$

was used as a parameter selection criterion in [1,2]. Later, we will be concerned with this measurement criterion as well but first we continue in a general manner and discuss the use of the

Chebyshev radius relative to some semi-norm $|\cdot|$ on $\mathbb{R}^p$ as means for parameter selection. Thus, we consider the quantity

$$r(U(y)) := \min\ \{\max\{|\mu - \nu| : \nu \in U(y)\} : \mu \in \mathbb{R}^p\} \tag{2.7}$$

which is the Chebyshev radius of $U(y)$. The number $r(U(y))$ measures the least error possible in using *one* parameter selection $\hat{\mu} \in \mathbb{R}^p$ which is chosen so that

$$\max\ \{|\hat{\mu} - \nu| : \nu \in U(y)\} = r(U(y)). \tag{2.8}$$

The parameter vector $\hat{\mu}$ is called the Chebyshev center of $U(y)$ (relative to $|\cdot|$). In the case that $|\mu| := |\mu_i|$, for some i, $1 \le i \le N$, in (2.7) above,

$$r(U(y)) = \frac{1}{2} \text{ length } PUI_i$$

and $\hat{\mu}$ is any vector in $\mathbb{R}^p$ such that $\hat{\mu}_i = \frac{1}{2}(\mu_i^m + \mu_i^M)$.

It is hard to determine the Chebyshev center and radius of $U(y)$, however, there are some general observations to be made. For instance, if there is some $\tilde{\mu}$ such that $y = \Lambda\tilde{\mu}$ (as is always the case when $N = p$ and Λ is nonsingular) then $\tilde{\mu}$ is the Chebyshev center of $U(y)$, its radius is *independent* of $\tilde{\mu}$ and is given by

$$r(U(\Lambda\tilde{\mu})) = \max\ \{|\mu| : \|\Lambda\mu\| \le 1\}. \tag{2.9}$$

To see this, we note that $\mu \in U(y)$ if and only if $\|\Lambda(\tilde{\mu} - \mu)\| \le 1$. Hence, for any $\hat{\mu} \in \mathbb{R}^p$ with $\|\Lambda\hat{\mu}\| \le 1$ and any $\mu \in \mathbb{R}^p$

$$\begin{aligned} &\max\{|\mu - \nu| : \nu \in U(y)\} \\ &\ge \frac{1}{2}(|\mu - (\tilde{\mu} - \hat{\mu})| + |\mu - (\tilde{\mu} + \hat{\mu})|) \\ &\ge |\hat{\mu}|. \end{aligned} \tag{2.10}$$

Similarly, for any $\nu \in U(y)$

$$|\tilde{\mu} - \nu| \le \max\{|\mu| : \|\Lambda\mu\| \le 1\}$$

since $\|\Lambda(\tilde{\mu} - \nu)\| \le 1$ which establishes equation (2.9).

When $|\mu| = |\mu_i|$, formula (2.9) has another interpretation: If we let $\Lambda^1, \ldots, \Lambda^p \in \mathbb{R}^N$ be the columns of the matrix Λ then

$$r(U(y)) = 1/\text{dist}\,(\Lambda^i, \text{ span } \{\Lambda^j : j \ne i\}).$$

Here dist $(\Lambda^i, \text{ span } \{\Lambda^j : j \ne i\})$ is the error in approximating Λ^i by linear combinations of the vectors $\Lambda^1, \Lambda^2, \ldots, \Lambda^{i-1}, \Lambda^{i+1}, \ldots, \Lambda^p$, that is,

$$= \min \left\{ \|\Lambda^i - \sum_{j \ne i} y_j \Lambda^j\| : (y_1, \ldots, y_{i-1}, y_{i+1}, \ldots, y_p) \in \mathbb{R}^{p-1} \right\}.$$

When the norm which measures the size of the error vector is a Hilbert space norm, that is, comes from an inner product the Chebyshev radius and center of $U(y)$ are easily identifiable. We state this useful fact, as well as (2.9), as

Theorem 2.1. Let Λ *be* $N \times p$ *matrix and* y *a vector in* $\mathbb{R}^N$. *Then*

i) *the Chebyshev center of* $U(\Lambda\tilde{\mu})$ *is* $\tilde{\mu}$ *and its radius is*

$$r(U(\Lambda\tilde{\mu})) = \max\{\, |\mu| : \|\Lambda\mu\| \le 1\}.$$

ii) *Suppose* $\|\cdot\|$ *is a Hilbert space norm and* $P_\Lambda: \mathbb{R}^N \to \text{span}\,\{\Lambda^1, \ldots, \Lambda^p\}$ *is the orthogonal projection of* $\mathbb{R}^N$ *onto span* $\{\Lambda^1, \ldots, \Lambda^p\}$. *Then for any* $y \in \mathbb{R}^N$ *the Chebyshev radius of* $U(y)$ *is given by*

$$r(U(y)) = \sqrt{1 - \|Q_\Lambda y\|^2}\ \max\ \{\, |\mu| : \|\Lambda\mu\| \le 1\}$$

where $Q_\Lambda y := \ y - P_\Lambda y$ *and the Chebyshev center is any* $\hat{\mu} \in \mathbb{R}^p$ *where*

$$\Lambda\hat{\mu} = P_\Lambda y.$$

Proof: We have already proved the first claim. For the second claim we use the fact that

$$\|\Lambda\mu\|^2 \le 1 - \|y - P_\Lambda y\|^2 = 1 - \|Q_\Lambda y\|^2$$

is equivalent to the fact that

$$\|y - P_\Lambda y + \Lambda\mu\| \le 1.$$

Consequently, $\mu \in U(y)$ if and only if $\|\Lambda(\hat{\mu} - \mu)\| \le 1 - \|Q_\Lambda y\|^2$. Now, ii) follows easily from the same idea used to prove i).

As an example of Theorem 1.1 we consider the parameter estimation problem

$$\begin{aligned} y_i &= \sum_{i=1}^{p} \Lambda_{ij}\mu_j + \varepsilon_i, \qquad i = 1, \ldots, N, \\ &\sum_{j=1}^{p} \varepsilon_j^2 \le \sigma^2. \end{aligned} \tag{2.11}$$

where Λ has rank p. In this case,

$$P_\Lambda y = \Lambda\hat{\mu}$$

where $\hat{\mu}$ solves the normal equation

$$(y, \Lambda^k) = \sum_{j=1}^{p} \hat{\mu}_j(\Lambda^k, \Lambda^j), \quad j = 1, \dots, p$$

and

$$(x, y) := \sum_{i=1}^{N} x_i y_i, \quad x, \ y \in \mathbb{R}^N.$$

Note that the estimate $\hat{\mu}$ for the model (2.11) depends on all data. In the remainder of this section we will contrast this property with the case of errors constrained by the condition $\|\varepsilon\|_\delta \leq 1$, that is,

$$|\varepsilon_i| \leq \delta_i, \quad i = 1, \dots, N.$$

We will identify a class of matrices Λ and data y for which only p components of the data vector y are necessary to determine the optimal parameter selection.

As a preliminary observation we mention the following fact (a related statement was made in [1]). We suppose that the matrix Λ has all its $r \times r$ minors, $r = p - 1$, nonzero. Let $\tilde{\mu}^i \in \mathbb{R}^s$ be any parameter selection which satisfies $\tilde{\mu}_i^i = \mu_i^M$, for some i, $1 \leq i \leq N$ then the set

$$E(\tilde{\mu}^i) := \left\{ k\colon |y_k - \sum_{j=1}^{p} \Lambda_{kj} \tilde{\mu}_j^i| = \delta_k \right\} \tag{2.12}$$

consists of at least p indices. The argument is standard: if $|E(\tilde{\mu}^i)| :=$ cardinality of $E(\tilde{\mu}^i) < p$ then there is a nonzero vector $v \in \mathbb{R}^p$ such that $(\Lambda v)_k = 0$ for all $k \in E(\tilde{\mu}^i)$. Since Λ has only nonsingular $r \times r$ minors, $r = p - 1$, all components of v are nonzero and so, in particular $v_i \neq 0$. Furthermore, by construction the vector $\hat{\mu} = \tilde{\mu}^i + tv$ is in $U(y)$ for all $|t| \leq t_0$, where $t_0 > 0$ is sufficiently small. But this contradicts the fact that $\hat{\mu}_i \leq \tilde{\mu}_i^i$ and so $|E(\tilde{\mu}^i)| \geq p$.

The argument above can be improved to obtain more information for an important class of linear models which we shall now describe.

Definition 2.1. An $N \times p$ matrix Λ is said to be strictly totally positive (STP) if for all $1 \leq i_1 < \cdots < i_n \leq N$, $1 \leq j_1 < \cdots < j_n \leq p$

$$\Lambda\begin{pmatrix} i_1, \dots, i_n \\ j_1, \dots, j_n \end{pmatrix} := \det_{\ell, k=1, \dots, n} \Lambda_{i_\ell j_k} > 0.$$

As an example we mention that for any $0 < t_1 < \cdots < t_N$ the matrix $\Lambda_{ij} := t_i^j$ $j = 0, 1, \dots, p-1, i = 1, \dots, N$ is STP.

The reason that this notion is useful in the present context is the following fact: Given any nonempty disjoint sets $I_1, \dots, I_k \subseteq \{1, \dots, N\}$ such that all elements of I_ℓ are less than all elements of I_r, for $\ell < r$ and $1 \leq k < p$. Then for any i, $1 \leq i \leq p$ there exists a vector $v_0 \in \mathbb{R}^p$ such that

$$(-1)^{r-1}(\Lambda v_0)_\ell \geq 0, \quad \ell \in I_r,\ r = 1, \dots, k$$

with $(v_0)_i > 0$. Thus the coordinates of the vector Λv_0 have the same signs on each group I_r, and alternates between consecutive groups I_r, I_{r+1}. Such a vector is easy to construct. For instance, pick any $1 \leq j_1 < \cdots < j_k \leq N$ with $i = j_r$, for some odd integer r, $1 \leq r \leq k$ and define $i_\ell = \max\ \{k: k \in I_\ell\}$ then $v_0 \in \mathbb{R}^p$ defined by

$$(\Lambda v_0)_\ell = \frac{\Lambda\begin{pmatrix}\ell, i_1, \dots, i_{k-1} \\ j_1, j_2, \dots, j_k\end{pmatrix}}{\Lambda\begin{pmatrix}i_1, \dots, i_{k-1} \\ j_2, \dots, j_k\end{pmatrix}}$$

has the required properties. We use the vector v_0 as follows: Partition $E(\tilde{\mu}^i)$, defined in (2.12) into disjoint groups $I_1, I_2, \dots, I_k$ as above where on each set I_ℓ, $(y - \Lambda\tilde{\mu}^i)_\ell$ has a fixed sign. Suppose $k < p$ and assume in the first group I_1, just for definiteness that $(y - \Lambda\tilde{\mu}^i)_\ell$, $\ell \in I_1$, is positive. Then the vector, $\mu = \tilde{\mu}^i + tv_0$ for $0 \leq t < t_0$, where $t_0 > 0$ is sufficiently small is still in $U(y)$. Again, this is a contradiction to the fact that $\mu_i \leq \tilde{\mu}_i$ and so $k \geq p$. This means that for any $y \in \mathbb{R}^N$ there is a parameter vector $\tilde{\mu}^i \in \mathbb{R}^p$ such that

$$y_\ell - \delta_\ell \leq \sum_{j=1}^{p} \Lambda_{\ell j}\tilde{\mu}_j^i \leq y_\ell + \delta_\ell, \quad \ell = 1, \dots, N \tag{2.13}$$

and that for at least p indices $i_1 < \cdots < i_p$ equality is achieved *alternately* in (2.13). Now to obtain more information about the sign pattern of the components of $\tilde{\mu}^i$, we assume, for simplicity that $0 \in \operatorname{int} U(y)$ that is, $|y_j| < \delta_j$, $j = 1, 2, \dots, N$. Then it is clear that $\tilde{\mu}_i^i = \mu_i^M > 0$. Arguing with μ_i^m we can find another vector $\underset{\sim}{\mu}^i$ satisfying (2.13) which again achieves equality alternatively at least p times in (2.13) but now $\underset{\sim}{\mu}_i^i = \mu_i^m < 0$. To proceed further, we appeal to the following fact: Let $S^-(x)$ = the number of sign changes in the components $x_1, \dots, x_N$ of $x = (x_1, \dots, x_N) \in \mathbb{R}^N$ where the zero components are disregarded, then we have

Lemma 1.1. $S^-(\Lambda\mu) \leq S^-(\mu)$. *Furthermore, if* $S^-(\Lambda\mu) = S^-(\mu)$ *then the first nonzero component of* μ *has the same sign as the first nonzero component of* $\Lambda\mu$.

For a proof of this important fact, see, for instance, Pinkus [9, pp. 47]. As a consequence of this lemma we obtain

$$S^-(\Lambda\underset{\sim}{\mu}^i) = S^-(\Lambda\tilde{\mu}^i) = S^-(\tilde{\mu}^i) = S^-(\underset{\sim}{\mu}^i) = p - 1$$

and therefore $(-1)^{\ell+i+1}\underset{\sim}{\mu}_\ell^i > 0$, $(-1)^{\ell+i}\tilde{\mu}_\ell^i > 0$, $\ell = 1, \dots, p-1$. Moreover, the vectors $\Lambda\underset{\sim}{\mu}^i$, $\Lambda\tilde{\mu}^i$ must have opposite orientation. By this we mean one of them achieves equality in (2.13) first from below and the other from above.

We record this observation below in

Theorem 2.2. Let Λ be an $N \times p$ STP matrix $p \leq N$. Given any vectors a, $b \in \mathbb{R}^N$ such that $a_i < 0$, $b_i > 0$, $i = 1, \dots, N$, there exist two vectors μ^+, $\mu^- \in \mathbb{R}^p$ such that

$$a_i \leq \sum_{j=1}^{p} \Lambda_{ij}\mu_j^{\pm} \leq b_i, \quad i = 1, 2, \dots, N. \tag{2.14}$$

Moreover, equality holds in (2.14) both for $\Lambda\mu^+$, $\Lambda\mu^-$ alternately for at least p components and $\Lambda\mu^+$, $\Lambda\mu^-$ have opposite orientation, specifically $\Lambda\mu^-$ first touches a and $\Lambda\mu^+$ touches b.

We also have demonstrated that any parameter vector corresponding to any endpoint of PUI_i must be a vector with the properties described by Theorem 2.2. Specifically, we have

Corollary 2.1. Let Λ be an $N \times p$ STP matrix, $p \leq N$. For any data vector $y \in \mathbb{R}^p$, any error vector $\delta \in \mathbb{R}^N$ with $|y_i| < \delta_i$, $i = 1, \dots, N$, and any k, $1 \leq k \leq N$ the upper (lower) endpoint of the interval PUI_k is either a μ^+ or μ^- vector described by Theorem 2.2 for $a = y - \delta$ and $b = y + \delta$.

Generally, for any data vector y the sets $E(\tilde{\mu}^i)$, $E(\underset{\sim}{\mu}^i)$ corresponding to endpoints of PUI_i consists of more than p indices. However, we will next describe a class of data for which not only do $E(\tilde{\mu}^i)$ and $E(\underset{\sim}{\mu}^i)$ contain exactly p indices but are in fact more or less *independent* of i.

For this purpose, we note the following properties of vectors $\mu^{\pm}$ of Corollary 2.1. There are indices $1 \leq i_1^{\pm} < \dots < i_p^{\pm} \leq N$ such that

$$\sum_{j=1}^{p} \Lambda_{i_\ell^+ j}\mu_j^+ = \begin{cases} y_{i_\ell} + \delta_{i_\ell}, & \ell \text{ odd} \\ y_{i_\ell} - \delta_{i_\ell}, & \ell \text{ even} \end{cases}$$

$$\sum_{j=1}^{p} \Lambda_{i_\ell^- j}\mu_j^- = \begin{cases} y_{i_\ell} - \delta_{i_\ell}, & \ell \text{ odd} \\ y_{i_\ell} + \delta_{i_\ell}, & \ell \text{ even.} \end{cases}$$

Hence, since Λ is STP we have $sgn\, \mu_j^- = (-1)^j$ and $sgn\, \mu_j^+ = (-1)^{j+1}$, $j = 1, 2, \dots, p$.

From these two vectors, we form for each k, two vectors

$$\tilde{\mu}^k := \begin{cases} \mu^-, & k \text{ even} \\ \mu^+, & k \text{ odd} \end{cases}$$

and

$$\underset{\sim}{\mu}^k := \begin{cases} \mu^-, & k \text{ odd} \\ \mu^+, & k \text{ even.} \end{cases}$$

Therefore, in particular, $\tilde{\mu}_k^k = \max\{\mu_k^-, \mu_k^+\} > 0$ and $\underset{\sim}{\mu}_k^k = \min\{\mu_k^-, \mu_k^+\} < 0$. Also, it is easy to check the "orientation" of the vectors $y - \Lambda\tilde{\mu}^k$ and $y - \Lambda\underset{\sim}{\mu}^k$ are $(-1)^k$ and $(-1)^{k+1}$, respectively, that is, the first component of these vectors which touches the corresponding component of the error vector δ has sign $(-1)^k$ and $(-1)^{k+1}$, respectively.

Corollary 2.2. Suppose the data vector $y \in \mathbb{R}^N$ has the property that the $N \times (p+1)$ matrix

$$\Lambda_k(y) := [\Lambda^1, \dots, \Lambda^{k-1}, y, \Lambda^k, \dots, \Lambda^p]$$

is totally positive (i.e. has all nonnegative minors) then

$$PUI_k = [\underset{\sim}{\mu}_k, \widetilde{\mu}_k].$$

Proof: We will only prove that $\widetilde{\mu}_k = \mu_k^M$; the proof that $\underset{\sim}{\mu}_k = \mu_k^m$ is similar. Thus, we let μ be any vector in $U(y)$ and want to show $\mu_k \leq \widetilde{\mu}_k$. Suppose to the contrary that $\widetilde{\mu}_k < \mu_k$. We define $\lambda := \widetilde{\mu}_k / \mu_k$ and consider the vector

$$e = (1-\lambda)y - \Lambda(\widetilde{\mu}^k - \lambda\mu) = y - \Lambda\widetilde{\mu}^k - \lambda\,(y - \Lambda\mu) := \Lambda_k(y)v, \quad v \in \mathbb{R}^{p+1}.$$

Since $0 < \lambda < 1$, the vector e has at least $p-1$ sign changes. Moreover, the vector $v \in \mathbb{R}^{p+1}$ has at most $p-1$ sign changes since it has at least one zero component and $v_k > 0$. Thus by hypothesis we conclude that both vectors have exactly $p-1$ sign changes. Since the vector e has orientation $(-1)^k$, it follows that v has the same orientation. This contradiction proves the corollary.

Remark 2.1. Much of what we said in Theorem 2.2 and Corollary 2.2 can be extended to the case that the parameter vector lies in an (infinite dimensional) L^∞ - space of some compact interval. This case deserves further study. For related investigations, see Micchelli [5]; also, the survey article Micchelli and Rivlin [6] contains a discussion of optimal sampling schemes for standard function classes.

3. p-WIDTHS UNDER STOCHASTIC ERRORS

In our previous discussion of the parameter estimation model

$$y = x + \varepsilon, \quad x = \Lambda\mu, \quad \mu \in \mathbb{R}^p$$
$$\Lambda: \mathbb{R}^p \to \mathbb{R}^N, \tag{3.1}$$

an $N \times p$ matrix Λ was specified in advance and then good bounds for μ were obtained in various cases from available data y. The selection of the matrix was assumed to be specified by the application environment. In this section, we consider the situation when the true signal x is only constrained to lie in some set $\mathscr{S} \subseteq X$, and therefore may depend nonlinearly on some parameter space. We have in mind cases where instead of assuming x has for instance a polynomial trend, say, we may only know x is "close" to a polynomial. Therefore it is perhaps better to assume only that some derivative of x is "small". Hence, we have in mind sets $\mathscr{S}$ which are not linear spaces, as in (3.1).

In this context, we ask what linear parameter model with p degrees of freedom is the best estimate for the full set $\mathscr{S}$. This leads us to two notions of p-widths suitable for the analysis of estimation under error. For background material on p-widths (without errors) we recommend Pinkus [9].

In this section, we consider the case of stochastic errors and present the solution of one model problem for which we can compute the stochastic p-width and identify an optimal parameter model. Our discussion of p-widths for deterministic errors is given in the last section. The results of Melkman and Micchelli [4] will be used to obtain an optimal parameter model with p degrees of freedom under deterministic errors.

We begin our description of stochastic p-width. The situation is the following: an $N \times N$ positive definite symmetric matrix Σ is given and is assumed to represent the covariance matrix for mean zero random noise, that is,

$$E\, \varepsilon_i \varepsilon_j = \Sigma_{ij}, \quad i, j = 1, 2, \dots, N.$$

The set $\mathscr{S}$ is determined by an $N \times N$ matrix S by means of the equation

$$\mathscr{S} := \{x \colon \|Sx\| \le 1, \quad x \in \mathbb{R}^N\}$$

where $\|\cdot\| \colon \mathbb{R}^N \to \mathbb{R}$ is some norm on $\mathbb{R}^N$.

Definition 3.1. The p-width of $\mathscr{S}$ in $\mathbb{R}^N$ relative to the covariance matrix Σ is defined as

$$s_p^2(\mathscr{S}; \Sigma) = \inf_{\Lambda_p} \sup_{x \in \mathscr{S}} E(dist^2(x + \varepsilon, \Lambda_p))$$

where Λ_p is any linear space of dimension $\le p$ contained in $\mathbb{R}^N$ and

$$dist(x, \Lambda_p) = \inf_{y \in \Lambda_p} \|x - y\| \,;$$

any subspace Λ_p^0 which achieves the infinum above is called an optimal subspace.

In general, we cannot identify $s_p(\mathscr{S}; \Sigma)$, however, when $\|x\|$ is any *quadratic norm on* $\mathbb{R}^N$, which for simplicity we assume is $(x \cdot x)^{1/2}$ and $\mathscr{S}$, Σ *commute* we have

Theorem 3.1. Suppose that there exists a set of orthonormal vectors $\{x^1, \dots, x^N\} \subseteq \mathbb{R}^N$, $(x^i, x^j) = \delta_{ij}$ such that

$$S^T S x^i = \lambda_i x^i, \quad i = 1, 2, \dots, N$$

$$\Sigma x^i = \sigma_i x^i, \quad i = 1, 2, \dots, N$$

for some constants $0 < \lambda_1 \le \cdots \le \lambda_N$, $0 < \sigma_1 \le \cdots \le \sigma_N$. Then $\Lambda_p^0 := \{x^1, \dots, x^p\}$ is an optimal subspace for $s_p(\mathscr{S}; \Sigma)$ and

$$s_p^2(\mathscr{S}; \Sigma) = \lambda_{p+1}^{-1} + \sum_{i=p+1}^{N} \sigma_i. \tag{3.2}$$

Proof: First we observe that for any $N \times N$ matrix B we have

$$E(\|B(x+\varepsilon)\|^2) = E(\|Bx\|^2 + 2(Bx,\ B\varepsilon) + \|B\varepsilon\|^2)$$

$$= \|Bx\|^2 + \text{ trace } B\Sigma B^T.$$

Therefore, if Q_{Λ_p} is the orthogonal projection of $\mathbb{R}^N$ onto $\Lambda_p^{\perp} := \{x: (x, y) = 0,\ \forall\, y \in \Lambda_p\}$ then

$$\begin{aligned} &s_p^2(\mathcal{S};\ \Sigma) \\ &= \min_{\Lambda_p} \max_{x \in \mathcal{S}} E\{\|Q_{\Lambda_p}(x+\varepsilon)\|^2\} \\ &= \min_{\Lambda_p} \max_{x \in \mathcal{S}} \{\|Q_{\Lambda_p} x\|^2 + \text{ trace } Q_{\Lambda_p} \Sigma Q_{\Lambda_p}^T\} \\ &= \min_{\Lambda_p}\{\max_{x \in \mathcal{S}} \|Q_{\Lambda_p} x\|^2 + \text{ trace } \Sigma Q_{\Lambda_p}\}. \end{aligned}$$

First we obtain an upper bound for $s_p^2(\mathcal{S};\ \Sigma)$. For this purpose, we let x be any vector in $\mathbb{R}^N$ such that $\|Sx\| \le 1$. Writing x as

$$x = \sum_{i=1}^{N} d_i x^i, \quad d_i = (x, x^i), \quad i = 1, \ldots, N$$

we get $\|Sx\|^2 = \sum_{i=1}^{N} |d_i|^2 \lambda_i$. On the other hand, for $\Lambda_p^0 = span\,\{x^1, \ldots, x^p\}$ we have

$$Q_{\Lambda_p^0} x = \sum_{j=p+1}^{N} (x, x^j)\, x^j = \tilde{Q} x \tag{3.3}$$

where $\tilde{Q}$ is the $N \times N$ matrix

$$\tilde{Q}_{\ell m} := \sum_{j=p+1}^{N} x_\ell^j x_m^j, \quad \ell,\ m = 1, \ldots, N. \tag{3.4}$$

Thus it follows that

$$\begin{aligned} \lambda_{p+1} \|Q_{\Lambda_p^0} x\|^2 &= \lambda_{p+1} \sum_{i=p+1}^{N} |d_i|^2 \\ &\le \sum_{i=p+1}^{N} |d_i|^2 \lambda_i \le \|Sx\|^2 \le 1. \end{aligned}$$

Similarly, using (3.3) we get

$$\text{trace}\, \Sigma Q_{\Lambda_p^0}$$

$$= \sum_{i=1}^{N} \sum_{\ell=p+1}^{N} \sigma_\ell x_i^\ell x_i^\ell$$

$$= \sum_{\ell=p+1}^{N} \sigma_\ell .$$

Therefore $s_p^2(\mathscr{S}; \Sigma) \leq \lambda_{p+1}^{-1} + \sum_{\ell=p+1}^{N} \sigma_\ell$.

Now, for the lower bound we let Λ_p be any subspace of dimension $\leq p$ of $\mathbb{R}^N$ and choose a y of norm one in $\Lambda_{p+1}^0 \cap \Lambda_p^\perp$, that is, we may write

$$y = \sum_{i=1}^{p+1} d_i x^i, \quad d_i = (y, x^i), \quad i = 1, \dots, p+1.$$

Consequently, $1 = \|y\|^2 = \sum_{i=1}^{p+1} |d_i|^2$ and $Q_{\Lambda_p} y = y$. This gives us

$$\|Sy\|^2 = \sum_{i=1}^{p+1} \lambda_i |d_i|^2 \leq \lambda_{p+1} \sum_{i=1}^{p+1} |d_i|^2 \leq \lambda_{p+1}$$

and so

$$\max_{x \in \mathscr{S}} \|Q_{\Lambda_p^0} x\|^2 \geq \|Q_{\Lambda_p} (\lambda_{p+1}^{-1/2} y)\|^2$$

$$= \lambda_{p+1}^{-1}.$$

Furthermore, whenever $\mathbb{R}^N = \text{span}\ \{v^1, \dots, v^n\}$, $(v^i, v^j) = \delta_{ij}$, $i, j = 1, \dots, N$ and $\Lambda_p = \text{span}\ \{v^1, \dots, v^p\}$, we have

$$\text{trace}\, \Sigma Q_{\Lambda_p} = \sum_{i=p+1}^{N} (v^i, \Sigma v^i)$$

which is

$$\geq \sum_{i=p+1}^{N} \sigma_i,$$

by Ky Fan's inequality, see for instance Marshall and Olkin [3].

Remark 3.1. It would be interesting to know how to determine $s_p^2(\mathscr{S};\ \Sigma)$, in general. Specifically, whether or not in a Hilbert space, the spectral data for the pencil of matrices $\lambda\Sigma + \mu S^T S$ determine $s_p^2(\mathscr{S}; \Sigma)$.

Next we consider an important special case of Theorem 3.1. In particular, we consider the estimation problem for N-periodic sequences $\{x_i: i \in \mathbb{Z}\}$, $x_i = x_{i+N}$, in the stationary model

$$y_i = \sum_{j=0}^{N-1} s_{i-j} x_j + \varepsilon_i, \quad i \in \mathbb{Z}$$

where

$$E\, \varepsilon_i \varepsilon_j = \sum_{\ell=0}^{N-1} b_{i-\ell} b_{j-\ell}$$

and both $\{s_i: i \in \mathbb{Z}\}$ and $\{b_i: i \in \mathbb{Z}\}$ are N-periodic sequences. We let $\omega = e^{2\pi i/N}$ and $(x^\ell)_k := \omega^{k\ell}$, $k, \ell = 0, 1, \dots, N-1$. Then $(x^\ell, x^r) = N\delta_{\ell r}$ and

$$\left.\begin{aligned} S^T S x^\ell &= |P_s(\omega^\ell)|^2 x^\ell \\ \Sigma x^\ell &= |P_b(\omega^\ell)|^2 x^\ell \end{aligned}\right\}, \quad \ell = 1, \dots, N$$

where

$$P_s(z) = \sum_{j=0}^{N-1} s_j z^j$$

and

$$P_b(z) = \sum_{j=0}^{N-1} b_j z^j.$$

Therefore $\Lambda_p^0 = \{x^0, \dots, x^{p-1}\}$ is the optimal parameter model (over $\mathbb{C}^N$ = complex N-space) with p degrees of freedom.

4. p-WIDTHS UNDER DETERMINISTIC ERRORS

In this section we consider the following

Definition 4.1. Let $\mathscr{S}$, $\mathscr{E}$ be prescribed subsets of some normed linear space X. Then we set

$$d_p(\mathscr{S};\ \mathscr{E}) = \inf_{\Lambda_p} \sup_{\substack{x \in \mathscr{S} \\ \varepsilon \in \mathscr{E}}} \inf_{g \in \Lambda_p} \|x + \varepsilon - g\|.$$

Notice the set $\mathscr{E}$ determines the additive noise in the model

$$y = x + \varepsilon, \quad x \in \mathcal{S}, \quad \varepsilon \in \mathcal{E}.$$

In the usual definition of p-width $\mathcal{E} = \phi$. However, even in the general case, we see the clear parallel between ordinary p-width of $\mathcal{S}$ (when $\mathcal{E} = \phi$) and the p-width of $\mathcal{S} + \mathcal{E}$.

In general, it is difficult to compute $d_p(\mathcal{S}; \mathcal{E})$, however, in Hilbert spaces we will be able to identify $d_p(\mathcal{S}; \mathcal{E})$ as well as find an optimal subspace. The basis of our analysis is the following proposition from Melkman and Micchelli [4].

Proposition 4.1. Let $\|x\|_i^2$, $i = 0, 1, 2$ be quadratic norms on some linear space X. Then

$$\sup \{\|x\|_0^2 : \|x\|_1 \le 1, \ \|x\|_2 \le 1\}$$

$$= \min_{0 \le \lambda \le 1} \sup \{\|x\|_0^2 : \lambda \|x\|_1^2 + (1 - \lambda)\|x\|_2^2 \le 1\}.$$

Although it is not essential, we will consider only the case $X = \mathbb{R}^N$ so as to parallel the notation of Section 3. In this case, the following consequence of Proposition 4.1 will be used.

Corollary 4.1. Let A, B, C be symmetric positive definite matrices. Then

$$\max \{(Ax, x) : (Bx, x) \le 1, \ (Cx, x) \le 1\}$$

$$= \min_{0 \le \lambda \le 1} \max \{(Ax, x) : \lambda (Bx, x) + (1 - \lambda)(Cx, x) \le 1\}$$

To proceed further we need the following lemma.

Lemma 4.1. Let A, B be $N \times N$ nonsingular symmetric matrices and define the $N \times 2N$ matrix

$$H := [A : B].$$

Then $H^T H$ has zero as an eigenvalue of multiplicity N and the remaining eigenvalues $\mu_1, \dots, \mu_N$ are the eigenvalues of matrix

$$V := A^2 + B^2.$$

Moreover, if $Vx^i = \mu_i x^i$, $i = 1, \dots, N$ then the eigenvectors of $H^T H$ corresponding to eigenvalues $\mu_1, \dots, \mu_N$ are given by

$$v^i = \begin{pmatrix} A x^i \\ B x^i \end{pmatrix}, \quad i = 1, \dots, N.$$

Proof: The proof begins by noting that

$$G := H^T H = \begin{pmatrix} A^2 & AB \\ BA & B^2 \end{pmatrix}.$$

We will transform H^TH by means of the matrix

$$X := \begin{pmatrix} I & I \\ 0 & -B^{-1}A \end{pmatrix}$$

whose inverse is given by

$$X^{-1} = \begin{pmatrix} I & A^{-1}B \\ 0 & -A^{-1}B \end{pmatrix}.$$

Since

$$(G - \lambda I)\, X = \begin{pmatrix} A^2 & 0 \\ BA & 0 \end{pmatrix} - \lambda X,$$

we get

$$X^{-1}(G - \lambda I)X$$
$$= \begin{pmatrix} A^2 + A^{-1}B^2A - \lambda I & 0 \\ -A^{-1}B^2A & -\lambda I \end{pmatrix} \tag{4.1}$$

from which it follows that $\det\,(G - \lambda I) = (-1)^n \lambda^n \det(V - \lambda I)$. This proves the first claim. For the second, we return to equation (4.1) which gives

$$X^{-1}GX \begin{pmatrix} A^{-1}x^i \\ -\mu_i^{-1}A^{-1}B^2x^i \end{pmatrix} = \mu_i \begin{pmatrix} A^{-1}x^i \\ -\mu_i^{-1}A^{-1}B^2x^i \end{pmatrix}.$$

Since

$$X \begin{pmatrix} A^{-1}x^i \\ -\mu_i^{-1}A^{-1}B^2x^i \end{pmatrix} = \begin{pmatrix} A^{-1}x^i - \mu_i^{-1}A^{-1}B^2x^i \\ \mu_i^{-1}Bx^i \end{pmatrix}$$
$$= \mu_i^{-1} \begin{pmatrix} Ax^i \\ Bx^i \end{pmatrix}$$

the lemma is proved.

Now, we consider the deterministic p-width problem for

$$\mathscr{E} = \{x : x \in \mathbb{R}^N,\ \|\Sigma^{-1}x\| \le 1\}$$

and, as before

$$\mathscr{S} = \{x : x \in \mathbb{R}^N,\ \|Sx\| \le 1\}$$

where both Σ and S are assumed to be nonsingular symmetric matrices.

For every $\lambda \in [0, 1]$ we introduce the strictly positive definite symmetric matrix

$$D_\lambda := \begin{cases} \lambda^{-1}\Sigma^2 + (1-\lambda)^{-1} S^{-2}, & 0 < \lambda < 1 \\ \Sigma^2, & \lambda = 1 \\ S^{-2}, & \lambda = 0 \end{cases}$$

We also require the eigenvalues $\gamma_1(\lambda) \geq \cdots \geq \gamma_N(\lambda) > 0$ and orthonormal eigenvectors $x^1(\lambda), \ldots, x^N(\lambda)$ of D_λ.

Theorem 4.1. There exists a $\delta \in [0, 1]$ such that

$$d_p^2(\mathscr{S}; \mathscr{E}) = \gamma_{p+1}(\delta)$$

and moreover $\Lambda_p^0 := \{x^1(\delta), \ldots, x^p(\delta)\}$ *is an optimal subspace.*

Proof: The proof combines Corollary 4.1 and Lemma 4.1 as follows:

$$\begin{aligned} d_p^2(\mathscr{S}; \mathscr{E}) &= \min_{\Lambda_p} \max_{\substack{\varepsilon \in \mathscr{E} \\ x \in \mathscr{S}}} \min_{y \in \Lambda_p} \|x + \varepsilon - y\|^2 \\ &= \min_{\Lambda_p} \max \{\|Q_{\Lambda_p}(x + \varepsilon)\|^2 : \|Sx\|^2 \leq 1,\ \|\Sigma^{-1}\varepsilon\| \leq 1\} \end{aligned}$$

which equals by the corollary

$$= \min_{0 \leq \lambda \leq 1} \min_{\Lambda_p} \max \{\|Q_{\Lambda_p}(x + \varepsilon)\|^2 : \lambda\|\Sigma^{-1}\varepsilon\|^2 + (1-\lambda)\|Sx\|^2 \leq 1\}$$

$$= \min_{0 \leq \lambda \leq 1} \min_{\Lambda_p} \max \left\{\left\|Q_{\Lambda_p}\left(\frac{S^{-1}}{\sqrt{1-\lambda}} x + \frac{\Sigma}{\sqrt{\lambda}} w\right)\right\|^2 : \|w\|^2 + \|x\|^2 \leq 1\right\}$$

However, by the ideas used to prove Theorem 3.1 we get that this equals

$$= \min_{0 \leq \lambda \leq 1} \sigma_{p+1}(\lambda) \tag{4.2}$$

where

$$K_\lambda := \left[\frac{S^{-1}}{\sqrt{1-\lambda}} ; \frac{\Sigma}{\sqrt{\lambda}}\right]$$

and $\sigma_{2N}(\lambda) \leq \cdots \leq \sigma_1(\lambda)$ are the singular values of $K_\lambda^T K_\lambda$, that is, the eigenvalues of $K_\lambda^T K_\lambda$. However, Lemma 3.1 identifies the singular values of K_λ and so (4.2) equals

$$= \min_{0 \leq \lambda \leq 1} \gamma_{p+1}(\lambda).$$

Finally, the identification of the optimal subspace is also as in the proof of Theorem 3.1. This completes the proof.

As a means of comparison, with Theorem 3.1, we consider the case of Theorem 4.1 when Σ and S commute. Hence they share common eigenvectors as in Theorem 3.1

$$S^2 x_i = \lambda_{p+1}^2 x^i$$

$$\Sigma^2 x^i = \sigma_i^2 x^i .$$

This implies that

$$\left(\frac{1}{1-\lambda} S^{-2} + \frac{\Sigma^2}{\lambda} \right) x^i = \left(\frac{\lambda_i^{-2}}{1-\lambda} + \frac{\sigma_i^2}{\lambda} \right) x^i$$

and since

$$\min_{0 \le \lambda \le 1} \left(\frac{\lambda_{p+1}^{-2}}{1-\lambda} + \frac{\sigma_{p+1}^2}{\lambda} \right) = (\lambda_{p+1}^{-1} + \sigma_{p+1})^2$$

we get

$$d_p^2(\mathscr{S}; \mathscr{E}) = \lambda_{p+1}^{-1} + \sigma_{p+1}$$

in this case.

References

1. G. Belforte, B. Bona, S. Frediani, Optimal sampling schedule with unknown but bounded measurement errors; Families of Linear Models, Proc. of 23rd IEEE Conference on Decision and Control, Las Vegas, 1984.

2. G. Belforte, B. Bona and S. Frediani, Optimal sampling schedule with replications for linear models with unknown-but-bounded errors, International Conference on Systems Research Informatics and Cybernetics, Baden-Baden, 1985.

3. A.W. Marshall and I. Olkin, Inequalities: Theory of Majorization and Applications, Academic Press, 1979.

4. A.A. Melkman and C.A. Micchelli, Optimal estimation of linear operators in Hilbert space from inaccurate data, SIAM Numer. Analysis, 16 (1979), 87-105.

5. C.A. Micchelli, Optimal estimation of smooth functions from inaccurate data, Journal of the Institute of Mathematics and its Applications, 23 (1979), 473-495.

6. C.A. Micchelli and T.J. Rivlin, Lectures on optimal recovery, Lecture Notes in Mathematics, #1129, ed. P.R. Turner, Springer Verlag, Heidelberg, 1985.

7. M. Milanese and G. Belforte, Estimation theory and uncertainty intervals evaluation in presence of unknown but bounded errors: linear families of models and estimators, IEEE Transactions on Automatic Control, Vol. AC-27, #7, 408-414, 1982.

8. M. Milanese and A. Vicino, Robust estimation and exact uncertainty intervals evaluation for nonlinear models, IMACS INT. Symp. "System Modeling and Simulation" Atraro, 1988.

9. A. Pinkus, n-Widths in Approximation Theory, Springer Verlag, Heidelberg, 1985.

HOW USEFUL IS NONADAPTIVE INFORMATION FOR ORDINARY DIFFERENTIAL EQUATIONS?

Bolesław Z. Kacewicz

Institute of Informatics, University of Warsaw
PKiN p.850, 00901 Warsaw, Poland

1. INTRODUCTION

We present an extended abstract of results concerning the solution of systems $z'(x) = f(x, z(x))$, $x \in [0,1]$, $z(0) = \eta$, where the function $f : [0,1] \times \Re^s \to \Re^s$ has r continuous bounded partial derivatives. We assume that available information about the problem consists of evaluations of n linear functionals at f. If an adaptive choice of these functionals is allowed, then the minimal error of an algorithm is of order $n^{-(r+1)}$, for any dimension s. If nonadaptive information is only used, the minimal error cannot be essentially less than $n^{-(r+1)/(s+1)}$. Thus, as far as the error is concerned, adaption is significantly better, and the advantage of using it grows with s. The costs of computing adaptive and nonadaptive information which supply an ϵ-approximation are compared for sequential and parallel computations. A complete statement of the results will appear in Kacewicz (1988).

2. FORMULATION OF THE PROBLEM

We consider the initial value problem

$$z'(x) = f(x, z(x)) \quad , x \in [0,1], \quad z(0) = \eta, \tag{2.1}$$

where $f : [0,1] \times \Re^s \to \Re^s$, $s \geq 1$, and $\eta \in \Re^s$. We assume that the function f belongs to the class F_r,

$$(2.2) \qquad F_r = \{f \in C^r([0,1] \times \Re^s): \quad f(x,z) = 0 \text{ for } z \notin D \text{ and}$$

$$\|\partial^i f(x,z)/\partial x^{i_0} \partial z_1^{i_1} \ldots \partial z_s^{i_s}\| \leq 1 \text{ for all } x \in [0,1], z \in \Re^s$$

$$\text{and } 0 \leq i_0 + i_1 + \ldots + i_s = i \leq r\},$$

where D is an open set in $\Re^s$ such that $\eta \in D$, and $r \geq 1$. The norm of $z = [z_1, \ldots, z_s]$ is meant here as $\|z\| = \max\{|z_i| : 1 \leq i \leq s\}$.

Information about $f \in F_r$ will be defined by linear functionals on $C^r = C^r([0,1] \times \Re^s)$. In what follows, we assume that we can compute $L(f)$ for any $f \in F_r$ and any linear $L : C^r \to \Re$.

We shall consider two classes of information which differ in whether or not one allows adaptive choice of successive functionals. The first class consists of *nonadaptive information* given by

$$(2.3) \qquad N(f) = [L_1(f), \ldots, L_n(f)],$$

where L_i are linear functionals on C^r. Nonadaptive information is thus defined by functionals which are given in advance, independently of any particular problem. This situation has certain advantages. Firstly, we need not select new functionals for different right-hand side functions f, which may be costly. Secondly, since all values $L_i(f)$ can be computed simultaneously, nonadaptive information is well suited for parallel computations, see Section 6.

Loosing the requirement that the functionals are given independently of f, we arrive to the concept of adaptive information. Let $L_1 : C^r \to \Re$ be linear, $f \in F_r$, and $y_1 = L_1(f)$. Suppose that $y_1, \ldots, y_{i-1}$ are given. Based on these values, we choose a linear functional $L_i(\cdot; y_1, \ldots, y_{i-1})$ on C^r and we set $y_i = L_i(f; y_1, \ldots, y_{i-1})$. *Adaptive information* is defined by

$$(2.4) \qquad N(f) = [y_1, \ldots, y_n],$$

for $f \in F_r$. Since the functionals L_i may now depend on a particular f, the class of adaptive information is wider than the class of nonadaptive information.

3. ADAPTIVE INFORMATION

Knowing information about f (adaptive or not) $y = N(f)$, we must somehow use it to compute an approximation to the solution z. The mapping $\Phi : N(F_r) \to C([0,1])$ is said to be an *algorithm* using N. Given y, the algorithm Φ supplies a continuous function $\Phi(y)$ which approximates z. The *error* of an algorithm Φ is measured by the worst approximation error in F_r,

$$e(\Phi, N) = \sup\{\|z - \Phi(N(f))\|_\infty : f \in F_r\}, \tag{3.1}$$

where z is the solution of (2.1) and $\|z\|_\infty = \sup\{\|z(x)\| : x \in [0,1]\}$.

The power of adaptive (nonadaptive) information is characterized by the *n-th minimal error* of an algorithm $r^a(n)$ $(r^{non}(n))$ given as

$$r^{a(non)}(n) = \inf_N \inf_\Phi e(\Phi, N), \tag{3.2}$$

where the right infimum is taken with respect to all algorithms using fixed adaptive (nonadaptive) information N, while the left infimum with respect to all adaptive (non-adaptive) information N of the form (2.4) ((2.3)).

Obviously, we have that $r^a(n) \le r^{non}(n)$, i.e., nonadaption can be at most as powerful as adaption. For many problems (such as, e.g., the approximation or integration problems) it holds $r^{non}(n) \le 2r^a(n)$, i.e., the quality of both types of information is essentially the same, see Traub and Woźniakowski (1980) pp. 47–50.

Our aim is to compare the n-th minimal errors $r^a(n)$ and $r^{non}(n)$ for the problem (2.1). We first recall the result concerning adaptive information (Kacewicz 1984):

THEOREM 3.1 *For any* $s \ge 1$,

$$r^a(n) = \Theta(n^{-(r+1)}), \qquad as \quad n \to \infty. \quad \blacksquare$$

By $f = \Theta(g)$ we mean that $f = O(g)$ and $g = O(f)$. Thus, the n-th minimal error is of order $n^{-(r+1)}$, no matter what the dimension s happens to be. The best information N^*, for which $\inf_\Phi e(\Phi, N^*) = \Theta(n^{-(r+1)})$, is based on the adaptive choice of the functionals, see Kacewicz (1984).

We now turn to nonadaptive information. Can the best information be nonadaptive?

4. NONADAPTIVE INFORMATION

The following theorem states that $r^{non}(n)$ is significantly greater than $r^a(n)$.

THEOREM 4.1 (Kacewicz, 1988)

$$r^{non}(n) \geq dn^{-(r+1)/(s+1)}, \quad n = 1, 2, \ldots \quad ,$$

where d is a positive constant independent of n. ∎

Comparing the results of Theorems 3.1 and 4.1 we see that adaption is considerably more powerful for initial value problems than nonadaption. The remarkable difference between these two types of information lies in the influence of the dimension s on the n-th minimal error. To understand the reason for this difference, we stress that the solution $z = z(x)$ of (2.1) is a one dimensional curve in $\Re^s$. Adaptive information can use this fact, by adjusting itself to a particular behavior of z (for a particular f). Therefore, to within a constant, $r^a(n)$ is independent of the dimension s.

This is not the case for information (2.3) which does not adapt itself to f. The same functionals must deal with all possible z, i.e., with all possible directions in $\Re^s$. Hence, the dependence of $r^{non}(n)$ on s is more significant than that of $r^a(n)$, as it concerns the speed of convergence as $n \to +\infty$, not only a constant. Recall that for some problems, such as the problem of approximating functions, even adaption does not us allow to get rid of the dimension (see Babenko, 1979).

5. COMPLEXITY FOR SEQUENTIAL COMPUTATIONS

In this section we shortly describe conclusions concerning the ϵ-complexity of the problem (2.1), i.e., the minimal cost of computing an ϵ-approximation to z. We assume that computations are sequential, i.e., that only one processor is available. For simplicity, we only consider the cost of computing information (2.3) or (2.4), and neglect the cost of combining it to get an approximation. Assume that the cost of (time needed for) computing $L(f)$ is c ($c > 0$), for any linear functional L and any $f \in F_r$. In this model of computation, denote by cost(Φ, N) the maximal cost of computing $\Phi(N(f))$, with respect to all $f \in F_r$.

Let $\epsilon > 0$. Our aim is to compute an ϵ-approximation to z for all $f \in F_r$, i.e., to find information N and an algorithm Φ such that $e(\Phi, N) < \epsilon$. The minimal cost of computing an ϵ-approximation

$$\text{comp}(\epsilon) = \inf\{\text{cost}(\Phi, N) : \quad \Phi, N \text{ such that } e(\Phi, N) < \epsilon\}$$

is called the ϵ- *complexity* of the problem (2.1). For a more detailed discussion of the model of computation, the concept of cost, as well as of the concept of ϵ-complexity, the reader is referred to Woźniakowski (1986), Sections 3.5 and 3.6.

Theorems 3.1 and 4.1 yield the following conclusion as to the behavior of ϵ-complexity:

COROLLARY 5.1 *For adaptive information*

$$\text{comp}(\epsilon) = \Theta(\epsilon^{-1/(r+1)}), \quad \textit{as} \quad \epsilon \to 0.$$

For nonadaptive information

$$\text{comp}(\epsilon) \geq K\epsilon^{-(s+1)/(r+1)}, \quad \textit{as} \quad \epsilon \to 0,$$

where K is a positive constant independent of ϵ. ∎

In both cases the ϵ-complexity of the problem (2.1) grows as a power of $1/\epsilon$, when $\epsilon \to 0$. If adaption is not allowed, this growth is significantly faster, and dependent on the dimension s. The larger s is, the greater is the advantage of using adaption in sequential computations.

6. PARALLEL COMPUTATIONS

The conclusion of the previous section as to the advantage of adaptive information need not be true if we could use parallel computations. For instance, if sufficiently many processors are available, nonadaptive information can be computed more efficiently than adaptive one. Indeed, devoting one processor to each of n functionals in (2.3), we could compute nonadaptive information with cost c (independent of n). At the same time, adaptive information (2.4) may still cost nc, as for the single processor. In this section we shortly discuss both information for parallel computations assuming that k processors are available.

We showed in Kacewicz (1988) how nonadaptive information can be used to solve (2.1). We defined there an algorithm Φ^* based on evaluations of a right hand side f at certain points independent of f. The error of Φ^* satisfies:

THEOREM 6.1 (Kacewicz, 1988) *For sufficiently large n it holds*

$$e(\Phi^*, N^*) \leq Cn^{-r/(s+1)},$$

where C is a constant independent of n. ∎

From Theorems 4.1 and 6.1 we have that

$$dn^{-(r+1)/(s+1)} \leq r^{non}(n) \leq Cn^{-r/(s+1)}. \tag{6.1}$$

Thus, there is a gap between a lower and upper bound. Recall that for linear adaptive information we have $r^a(n) = \Theta(n^{-(r+1)})$. If we, however, restrict a permissible class of information (2.4) to be only given by the values of f or its partial derivatives (such information is called *standard*), then $r^a(n) = \Theta(n^{-r})$, i.e., we loose one order of magnitude, see Kacewicz (1984). We may thus conjecture that for nonadaptive information $r^{non}(n) = \Theta(n^{-(r+1)/(s+1)})$ if arbitrary linear functionals are allowed in (2.3), and $r^{non}(n) = \Theta(n^{-r/(s+1)})$ if information (2.3) is standard.

Let $\epsilon > 0$. As in Section 5, we wish to compute an ϵ-approximation to the solution of (2.1). We restrict ourselves to standard information, and assume that it can be computed using k processors. Our aim is to compare the minimal costs of computing adaptive and nonadaptive information which give an ϵ-approximation. More specifically, let $\text{cost}(N, k, f)$ denote the cost of computing values of f or its derivatives in (2.3) or (2.4). As in Section 5 we assume that we need c $(c > 0)$ units of time to perform each such single evaluation, where c is independent of f and of a point at which evaluation is performed. Let $\text{cost}(N, k) = \sup\{\text{cost}(N, k, f) : f \in F_r\}$. We wish to compare quantities $P^a(\epsilon, k)$ and $P^{non}(\epsilon, k)$ given by

$$P^{a(non)}(\epsilon, k) = \inf\{\text{cost}(N, k) : \exists \Phi \text{ using } N \text{ such that } e(\Phi, N) < \epsilon\},$$

where the superscript 'a' or 'non' indicates that the infimum is taken with respect to all adaptive or nonadaptive information, respectively. The number $P^{a(non)}(\epsilon, k)$ is thus equal to the minimal cost of respective information which supplies an ϵ-approximation.

Comparing $P^{non}(\epsilon, k)$ with $P^{a}(\epsilon, k)$ we find under some assumptions that

$$P^{non}(\epsilon, k) < P^{a}(\epsilon, k) \text{ iff } k = \Omega(k(\epsilon)),$$

where $k(\epsilon)$ is some 'critical' number of processors. The notation $k = \Omega(l)$ has the usual meaning that $l = O(k)$. The constants in the Ω-notation in 'sufficiency' and 'necessity' above may be not the same. We now present bounds on $k(\epsilon)$. From $r^{a}(n) = \Theta(n^{-r})$, as $n \to +\infty$, and from (6.1) we get for small ϵ that

$$q_1 k_1(\epsilon) \leq k(\epsilon) \leq q_2 k_2(\epsilon),$$

where $k_1(\epsilon) = \lceil \epsilon^{-(s+1)/(r+1)+1/r} \rceil$, $k_2(\epsilon) = \lceil \epsilon^{-s/r} \rceil$ and q_1, q_2 are constants independent of ϵ, $q_1 > 0$.

Thus, if at least about $\lceil \epsilon^{-s/r} \rceil$ processors are available, nonadaptive information requires less computational effort to compute an ϵ-approximation. On the other hand, if the number of processors is less (within a constant) than $k_1(\epsilon)$, adaptive information is more efficient. Note that for $\max(r, s) \geq 2$, $k_1(\epsilon)$ goes to infinity as $\epsilon \to 0$, which yields the same for $k(\epsilon)$. Note also that if $r^{non}(n) = \Theta(n^{-r/(s+1)})$ is true for standard information, as conjectured above, then $k(\epsilon) = \Theta(\lceil \epsilon^{-s/r} \rceil)$, as $\epsilon \to 0$.

References

Babenko, K.I. (1979), ed. 'Theoretical Background and Constructing of Computational Algorithms for Mathematical-Phisical Problems', Nauka, Moscow (in Russian).

Kacewicz, B.Z. (1984), How to increase the order to get minimal-error algorithms for systems of ODE, Numer. Math. 45, 93–104.

Kacewicz, B.Z. (1988), Does adaption help for initial value problems?, to appear in J. Complexity.

Traub, J.F. and Woźniakowski, H. (1980), 'A General Theory of Optimal Algorithms', Academic Press, New York.

Woźniakowski, H. (1986), Information-based complexity, Ann. Rev.Comput.Sci. 1, 319–380.

FAST ALGORITHMS FOR THE COMPUTATION OF FIXED POINTS

K. Sikorski

Computer Science Department
University of Utah
Salt Lake City, UT 84112
USA

SUMMARY

We survey recent complexity results for the computation of fixed points of contractive functions and for the computation of the topological degree of Lipschitz functions in an arbitrary number of dimensions. We exhibit optimal or nearly optimal algorithms, i.e., algorithms which match or are close to the lower bounds on the cost of solving these problems.

In Section 1 we describe a Fixed Point Envelope (FPE) algorithm which we have shown to be the most efficient method for approximating fixed points of contractive univariate functions with using of the absolute and relat ive error criteria. In the multivariate case it is impossible to essentially improve the efficiency of the simple iteration whenever the dimension of the domain of contractive functions is large. For a moderate dimension we have developed a Fixed Point Ellipsoid algorithm which is much more efficient than the simple iteration for mildly contractive functions. This algorithm is based on the ellipsoid construction of Kchachiyan used for solving the linear programming problem.

In Section 2 we exhibit lower and upper bounds on the minimal number of function evaluations for the computation of the topological degree of Lipschitz functions defined on the unit cube in an arbitrary number of dimensions. We outline an algorithm to compute the degree. We stress that nonzero degree value implies that a function has a zero in that particular domain. Thus the degree computation can be used to determine existence of zeros of nonlinear functions in arbitrary domains.

1 Computation of Fixed Points

In this section we exhibit efficient algorithms for approximating fixed points of contractive nonlinear functions with the contracti ve factor $q < 1$. We study two different error criteria: absolute and relative.

The reader may find relevant literature on theory and numerical practice of computing fixed points and solving systems of nonlinear equations in e.g., Traub [1964], Scarf [1967], Ortega and Rheinboldt [1970], Eaves [1972, 1976], Todd [1976], Allgower and Georg [1980] and Garcia and Zangwill [1981]. Numerous applications of the fixed point computation for economic models, price equilibria, game theory, elasticity and catastrophe theory are listed in Garcia and Zangwill [1981] and Allgower and Georg [1980]. Most of the methods used to approximate fixed points are based on classical fixed point theorems, like the Banach contraction theorem, Brouwer, Schauder or Leray-Schauder, see the excellent review of Allgower and Georg [1980]. Contractive fixed point theorems (Banach) afford a constructive means of obtaining a sequence of points convergent to the unique fixed point, like for example the simple iteration algorithm defined by $z_{i+1} = f(z_i), i = 1, 2, \ldots$. The more general fixed point theorems did not until recently offer constructive algorithms for approximating fixed points. The constructive use of Brouwer's fixed point theorem was initiated by Scarf [19 67], Kuhn [1968], Hansen [1968], Eaves [1972] and Eaves and Saigal [1972], an d furnished a basis for the development of simplicial continuation and continuation methods, see Allgower and Georg [1980]. Recently (Sikorski and Wozniakowski [1987, 1989], and Hirsch and Vavasis [1987]) a serious effort was undertaken to develop fast algorithms for approximating fixed points. In our [1987] paper we have developed a Fixed Point Envelope (FPE) algorithm for approximating fixed points of contractive univariate functions with the use of a relative error criterion. We proved that the FPE algorithm minimizes the number of function evaluations needed to compute ϵ-approximation to the fixed point of any contractive function. Hirsch and Vavasis studied the residual error criterion for the Lipschitz class of functions with the constant $K > 1$ satisfying the Brouwer's fixed point theorem. They proved that any algorithm based on function evaluations must use an exponential number of these evaluations to compute close approximation to a fixed point of any such function.

We have demonstrated (Sikorski and Wozniakowski [1987]) that it is impossible to essentially improve the efficiency of the (Banach) simple iteration whenever the dimension of the domain of contractive functions is large. For a moderate dimension we have developed a Fixed Point Ellipsoid algorithm (Sikorski and Wozniakowski [1989])which we outline below. This algor ithm is much more efficient than the simple iteration for mildly contractive functions. It is based on the ellipsoid construction of Kchachiyan used to solve the linear programming problem. We have estimated that our algorithm needs at most $d^3 log(1/\epsilon) + d^4 log(1/(1-q))$ function evaluations to compute an ϵ-approximation to a fixed point in the absolute sense, where d is the dimension of the domain of functions. Thus our algorithm can be thousands times more effective (for q close to the simple iteration which needs $log(1/\epsilon)/log(1/q)$ function evaluation s to compute an ϵ-approximation. Taking for example $\epsilon = 10^{-8}$, $q = 1 - 10^{-5}$ and $d = 5$ the simple iteration will compute approximately $1.6 * 10^6$ function values to obtain the same accuracy of solut ion as our Ellipsoid algorithm obtains with using of only $1.7 * 10^3$ function evaluation s. Thus our algorithm is almost 1000 times more effective than the simple iteration for this data.

1.1 Formulation of the Problem

We consider the class of functions F:

$$F = \{f : B(0,1) \to B(0,1) : ||f(x) - f(y)|| \leq q||x - y||, q < 1\} \tag{1}$$

where $||.||$ is the second norm and B(0,1) a unit ball in the d-dimensional r eal space R^d. We are interested in computing an ϵ-approximation x^*, $\epsilon > 0$, to the fixed point $\alpha = \alpha(f)$, for any $f \epsilon F$ with using of the absolute (2) and the relative (3) error criteria, i.e.,

$$||x^* - \alpha|| \leq \epsilon \quad (absolute); \tag{2}$$

$$||x^* - \alpha||/||\alpha|| \leq \epsilon \quad (relative); \tag{3}$$

In the Sikorski and Wozniakowski [1987] paper we consider the relative error cri terion (3) and study algorithms based on function evaluations. The Banach contraction theorem yields a simple iteration algorithm defined as:

$$z_n = f(z_{n-1}), n = 1, 2, ..., \tag{4}$$

where z_0 is any point in B(0,1). Then

$$||z_n - \alpha|| \leq q^n ||z_0 - \alpha|| \tag{5}$$

Taking $z_0 = 0$, the relative error of the n-th approximation z_n is estimated by

$$||z_n - \alpha||/||\alpha|| \leq q^n \tag{6}$$

This bound is sharp, i.e., there exists a function f for which the relative error of z_n is equal to q^n. Thus to guarantee that the relative error is at most ϵ we must perform

$$n = n(\epsilon, q) = \lceil log(\frac{1}{\epsilon})/log(\frac{1}{q}) \rceil \tag{7}$$

steps which require $n(\epsilon, q)$ function evaluations. For many scientific applications the contraction factor q is very close to one. In this case the number of function evaluations of the simple iteration is huge. Taking for example $\epsilon = 10^{-6}$ and $q = 1 - 10^{-4}$, the number of function evaluat ion is roughly $0.9 * 10^5$.

Problem 1

Can we do better? That is, can we guarantee the same error estimate with using less function evaluations? Or what is the minimal number $m(\epsilon, q)$ of fun ction evaluations needed to approximate the fixed point of any f in F to with in ϵ ?

1.2 A Fixed Point Envelope Algorithm

In the 1987 paper we show that the solution to *Problem* 1 depends on the dimension d of the space R^d. For the univariate case (d=1) we show that $m(\epsilon, q)$ is much less than $n(\epsilon, q)$. We present a Fixed Point Envelope (FPE) algorithm which constructs a sequence x_n, n=1,2,.. of successive approximations to the fixed point $\alpha = \alpha(f)$ with the relative error $e_n = |x_n - \alpha|/|\alpha|$ satisfying t he inequality:

$$e_n \leq \frac{1+3q}{3+q} \frac{e_{n-1}}{1+\sqrt{1-e_{n-1}^2}}, \qquad e_1 \leq q. \tag{8}$$

Obviously $e_n \to 0$ as $n \to \infty$ and for $q \approx 1$ and large n we have $e_n \leq 0.5 * e_{n-1}$. Therefore, we have a linear convergenc e with the ratio 0.5, instead of q as in (5).

We have obtained the following bounds on $m(\epsilon, q)$, assuming that $\epsilon \leq 0.5$ and $1/3 < q < 1$:

$$\lfloor loglog(\frac{1}{1-q}) \rfloor + \lceil \frac{log(\frac{1}{2\epsilon})}{log(\frac{2+2q}{3q-1})} \rceil \leq m(\epsilon, q) \leq \lceil \frac{log(\frac{1}{2\epsilon})}{log(\frac{3+q}{1+3q}) + 0.9} \rceil + \lceil loglog(\frac{1}{1-q}) \rceil + 1 \tag{9}$$

Therefore, asymptotically as $\epsilon \to 0$, $m(\epsilon, q)$ does not depend on q. On the other hand, for fixed ϵ and $q \to 1^-$, $m(\epsilon, q)$ goes to infinity pathologically slowly, as $loglog(1/(1-q))$. We now compare $m(\epsilon, q)$ with $n(\epsilon, q)$ for $\epsilon = 10^{-4}$ and $q = 1 - 10^{-4}$. We have $m(\epsilon, q) \varepsilon [16, 18]$ and $n(\epsilon, q)/m(\epsilon, q) \geq 5000$. Thus our FPE algorithm is 5000 times more effective than the simple iteration for this data.

The Fixed Point Envelope algorithm relies on constructing two envelopes which interpolate the already computed function values. Then the set of all possible fixed points of functions which have the same values at all evaluation points is given by the interval [a, b], where a and b are fixed points of the envelopes. The best approximation is provided by the harmonic mean of a and b. The next evaluation p oint is chosen such that it minimizes the relative error for a worst possible function value. It is a zero of a quadratic polynomial. We stress that the FPE algorithm uses function evaluations at sequentially chosen points. In fact, we have also shown that n simultaneous function evaluations can not provide an ϵ-approximation with $\epsilon < q$ no matter how large n is. Thus the fixed point problem with the relative error criterion is an example of a nonlinear problem for which the sequential computation must be used.

The fixed point envelope algorithm using the relative error criterion can be summarized in the following flowchart:

The Fixed Point Envelope Algorithm FPE_r

Let $a_0 = 0, \ b_0 = 1, \ n = 0$;

$LOOP: \ n := n + 1$;

$t_n := \frac{4a_{n-1}b_{n-1}}{\sqrt{(a_{n-1}+b_{n-1})^2(1-q)^2+16a_{n-1}b_{n-1}q}+(1-q)(a_{n-1}+b_{n-1})}$;

$f_n := f(t_n)$;

$if \ f_n \geq t_n \ then$

$a_n := \frac{f_n+qt_n}{1+q}, \ b_n := min\left(\frac{f_n-qt_n}{1-q}, b_{n-1}\right)$;

$if \ f_n < t_n \ then$

$a_n := max\left(\frac{f_n-qt_n}{1-q}, a_{n-1}\right), \ b_n := \frac{f_n+qt_n}{1+q}$;

$x_n = \frac{2a_nb_n}{a_n+b_n}$;

$if \ (b_n - a_n)/(b_n + a_n) > \epsilon \ then \ go \ to \ LOOP$

$STOP: \ x_n \ is \ an \ \epsilon - approximation.$

For the multivariate case, if f is a contractive function of d variables, with $d \geq \lfloor log(1/\epsilon)/log(1/q) \rfloor$, then it is impossible to essentially improve the efficiency of the simple iteration. More precisely, using the recent result of Chou [1987], which is based on Nemirovsky and Yudin [1983], we conclude that

$$m(\epsilon, q) \geq 0.5n(\epsilon, q) - 1, \tag{10}$$

even if the class F consists of only affine contractive mappings.

In the next paper(Sikorski and Wozniakowski [1989]) we consider the absolute er ror criterion (2). For the univariate case we show that a version FPE_a of the FPE algorithm also minimizes the number of function evaluations needed to approximate the fixed point of any f in F. The FPE_a algorithm uses the same envelope construction as the FPE_r algorithm, however the next evaluati on point (and current best approximation) is provided by the midpoint of the interval of uncertainty. Thus the FPE_a is an envelope-bisection hybrid meth od. We show that the minimal number $m(\epsilon, q)$ of function evaluations is now given by:

$$m(\epsilon, q) = \lceil log(1/\epsilon)/log((1+q)/q) \rceil \leq \lceil log(1/\epsilon) \rceil. \tag{11}$$

Thus even for q=1, the FPE_a algorithm takes only $\lceil log(1/\epsilon) \rceil$ function evaluations to compute an ϵ-approximation to the fixed point.

The fixed point envelope algorithm FPE_a using the absolute error criterion can be summarized in the following flowchart:

The Fixed Point Envelope Algorithm FPE_a

Let $a_0 = 0,\ b_0 = 1,\ n = 0;$
$LOOP:\ n\ := n + 1\ ;$
$t_n\ := (a_{n-1} + b_{n-1})/2\ ;$
$f_n\ := f(t_n)\ ;$
$if\ f_n \geq t_n\ then$
$a_n\ := \frac{f_n + qt_n}{1+q}\ ,\ b_n\ := min\left(\frac{f_n - qt_n}{1-q},\ b_{n-1}\right)\ ;$
$if\ f_n < t_n\ then$
$a_n\ := max\left(\frac{f_n - qt_n}{1-q},\ a_{n-1}\right),\ b_n\ := \frac{f_n + qt_n}{1+q}\ ;$
$if\ (b_n - a_n)/2 > \epsilon\ then\ go\ to\ LOOP;$
$STOP:\ (a_n + b_n)/2\ is\ an\ \epsilon - approximation.$

What algorithm is minimizing the number of function evaluations in the multivariate case? As for the relative error criterion we have shown that when the dimension d is large, $d \geq \lfloor log(1/\epsilon)/log(1/q) \rfloor$, then the minimal number of function evaluations is bounded from below by roughly
$0.5\lfloor log(1/\epsilon)/log(1/q) \rfloor - 1$. Thus, the simple iteration algorithm becomes almost optimal also in this case. What algorithm is minimizin g the number of function evaluations for a moderate dimension d? This is an o pen research problem. We believe that the minimal number of function evaluations needed to compute an ϵ-approximation to a fixed point depends weakly on q through an additive term depending on $log(1/(1-q))$.

In what follows we outline a Fixed Point Ellipsoid Algorithm which is much more efficient than the simple iteration for a moderate dimension d.

1.3 A Fixed Point Ellipsoid Algorithm

As a basic tool for designing the ellipsoid algorithm we have been using the fol lowing lemma:

Lemma (Sikorski and Wozniakowski, 1989):

Let f be any function in F, as defined in (1), and let A be any set containing $\alpha(f)$. Let x be any point in $A \cap B(0,1)$. Then the fixed point $\alpha(f)$ belongs to $A \cap B(y,r)$, where $y = x + 1/(1-q^2)(f(x)-x)$, and $r = q/(1-q^2)||f(x)-x||$.

This lemma enables us to construct a sequence of ellipsoids convergent to the fixed point of any f in F. In what follows we outline the idea of our algorithm:

A Fixed Point Ellipsoid Algorithm - Idea

Let f be any function in the class F, as defined in (1). Let ϵ, q, and $\epsilon_i, i = 1, 2, ...d$ be given numbers, $\epsilon > 0$, $\epsilon_i > 0$, $0 \le q < 1$.

START

i := 0 ; $x_0 := 0$;

$E_0^d := B^d(0,1)$, i.e., the initial d-dimensional ellipsoid E_0^d is equal to the d-dimensional unit ball $B^d(0,1)$.

LOOP

Compute $f(x_i)$, and construct the smallest ellipsoid E_{i+1}^d whic h contains the set $Z = E_i^d \cap \{w \; : \; (w-x)^T(y-x) \ge 0\}$, wher e y and r are given in the above Lemma with $x = x_i$. We remark that the set Z contains the intersection $E_i^d \cap B^d(y,r)$.

The ellipsoid E_{i+1}^d is constructed with using of Kchahiyan's algorith m originally designed for solving the linear programming problem (see e.g. Osborne [1985, p.326])

i := i+1 ;

x_i := the center of the ellipsoid E_i^d ;

If the length of one (say k-th) axis of E_i^d is less than ϵ_d then go to DEFLATION ;

go to LOOP ;

DEFLATION

In this step we reduce the dimension of ellipsoids. Upon entering it we have com puted a_d an ϵ_d -approximation to the k-th component, α_k, of the fixed point $\alpha(f)$, i.e., $|a_d - \alpha_k| \, leq \epsilon_d$

$E_0^{d-1} := E_i^d \bigcap H$, where H is the d-1 dimensional hype rplane going through x_i and orthogonal to the k-th axis of E_i^d .

Remark: Now we modify the nonlinear transformation f by fixing the k-th coordin ate to be equal to a_d and obtain a new f : $B^{d-1}(0,1) \to B^{d-1}(0,1)$ contractive with the same factor q (for details see Sikorski a nd Wozniakowski [

d := d-1; $x_0 := x_i$, i := 0 ;

If $d > 0$ go to LOOP;

STOP

(The point $a = (a_1, a_2, ..., a_d)$ is an ϵ-approximation to the fixed point $\alpha(f)$, i.e., $||a - \alpha(f)|| \leq \epsilon$).

Remark: It is essential to choose proper termination parameters ϵ_i , such that the computed approximation is within ϵ from the fixed point. In our first attempt we have been able to find the values of ϵ_i -s which guarantee at most roughly $d^3 log(1/\epsilon) + d^4 log(1/(1-q))$ funct ion evaluations to compute the ϵ - approximation to $\alpha(f)$ for any f in F. This estimate shows that our algorithm can be thousands times more effective than the simple iteration for q close to 1. We are currently implementing this algori thm and will be performing extensive numerical tests.

The following open problems regarding this algorithm and the fixed point computation remain to be solved:

1. Find an optimal choice of ϵ_i -s minimizing in our algorithm the number of function evaluations needed to compute an ϵ -approximation to the fixed point of any f in F.

2. Find the minimal number or a lower bound on the minimal number of function evaluations necessary to compute an ϵ -approximation to the fixed poi nt of any f in F.

3. Find out whether the Ellipsoid algorithm is almost optimal for small dimensio n d, i.e., whether it almost minimizes the number of function evaluations.

4. Analyse the average number of function evaluations necessary to solve our problem. The average number is defined here with respect to a given probability measure on F, like for example the Gaussian distribution (see Traub, Wasilkowski, Wozniakowski [1988] for a general formulation of the average ca se analysis) .

2 Computation of the Topological Degree

In this section we consider the problem of computing the topological degree $deg(f, C)$ of Lipschitz functions defined on the unit cube $C = [0,1]^d$ in d dimensions. The crucial property of the degree, expressed by the Kronecker's theorem, is the following: if the degree of f is not zero on some domain D then the function f has a zer o in D. Thus the degree value can be used as an existential test for zeros as well as in an al domain, compute the degree (if it is well defined) for the smaller domains, cho ose a subdomain with non-zero degree, e.t.c. In this way we would construct a sequence of domains with decreasing diameters convergent to a zero of f. Thi s idea was invest

We consider the following class G of functions:

$$G = \{f \; : \; C \rightarrow R^d \; : ||f(x) - f(y)||_\infty \leq K||x - y||_\infty, \tag{12}$$

$$||f(x)|| \geq b > 0, \; for \; every \; x \varepsilon \partial C\}$$

where ∂C is the boundary of C.

Since the degree is uniquely defined by the function values on the boundary of C, we assume that arbitrary sequential evaluations of function values on ∂C are allowed. In Boult and Sikorski [1986a] we show the following bounds on the minimal number $m(deg, G)$ of function evaluations to compute the degree of any f in G.

$$n_{low} \leq m(deg, G) \leq n_{up},$$

$$n_{low} \approx 2d(K/(8b))^{d-1}, \tag{13}$$

$$n_{up} \approx 2d(K/(2b))^{d-1},$$

whenever $K/(8b) \geq 1$.

Note that if $K/(2b) < 1$ then the functions in G do not have zeros which implies that the degree is zero for every f. The case $1 \leq K/(2b) < 4$ is open. For the two dimensional case we have obtained a stronger result (Boult and Sikorski [1985]) :

$$m(deg, G) = 4\lfloor K/(4b) \rfloor, \quad whenever\ K/(4b) \geq 1. \tag{14}$$

In what follows we outline an algorithm to compute the degree of any f in G. This algorithm was originally designed by Kearfott [1979] (compare also Stynes [1979, 1980]) and was implemented in current form by Boult and Sikorski [1986 b]. The algorithm uniformly subdivides ∂C into small d-1 dimen sional cubes and then uses function evaluations at all vertices in this subdivision. More precisely, subdivide each d-1 dimensional face of C into M^{d-1} equal cubes of diameter R=1/M , where M=$\lfloor K/(2b) + 1 \rfloor$. In this way we obtain a subdivision of ∂C into $2dM^{d-1}$ cubes C_i of diameter R :

$$\partial C = \bigcup_{i=1}^{2dM^{d-1}} C_i.$$

Let then subdivide each C_i into (d-1)! d-1 dimensional simplices as describ ed in Jeppson [1972]. This forms a simplicial subdivision of ∂C into $2dM^{d-1}(d-1)!$ simplices,

$$\partial C = \sum_{j=1}^{L} t_j S_j, \quad t_j = \pm 1, \ L = 2dM^{d-1}(d-1)!\,.$$

Let $S = [V_1, ..., V_d]$ be any d-1 dimensional simplex in R^d with vertices $V_1, ..., V_d$ The range matrix $R(S, f)$ associated with S and $f \varepsilon G$ is defined as:

$$R(S, f) = [r_{i,j}]_{i,j=1}^{n},$$

where $r_{i,j} = sgn(f_j(V_i))$, and

$$sgn(x) = \begin{cases} 1 & \text{if } x \geq 0, \\ 0 & \text{if } x < 0. \end{cases}$$

The matrix $R(S, f)$ is called feasible if and only if

$$r_{i,j} = 1 \ for\ all\ i \geq j,$$

$$r_{i,i+1} = 0 \ for\ i = 1, ..., d-1.$$

Define the parity of $R(S, f)$ by

$$Par(R(S, f)) = \begin{cases} 1 & \text{if } R(S,f) \text{ is feasible after an even permutation of rows,} \\ -1 & \text{if } R(S,f) \text{ is feasible after an odd permutation of rows,} \\ 0 & \text{otherwise.} \end{cases}$$

The parity can be easily computed with roughly $d^2/2$ comparisons. The topological degree deg(f,G) is now given by (see Kearfott [1979] and Boult and Sikorski [1986 a]) :

$$deg(f,G) = \sum_{j=1}^{L} Par(R(t_j S_j, f)) \tag{15}$$

This algorithm uses n_{up} function evaluations, i.e., establishes the upper bound in (13). It has been implemented in Boult and Sikorski [1986 b], where several numerical tests are presented. A two dimensional version of the algorithm using exactly the minimal number $m(deg, G)$ of function evaluations has been developed and implemented in Boult and Sikorski [1985].

Bibliography

Allgower, E., and Georg, K. (1980), Simplicial and continuation methods for approximating fixed points and solutions to systems of equations, SIAM Rev. 22(1), 28-85.

Boult, T., and Sikorski, K. (1985), Complexity of computing topological degree of Lipschitz functions in two dimensions, Tech. Rep., Computer Science Department, Columbia University.

Boult, T., and Sikorski, K. (1986a), Complexity of computing topological degree of Lipschitz functions in N-dimensions, Journal of Complexity 2, 44-59.

Boult, T., and Sikorski, K. (1986b), A Fortran subroutine for computing topological degree of Lipschitz functions, submitted for publication.

Chou, D. (1987), On the optimality of Krylov information, J. Complexity 3, 26-40.

Eaves, B.C. (1972), Homotopies for computation of fixed points, SIAM Rev. 3(1), 1-22.

Eaves, B.C. (1976), A short course in solving equations with PL homotopies, SIAM-AMS Proc. 9, 73-143.

Eaves, B.C., and Saigal, R. (1972), Homotopies for computation of fixed points on unbounded regions, Math. Programming, 3(2), 225-237.

Eiger, A., Sikorski, K., and Stenger, F. (1984), A bisection method for systems of nonlinear equations, ACM ToMS 10, No. 4, 367-377.

Garcia, C.B., and Zangwill, W.I. (1981), "Pathways to Solutions, Fixed Points and Equilibria", Prentice-Hall, Englewood Cliffs, NJ.

Hansen, T. (1968), On the approximation of a competitive equilibrium, Ph.D. thesis, Yale University.

Harvey, C. and Stenger, F. (1976) A two dimensional analogue to the method of bisections for solving nonlinear equations, Quart. Appl. Math., 351-367.

Hirsch, M.D., and Vavasis, S. (1987), Exponential lower bounds for finding Brouwer fixed points, submitted for publication.

Jeppson, M. M. (1972), A search for the fixed points of a continuous mapping, in "Mathematical Topics in Economic Theory and Computation" (R.H. Day and S.M . Robinson Eds.), SIAM, Philadelphia, 122-129.

Kearfott, R.B. (1977), Computing the Degree of Maps and a Generalized Method of Bisection, Doctoral dissertation, University of Utah.

Kearfott, R.B. (1979), An efficient degree computation method for a generalized method of bisection, Numer. Math. 32, 109-127.

Kuhn, H.W. (1968), Simplicial approximation of fixed points, Ibid., 61, 1238-1242.

Nemirovsky, A.S., and Yudin, D.B. (1983), "Problem Complexity and Method Efficiency in Optimization", Wiley, New York; translated from "Slozhnost Zadach i Effektivnost Metodov Optimizatsii", Nauka, Moscow, 1979.

Ortega, J.M., and Rheinboldt, W.C. (1970), "Iterative Solution of Nonlinear Equations in Several Variables", Academic Press, New York.

Osborne, M.E. (1985), "Finite Algorithms in Optimization and Data Analysis", John Wiley & Sons.

Prufer, M., and Siegberg, H.W. (1980), On Computational Aspects of Topological D egree in R^n, Sonderforschungsbereich 72, Approximation und Optimierung, Universitat Bonn, preprint No. 252.

Scarf, H. (1967), The approximation of fixed points of a continuous mapping, SIAM J.Appl.Math., 15(5), 1328-1343.

Sikorski, K. (1982), Bisection is optimal, Numer. Math. 40, 111-117.

Sikorski, K. (1985), Optimal solution of nonlinear equations, J.Complexity, 1, 197-209.

Sikorski, K., and Wozniakowski, H. (1987), Complexity of fixed points I, J.Complexity, 3, 388-405.

Sikorski, K., and Wozniakowski, H. (1989), Absolute error criterion for the computation of fixed points, in progress.

Stenger, F. (1975), Computing the topological degree of a mapping in R^n, Numer. Math. 25, 23-38.

Stynes, M. (1979), An algorithm for numerical calculation of the topological degree, Appl. Anal. 9, 63-77.

Stynes, M. (1981), On the construction of sufficient refinements for computation of topological degree, Numer. Math. 453-462.

Todd, M.J. (1976), "The Computation of Fixed Points and Applications", Springer Lecture Notes in Economics and Mathematical Systems, 124, Springer-Verlag, New York.

Traub, J.F. (1964), "Iterative Methods for the Solution of Equations", Prentice Hall, Englewood Cliffs, NJ.

Traub, J.F., Wasilkowski, G.W. and Wozniakowski, H. (1988), "Information Based Complexity", Academic Press, New York.

BOUNDING TECHNIQUES FOR MODEL-STRUCTURE SELECTION

J.P. Norton

School of Electronic and Electrical Engineering
University of Birmingham, P.O.Box 363
Birmingham U.K., B15 2TT

ABSTRACT

Structure-selection methods for regression-type models are discussed. Selection is based on parameter bounds, obtained by plotting in parameter space known deterministic bounds on the error between model output and observed output. One method examines the effect of imposing bounds on the sample autocorrelation of the errors, another detects near-degeneracy of the parameter bounds, and two methods aim to delete whichever parameter or combination of parameters is least well defined by the observations. The last two methods have close parallels with principal-component analysis and singular-value decomposition.

1. INTRODUCTION

As an alternative to point parameter estimation, the computation of model parameter bounds has received considerable attention in recent years. Norton (1987) and Walter (1988) review algorithms for parameter-bounding and explain its motivation. Briefly, the appeal of parameter bounding is that it does not rely on the availability of a probabilistic description of the uncertainty affecting the model, nor does it presuppose any criterion for optimality. It simply delineates the range of parameter values yielding model-output values within specified ranges about the observed output samples.

In applications requiring unique parameter estimates, some subsidiary extraction of estimates must then be performed. However, bounds on the parameters are exactly what is needed in many, indeed arguably most, applications. Examples are predictions of the range of possible outputs, worst-case (toleranced) control design, use of models to distinguish two or more types of behaviour, and exploration of the properties of the records to which the model is fitted.

The prior information required for parameter bounding (sometimes called "membership set estimation", which is pleonastic and misleading) consists only of the bounds on model-output error. These bounds may come from background knowledge of the sources of error, or may merely state the performance demanded of the model. Conversely, the object of parameter bounding may be to find out how accurately a model with a given structure can reproduce the observed output.

This paper considers selection of a regression-type scalar-output model structure

$$y_t = \underline{\varphi}_t^T \, \underline{\theta} + e_t \qquad t = 1,2, \ldots N \tag{1.1}$$

to fit the observed output sequence $\{y\}$ with error bounded by

$$r_t^l \leq e_t \leq r_t^u \tag{1.2}$$

With the regressor vector $\underline{\varphi}_t \in \mathbb{R}^p$ known, each observation y_t yields bounds

$$y_t - r_t^u \leq \underline{\varphi}_t^T \, \theta \leq y_t - r_t^l \tag{1.3}$$

on the parameter vector $\underline{\theta}$. They are hyperplanes, and some subset of the 2N such hyperplanes given by N observations constitute the active bounds making up the (p-1) faces of a polytope $\mathcal{P}_N$ which contains all $\underline{\theta}$ satisfying (1.1) and (1.2). Unless p and N are fairly small, the active-bound polytope may be so complicated that a simplified and approximate representation has to be used. The most popular choices are ellipsoids (Schweppe, 1968; Fogel and Huang, 1982)

$$\mathcal{E}_t = \{\underline{\theta} \mid (\underline{\theta} - \hat{\underline{\theta}})^T P_t^{-1} (\underline{\theta} - \hat{\underline{\theta}}_t) \leq 1\} \tag{1.4}$$

or boxes (Milanese and Belforte, 1982)

$$\mathcal{B}_t = \{\underline{\theta} \mid a_{it}^l \leq \theta_i \leq a_{it}^u \, , \quad i = 1,2, \ldots p\} \tag{1.5}$$

Both having the advantage of not becoming more complicated as t increases.

The bounding philosophy simplifies model-structure selection conceptually, compared with least-squares estimation or probabilistic parameter estimation. In the latter two approaches, selection is a compromise between model complexity and explanatory power. Some weighted function of both has to be optimized, as in the AIC, or a measure of the badness of the model has to be compared with a complexity-dependent threshold, as in F-testing. This dual simultaneous choice is split, in bounding, into prior specification of the explanatory power (output-error bounds) then acceptance of the simplest model satisfying the specification.

Four methods of structure selection for models of the form (1.1) will be suggested. One, described in section 2, picks the simplest model (smallest p) capable of satisfying both (1.2) and bounds on the sample autocorrelations of $\{e\}$ over a range of lags. In other words, the criterion for model acceptability is smallness and lack of structure (i.e. near-whiteness) of its residuals. The other three selection methods are based on the shape of $\mathcal{P}_N$ or its approximations. In section 3, it is assumed that the observations are generated by one of a family of processes indexed by p. For example, $\underline{\varphi}_t$ might consist of successive samples of the same input. The correct model order is found by comparing the reductions in hypervolumes of $\mathcal{P}_N$ or its approximations from their initial values, for the candidate models. Sections 4 and 5 present two techniques suggested by principal-component analysis and singular-value decomposition in least-squares estimation. They aim to delete the least well defined, least effective parameter or combination of parameters, and are well suited to model reduction.

2. IMPOSITION OF NOISE-WHITENESS BOUNDS

A suitable model structure can be found, in principle, by computing the feasible parameter set $\mathcal{P}_N$ for successively more complicated candidate models, stopping as soon as a non-empty $\mathcal{P}_N$ is found. That is, we accept the simplest model which does not conflict with the observations and specified error bounds. The practical drawback of this straightforward procedure is its sensitivity to the assumed values of the output-error bound. If they are a little smaller than the actual extreme values of the observation noise, even a model structure corresponding exactly to the process generating the observations will be rejected. Conversely, too-wide error bounds may lead to acceptance of a model which has systematic output error not present in the output of one of the candidate models.

A possible remedy is to supply more prior information, in the form of bounds on the time-structure of the output errors. Such information should prevent most types of systematic error, but may not discriminate against all unsatisfactory features of the error sequence, particularly in the presence of non-stationarity (Norton, 1986). The noise whiteness bounds are :

$$\left|\frac{\rho_i}{\rho_o}\right| \leq s_i \;, \qquad i = 1, 2, \ldots k \tag{2.1}$$

where

$$\rho_i = \frac{1}{N-i} \sum_{t=1}^{N-i} e_t \, e_{t+i} \qquad i = 0, 1, \ldots k \tag{2.2}$$

Details of how such bounds can be combined with ellipsoidal or polytope feasible parameter sets $\mathcal{E}_N$ or $\mathcal{P}_N$ are provided by Veres and Norton (1989), and are summarised briefly here. The basic idea is to check whether $\mathcal{E}_N$ or $\mathcal{P}_N$ intersects all the sets of parameter values satisfying the whiteness bounds (2.1). For computational simplicity ρ_o is replaced by its infimum $\bar{\rho}_o$ over $\mathcal{E}_N$ or $\mathcal{P}_N$, rather than being computed with $\underline{\theta}$ as its argument. The effect is to tighten the whiteness bounds. Ordinary least squares supplies $\bar{\rho}_o$ (and the corresponding $\underline{\theta}$, if desired). The set of parameter values satisfying (2.1) is then the intersection of

$$\mathcal{R}_i = \{\underline{\theta} \mid (\underline{y}_N^{(i)} - \Phi_N^{(i)} \underline{\theta})^T (\underline{y}_N^{(i)'} - \Phi_N^{(i)'} \underline{\theta}) \leq \frac{N-i}{N} \bar{\rho}_o s_i \} \quad i = 1, 2, .. k \tag{2.3}$$

where $\underline{y}_N^{(i)}$ and $\underline{y}_N^{(i)'}$ are respectively the first and last N-i elements of $\underline{y}_N$, and $\Phi_N^{(i)}$ and $\Phi_N^{(i)'}$ are the first and last N-i rows of Φ_N .

For an ellipsoidal feasible parameter set $\mathcal{E}_N$, (1.4) may be rewritten for $t = N$ as

$$\mathcal{E}_N = \{\underline{\theta} \mid (L^T(\underline{\theta} - \hat{\underline{\theta}}_N))^T (L^T(\underline{\theta} - \hat{\underline{\theta}}_N)) \leq 1\} \tag{2.4}$$

where L is the Choleski factor of P_N^{-1}. Hence we can determine whether $\mathcal{E}_N$ intersects $\mathcal{R}_i$ by checking whether the distance of $L^T \hat{\underline{\theta}}_N$ from $\mathcal{R}_i$ in $L^T \underline{\theta}$ - space is greater than 1. The Lagrange multiplier method allows us to minimise $(L^T(\underline{\theta} - \hat{\underline{\theta}}_N))^T (L^T(\underline{\theta} - \hat{\underline{\theta}}_N))$ on the boundary of each $\mathcal{R}_i$ in turn, and we reject the model if at any i the result is greater than unity.

If alternatively we employ a polytope feasible parameter set $\mathcal{P}_N$, the same idea can be applied. The polytope can be expressed as the set of convex combinations of its vertices $\underline{\theta}_1$ to $\underline{\theta}_n$:

$$\mathcal{P}_N = \{\underline{\theta} \mid \underline{\theta} = \sum_{j=1}^{n} \lambda_j \underline{\theta}_j , \sum_{j=1}^{n} \lambda_j = 1, \lambda_j \geq 0, j = 1, 2, \ldots n\} \qquad (2.5)$$

and each $\mathcal{R}_i$ then written as a quadratic in the λ's. The problem is thus reduced to quadratic programming to check the minimum of $|\rho_i/\bar{\rho}_o|$ over the polytope, subject to unity sum and non-negativity of the λ's. Again the Lagrange multiplier technique supplies a means, transforming the problem into one equivalent to that of finding a feasible point in linear programming. Computation is shortened by performing the quadratic programming solution first over the vertices of $\mathcal{R}_i$, then over its edges, 2-faces,.. stopping as soon as a feasible point is found. Results of tests on artificial records can be found in Veres and Norton (1989a).

A special case worth noting is a power bound on the error sequence $\{e\}$, requiring $\underline{\theta}$ to belong to

$$\mathcal{R}_o = \{\underline{\theta} \mid \frac{1}{N}(\underline{y}_N - \Phi_N\underline{\theta})^T(\underline{y}_N - \Phi_N\underline{\theta}) \leq W\} \qquad (2.6)$$

which can be rewritten as an ellipsoidal set $\mathcal{E}_o$ with centre

$$\hat{\underline{\theta}}_o = (\Phi_N^T \Phi_N)^{-1} \Phi_N^T \underline{y}_N \qquad (2.7)$$

and describing matrix P_o such that

$$P_o^{-1} = \Phi_N^T \Phi_N / (NW - \bar{\rho}_o) \qquad (2.8)$$

The power bound is simply employed as the starting ellipsoid for recursive updating of the feasible parameter set.

3. MODEL-STRUCTURE TERMS USING SHAPE OF FEASIBLE-PARAMETER SET

Inadequacy of a tentative model structure may show up in several different ways. One, time-structure of the model-output errors, has been discussed in section 2. Another, particularly relevant to parameter bounding, is degeneracy of the feasible-parameter set. If a model is overparameterized, its parameters could be equality-constrained without significantly affecting its performance. Geometrically, this implies that all feasible values correspond to points in some subspace of the parameter space employed. In the simplest case, a p-polytope bounding the feasible values might degenerate to a (p-1)-polytope, because a linear relation existed between the p parameters. Underparameterization is also detectable, if severe enough, by noticing that the set of feasible parameter values shrinks to nothing as the observations are processed.

In practice, we are interested not in detecting total degeneracy, but in measuring and comparing the extent to which the feasible-parameter sets for candidate models approach degeneracy. Many possibilities exist. For example, we could compute the ratio of the lengths of the longest and shortest, or average, axes of $\mathcal{P}_N$ or $\mathcal{E}_N$. One of the simplest possibilities, which has received some theoretical attention and seems to work well in simulations, is to compare the reduction in volume of the feasible parameter set (expressed as the ratio of final to initial volume) for candidate models (Veres and Norton, 1989b). For both under- and over-parameterized models, the volume tends to zero as the number of observations increases, under mild assumptions on the sequences $\{\underline{\varphi}\}$ and $\{e\}$; the model structure test is to accept the structure with smallest relative reduction in volume.

A statistical justification can be supplied by a Bayesian argument, assuming uniform distribution of $\{e\}$ and uniform prior probability densities for the parameters. However, consistency of the volume-reduction criterion can be proven under much less restrictive conditions (Veres and Norton, 1989b). An informal account of those conditions now follows. If (i) $\{e\}$ is uniformly heavy-tailed, i.e. there is positive probability of e_t being within any specified range of its bound, and (ii) $\{\underline{\varphi}\}$ is omnidirectional, i.e. the probability that the projection of $\underline{\varphi}_t$ in any specified direction exceeds a specified value is positive at all times, then $\mathcal{P}_N$ is uniformly potentially consistent, i.e. has a positive probability, as N tends to infinity, of excluding, at infinitely many points in time, all parameter values other than that generating the record. If, in addition, the sequence $\{[e\ \underline{\varphi}^T]^T\}$ is asymptotically independent, then the model structure giving the smallest volume reduction, tends, almost surely, to the structure generating the records.

Two comments about this statistical analysis of a bound-based test are in order. First, we are not excluded from statistical analysis by adopting a bound description of uncertainty; we do, of course, have to make additional assumptions in order to allow results to be derived about average behaviour of bounding algorithms and bound-based tests. Second, the natural accompaniment of an entirely bound-based computation would be a statement of worst-case behaviour of the algorithm and/or structure test.

4. PARAMETER-BOUNDING COUNTERPART OF PRINCIPAL-COMPONENT ANALYSIS

Principal-component analysis (Wetherill, 1986) is based on modal analysis of the normal matrix $\Phi^T\Phi$ of the regression modal

$$\underline{y} = \Phi\,\Theta + \underline{e} \qquad (4.1)$$

deriving from model (1.1). If the real, positive eigenvalues of $\Phi^T\Phi$ are $\lambda_1 > \lambda_2 > \ldots > \lambda_p$, and they correspond to orthonormal eigenvectors $\underline{m}_1, \underline{m}_2, \ldots \underline{m}_p$, then for white, zero-mean noise $\underline{e}$ with covariance $\sigma^2 I$, the ordinary-least-squares estimate $\hat{\underline{\Theta}}$ has covariance

$$\operatorname{cov} \hat{\underline{\Theta}} = \sigma^2 (\Phi^T\Phi)^{-1} = \sigma^2 M \Lambda^{-1} M^T = \sigma^2 \sum_{i=1}^{p} \lambda_i^{-1}\, \underline{m}_i\, \underline{m}_i^T \qquad (4.2)$$

where M is $(\underline{m}_1, \underline{m}_2 \ldots \underline{m}_p)$ and Λ is diag $(\lambda_1, \lambda_2, \ldots, \lambda_p)$. Hence, roughly speaking, any small λ_i and algebraically-large element of $\underline{m}_i$ make a large contribution to cov $\hat{\underline{\Theta}}$. Moreover

$$\| \varphi \underline{m}_i \|^2 = \underline{m}_i^T M \Lambda M^T \underline{m}_i = \lambda_i \qquad (4.3)$$

so if the smallest eigenvalue λ_p is very small, a linear combination $\varphi\underline{m}_p$ of the columns of the regressor matrix is small, i.e. the model contains a near-redundancy. It seems reasonable, therefore, to delete parameter Θ_j from the model, where m_{jp} is the algebraically largest element of the eigenvector $\underline{m}_p$ associated with the smallest eigenvalue λ_p.

To find a parameter-bounding counterpart, consider ellipsoid $\mathcal{E}_N$. Its axes are the eigenvectors $\underline{n}_1$ to $\underline{n}_p$ of P_N^{-1} and the square roots of the corresponding eigenvalues μ_1 to μ_p are the reciprocals of the semi-axis lengths. Thus deletion of Θ_j where n_{jp} is the algebraically largest element of $\underline{n}_p$ and μ_p the smallest eigenvalue of P_N^{-1}, is deletion of the parameter whose co-ordinate axis is closest in direction to the longest axis of $\mathcal{E}_N$. The parallel with the same procedure in least-squares estimation is completed by noticing that P_N plays a similar part, by showing the size of $\mathcal{E}_N$ and hence the uncertainty in $\underline{\theta}$, to that played by the covariance $\sigma^2 (\Phi^T\Phi)^{-1}$ of the least-squares estimate of $\hat{\underline{\theta}}$. We conclude that μ_1 to μ_p may be compared with scaled versions of λ_1 to λ_p and $\underline{n}_1$ to $\underline{n}_p$ with $\underline{m}_1$ to $\underline{m}_p$.

The idea of deleting the co-ordinate closest to the longest axis can be applied to non-ellipsoidal parameter bounds, provided the longest axis can be found. For example, the longest axis of a polytope bound may be found by exhaustive comparison of the distances between pairs of vertices. Such a computation will be acceptable wherever the calculations to locate the vertices are acceptable.

5. PARAMETER-BOUNDING COUNTERPART OF SINGULAR-VALUE DECOMPOSITION

Singular-value decomposition factorizes Φ in (4.1) into USV^T, where U is an $N \times p$ orthogonal matrix, V^T is $r \times p$ and orthogonal and S is a full-rank, diagonal $r \times r$ matrix of the same rank as Φ. If we define $\underline{\eta}$ as $SV^T\underline{\theta}$ then

$$\underline{y} = U\underline{\eta} + \underline{e} \tag{5.1}$$

and, as U is orthogonal, the least-squares estimate of $\underline{\eta}$ and the resulting least-squares estimate of $\underline{\theta}$ are

$$\hat{\underline{\eta}} = U^T\underline{y} \quad , \quad \hat{\underline{\theta}} = VS^{-1}\,\hat{\underline{\eta}} \tag{5.2}$$

Now

$$\eta_i = s_i\,\underline{v}_i^T\underline{\theta} \tag{5.3}$$

where s_i, element (i,i) of S, is the ith singular value of Φ, and $\underline{v}_i$ is column i of V. With $\underline{v}_i^T\underline{v}_i$ unity, η_i/s_i is the orthogonal projection of $\underline{\theta}$ into $\underline{v}_i$, so if we delete η_i from $\underline{\eta}$ we are reducing $\underline{\theta}$ space to the space orthogonal to $\underline{v}_i$. In least-squares model reduction, the smallest of the real, positive singular values $s_1 > s_2 > \ldots > s_r$ is found and η_r deleted. As U is $\Phi V S^{-1}$ and deletion of η_r removes the influence of column r of U from (5.1), the deletion removes a component $\Phi\underline{v}_r/s_r$ from the original regression equation (4.1).

The parameter-bounding counterpart is easily found; since

$$\Phi^T\Phi = VS^2V^T \tag{5.4}$$

we see that s_i^2 is eignevalue i of $\Phi^T\Phi$, and $\underline{v}_i$ is eigenvector i. Substituting P_N^{-1} for $(\Phi^T\Phi)^{-1}/\sigma^2$, as in section 4, we can identify the half-length $1/\mu_r^{1/2}$ of the longest axis of $\mathcal{E}_N$ with $1/s_r$. Removal of η_r and $\Phi\,\underline{v}_r/s_r$ corresponds to removal of the projections onto the longest axis of the normals $\underline{\varphi}_1, \underline{\varphi}_2, \ldots \underline{\varphi}_N$ to the hyperplane bounds (1.3). $\mathcal{E}_N$ is thereby projected onto the $(p-1)$ space orthogonal to its longest axis, yielding another ellipsoid.

For a polytope $\mathcal{P}_N$, projection onto the parameter subspace orthogonal to the longest axis is straightforward once that axis has been found. The idea could be extended to other shapes of parameter bounds by computing and projecting extreme points in directions orthogonal to the longest axis. Computational expense is the limiting factor in more complicated cases.

6. CONCLUSIONS

Several approaches to the selection of structures for parameter-bounding models have been described. They illustrate two important points, namely that methods in regression analysis have quite direct parameter-bounding counterparts (but geometrically rather than algebraically motivated), and that geometrical ideas of great simplicity suggest selection methods for parameter-bounding models.

7. REFERENCES

E.Fogel and Y.F.Huang (1982) On the value of information in system identification-bounded noise case, Automatica, 18, 229-238.

M.Milanese and G.Belforte (1982) Estimation theory and uncertainty intervals evaluation in the presence of unknown but bounded errors: linear families of models and estimators, IEEE Trans.Autom.Control, AC-27, 408-414.

J.P.Norton (1987) Identification and application of bounded-parameter models, Automatica, 23, 497-507.

F.C.Schweppe (1968) Recursive state estimation : unknown but bounded errors and system inputs, IEEE Trans.Autom.Control, AC-13, 22-28.

S.M.Veres and J.P.Norton (1989a) Structure identification of parameter-bounding models by use of noise-structure bounds, Int.J.Control, to appear.

S.M.Veres and J.P.Norton (1989b) Consistency of parameter-bounding algorithms, in preparation.

E.Walter and H.Piet-Lahanier (1988) Estimation of parameter bounds from bounded-error data : a survey, Proc.12th IMACS World Congress, Paris, 467-472.

G.B.Wetherill, P.Duncombe, M.Kenward, J.Kollerstrom, S.R.Paul and B.J.Vowden. Regression Analysis with Applications, Chapman and Hall, London and New York, 1986, Chapter 4.

ROBUST LINEAR AND NONLINEAR PARAMETER ESTIMATION IN THE BOUNDED-ERROR CONTEXT

Eric Walter and Hélène Piet-Lahanier

Laboratoire des Signaux et Systèmes
CNRS-SUPELEC
Plateau de Moulon
91192 Gif-sur-Yvette Cedex
France

INTRODUCTION

When estimating the parameters of a model from experimental data, one usually assumes that the error between the measurements and model outputs can be characterized as a stochastic process whose statistics are either known or expressed as a function of parameters to be estimated. There are, however, situations where such a hypothesis cannot be considered as satisfactory. A first example is when nothing is known about the type of distribution of the error and too few data points are available to make it possible to check any statistical assumption on the error from examination of the residuals. A second example is when the essential part of the error between the model outputs and measurements corresponds to the use of a simplified model (e.g. low order linear ordinary differential equation when the system studied is known to be nonlinear and distributed). The error is then deterministic by nature and not suitably described as random.

Following the work of Schweppe (1968, 1973) and Witsenhausen (1968), growing attention has been devoted to a somewhat cruder description of the uncertainty. In this approach, prior upper and lower bounds are assumed to be available for the error but nothing is supposed to be known about the distribution of the error between these bounds. One is then interested in characterizing the set of all values of the parameter vector that are consistent with the model structure, experimental data and bounds on the error. Various methods have been developed during the last decade for characterizing this set. When the model output is linear in the parameters, three types of approach have been proposed, namely ellipsoidal outer bounding (Fogel and Huang, 1982), orthotopic outer bounding (Milanese and Belforte, 1982) and exact description (Walter and Piet-Lahanier, 1987). When the model output is nonlinear in the parameters, various approaches have also been proposed, using a direct characterization of the boundary (Norton, 1986), a scanning of the parameter space (Fedra et al., 1981; Smit, 1983), linearizations (Belforte and Milanese, 1981) or the determination of isocriteria (Walter and Piet-Lahanier, 1986). A more detailed view of the state of the art can be found in the survey by Milanese in this volume.

If proper precautions are not taken, bounded-error estimators are not robust to outliers, i.e. to points where the actual error is larger (possibly much larger) than what was assumed when specifying the error bounds. Such outliers may result from mistakes committed during the collection or manipulation of the data, but also from overoptimistic error bounds. The purpose of the present paper is to address the robustness to outliers of a recently developed approach, which can be applied to both linear and nonlinear models.

OUTLIER MINIMAL NUMBER ESTIMATOR

For reasons which will become apparent, the estimator considered here has been called Outlier Minimal Number Estimator (OMNE) (Walter and Piet-Lahanier, 1986). Let us present it briefly. First an *error* $e(k, \underline{\theta})$ must be defined. This is usually an output error

$$e(k, \underline{\theta}) = y_d(k) - y_m(k, \underline{\theta}), \quad k=1, \ldots, N, \tag{1}$$

where $y_d(k)$ is the kth scalar datum and y_m is the output of a deterministic model depending on a p-dimensional vector $\underline{\theta}$ of real parameters to be estimated. Input or generalized errors could, however, also be used if appropriate (see an example in (Piet-Lahanier et al., 1989)). For $\underline{\theta}$ to be acceptable, the error must lie between bounds e_{min} and e_{max}, given *a priori*,

$$e_{min}(k) \leq e(k, \underline{\theta}) \leq e_{max}(k), \quad k=1, \ldots, N. \tag{2}$$

Nothing else is assumed about it. The *membership set* (or posterior feasible parameter set) S is then defined as

$$S = \Theta \cap \{\underline{\theta} \,;\, e_{min}(k) \leq e(k, \underline{\theta}) \leq e_{max}(k), \, k=1, \ldots, N\}, \tag{3}$$

where Θ is the prior feasible parameter set, which OMNE assumes to be specified as

$$\Theta = \{\underline{\theta} \,;\, \theta_{i_{min}} \leq \theta_i \leq \theta_{i_{max}}, \, i = 1, \ldots, p\}. \tag{4}$$

OMNE consists of two steps. The first is used to obtain a point within the membership set, while the second aims at exploring its boundary.

Reaching a Point Within S

During the first step, OMNE looks for a value $\hat{\underline{\theta}}$ of $\underline{\theta}$ maximizing the criterion

$$j(\underline{\theta}) = \frac{100}{N} \times \text{Card}\,\{k \in 1, \ldots, N;\, e_{min}(k) \leq e(k, \underline{\theta}) \leq e_{max}(k)\} \tag{5}$$

over Θ. This amounts to minimizing the number of data points considered as outliers, hence the name of the estimator. Assuming for the time being that there are no outliers, the optimal value of the criterion is 100% and any $\underline{\theta}$ such that $j(\underline{\theta}) = 100\%$ belongs to S. The specific difficulty of this optimization is that the gradient of the criterion with respect to $\underline{\theta}$ is zero wherever defined, which forbids the use of any classical local methods of nonlinear programming such as the gradient, Gauss-Newton or quasi-Newton algorithms. This reason, combined with the fact that the criterion may be multimodal, have led us to retain a global optimization method by adaptive random search (Bekey and Masri, 1983; Pronzato et al., 1984).

Exploring the Boundary

The membership set can alternatively be defined as

$$S = \Theta \cap \{\underline{\theta} \,;\, j(\underline{\theta}) = 100\%\}. \tag{6}$$

Any of the techniques developed for characterizing isocriteria in the parameter space (see e.g. (Richalet et al., 1971)) can therefore be used to characterize S during the second step of OMNE. Note that the isocriterion is then the set of interest itself, and not only its boundary as usual. We shall limit ourselves here to a brief description of the ideas underlying the algorithm we are using at present.

In any given direction $\underline{d}$ from $\hat{\underline{\theta}}$, a point $\underline{\theta}_b(\hat{\underline{\theta}},\underline{d})$ of the parameter space belonging to the boundary of S can be generated as follows. Let $\underline{\theta}_1(\hat{\underline{\theta}},\underline{d})$ be the point of the boundary of Θ reached when moving from $\hat{\underline{\theta}}$ in the direction $\underline{d}$. If $j(\underline{\theta}_1(\hat{\underline{\theta}},\underline{d})) = j(\hat{\underline{\theta}})$, then $\underline{\theta}_b(\hat{\underline{\theta}},\underline{d}) = \underline{\theta}_1(\hat{\underline{\theta}},\underline{d})$, else it is easy to find $\underline{\theta}_b(\hat{\underline{\theta}},\underline{d})$ with any desired precision by dichotomy between $\hat{\underline{\theta}}$ and $\underline{\theta}_1(\hat{\underline{\theta}},\underline{d})$. This algorithm can be visualized as analogous to the exploration of a cave with a torch. By pointing the torch from $\hat{\underline{\theta}}$ in the direction $\underline{d}$, we illuminate a point of the boundary of the cave. It is then necessary to change the direction and origin of the exploration so as to get a good idea of the extent of the cave and to avoid ignoring parts of it that may be hidden. The method described in (Walter and Piet-Lahanier, 1988) has been found on various test-cases to be much more efficient for pushing the $\underline{\theta}_b$'s as far apart as possible than the method described in (Lahanier et al., 1987). This becomes especially important when the number of parameters increases, because it allows one to avoid, at least in some measure, the curse of dimensionality.

If the number of parameters is smaller than or equal to three, a visual representation can be drawn of the set of points of the boundary of S thus obtained. When the number of parameters increases, various techniques can be used to give a more or less accurate description of the set. One may for example resort to principal component analysis, or estimate parameter uncertainty intervals by computing

$$\hat{\theta}_{i_{min}} = \underset{\{\underline{\theta}_b\}}{\mathrm{Min}}\ \theta_i \quad \text{and} \quad \hat{\theta}_{i_{max}} = \underset{\{\underline{\theta}_b\}}{\mathrm{Max}}\ \theta_i, \quad i=1, \ldots, p. \tag{7}$$

If the true uncertainty interval for parameter θ_i is denoted by $[\theta_{i_{min}}, \theta_{i_{max}}]$, one of course has

$$[\hat{\theta}_{i_{min}}, \hat{\theta}_{i_{max}}] \in [\theta_{i_{min}}, \theta_{i_{max}}], \quad i=1, \ldots, p, \tag{8}$$

so that we obtain *inner bounds* for the parameter uncertainty intervals.

Remarks

(i) Assuming that the model structure and error bounds are correct and that Θ contains the true value $\underline{\theta}^*$ for the parameters, there are two main reasons why the estimated parameter uncertainty intervals may not correspond exactly to the true ones. The first is that the membership set may present some narrow portions overlooked by the algorithm exploring its boundary. The second is that the membership set for nonlinear models may consist of several disconnected subsets which may not all be explored by the algorithm. This may be due to identifiability problems, which can be detected and accounted for by a prior study of the structural properties of the model (Walter et al., 1986), but it may have other causes not so easily detected. A new version of OMNE, capable of exploring such disconnected subsets, is being developed. The basic idea is simply to resume the optimization of the criterion (5) over Θ deprived of the smallest orthotopes containing the parts of S detected so far. If any $\hat{\underline{\theta}}$ such that $j(\hat{\underline{\theta}}) = 100\%$ is found, it is used as the starting point of a new exploration of the boundary.

(ii) In nonlinear estimation in the statistical framework, the Cramer-Rao inequality is often used to obtain a lower bound for the covariance of the error on $\underline{\theta}$. The analogy between this lower bound and the inner bounds for the parameter uncertainty intervals obtained with OMNE should not be pushed too far. In particular $[\hat{\underline{\theta}}_{i_{min}}, \hat{\underline{\theta}}_{i_{max}}]$ should tend to $[\theta_{i_{min}}, \theta_{i_{max}}]$ when the number of evaluations of the criterion tends to infinity, whereas the Cramer-Rao lower bound is only reached when the number of data points tends to infinity, an assumption not made here.

Dealing with Outliers

If the membership set turns out to be empty, this means either that Θ or the model structure are inadequate or that there are outliers in the data. In this section, the error is defined by (1) and Θ and the model structure are assumed to be correct, so that the data have been generated by a model $y_m(., \underline{\theta}^*)$, with $\underline{\theta}^* \in \Theta$. An outlier will then be any datum $y_d(k)$ such that $e(k, \underline{\theta}^*)$ does not satisfy (2). It may correspond not only to a measurement improperly performed (for example because of a sensor failure or erroneous reading) but also – and this is specific to the bounded-error approach to estimation – to overly optimistic hypotheses on the error bounds.

When outliers are to be feared, it is desirable to use estimation methods such that they perturb the estimates as little as possible (see e.g. Launer and Wilkinson, 1979). It is well known, for example, that least square estimation is not robust to outliers, as any very large deviation penalizes the criterion so much that the resulting least square estimate has nothing to do with the one that would have been obtained, had the outlier been detected and removed.

Since underestimating the noise bounds may create outliers even in the absence of any failed measurement, it is particularly important to assess the robustness properties of bounded-error estimators. In what follows we shall, somewhat schematically, distinguish *severe outliers* (which correspond to errors so large that together with the regular data they result in the emptiness of the membership set) and *mild outliers*. Surprising as it may sound, severe outliers will turn out to be easier to deal with than mild ones. Contrary to OMNE, most of the bounded-error estimators have not been designed specifically to deal with outliers. Ellipsoidal bounding algorithms may not even detect the presence of severe outliers. The orthotopic bounding and exact description algorithms would detect the presence of severe outliers but are unable to locate them in order to discard them. The technique suggested in (Norton, 1987), which amounts to removing the contribution to the boundary of S of all the data points in turn until S becomes non-empty, appears as exceedingly complex, especially if there are several outliers.

If the first step of OMNE finds a $\hat{\underline{\theta}}$ such that $j(\hat{\underline{\theta}}) < 100\%$, we may consider changing the model structure or adopting more pessimistic bounds for the error. We may, however, prefer to stick to our model structure and bounds and to consider any datum such that $e(k,\underline{\theta}^*)$ does not satisfy (2) as an outlier, whose effect on the membership set should be discarded. We can then define the *membership set at level* α as

$$S^{\alpha} = \Theta \cap \{\underline{\theta} ; j(\underline{\theta}) \geq \alpha\}, \tag{9}$$

so that S corresponds to S^{100}.

If there are only severe outliers, they can easily be detected and discarded by characterizing the membership set at level $j(\hat{\underline{\theta}})$ with the second step of OMNE. Provided that these outliers are not arranged in such a pattern that they can be described by the model structure chosen (a very unlikely event for which no solution can be provided), this procedure is robust even when there are more outliers than regular data points, an exceptionally good performance. If, on the other hand, there are mild outliers, the situation is not so propitious, for they will neither be detected nor discarded. Should they contribute to the boundary of the membership set at level $j(\hat{\theta})$, this set may no longer contain the true value for the parameters. Characterizing the membership set at level $j(\hat{\theta}) - 100 \frac{q}{N}$ will protect us against up to q occurrences of this situation, at the possible cost of rejecting some regular data and increasing the uncertainty on the parameters.

Remarks

(i) When the model output is linear in the parameters, the exact description or orthotopic outer bounding methods can be used to check that S is void and rule out the possibility that the global optimizer failed to detect a very small S.

(ii) It may happen that the data points rejected in the membership set at level $\alpha < 100$ do not always consider the same data points as outliers. This may result in S^{α} being non-connected and provides a further incentive for choosing a version of OMNE capable of dealing with such sets.

(iii) Prior information (if any) on the probability of the measurement error exceeding the assumed bounds can be used as a guideline for the choice of q.

EXAMPLE

Using a simulated example has the advantage that the model structure is known to be correct and the true value of each parameter is available for checking the results obtained. In order to make it easy to compare these results with those provided by other estimators, we have chosen a very simple model and give all the data used.

Table 1. Regular data set

t	y_d	ε
0.	0.97845024E+00	-0.21549774E-01
0.5	0.91775733E+00	0.12919909E-01
1.	0.76359284E+00	-0.55137943E-01
1.5	0.83734936E+00	0.96531123E-01
2.	0.66890925E+00	-0.14107943E-02
2.5	0.69519967E+00	0.88668980E-01
3.	0.60828614E+00	0.59474498E-01
3.5	0.48444057E+00	-0.12144732E-01
4.	0.53270918E+00	0.83380237E-01
4.5	0.37814140E+00	0.28428270E-01
5.	0.37381437E+00	0.59349239E-02
5.5	0.28107977E+00	-0.51791310E-01
6.	0.24459679E+00	-0.56597400E-01
6.5	0.23999761E+00	-0.32534171E-01
7.	0.24463543E+00	-0.19615411E-02
7.5	0.25536752E+00	0.32237351E-01
8.	0.21504229E+00	0.13145775E-01
8.5	0.12369311E+00	-0.58990408E-01
9.	0.11351015E+00	-0.51788736E-01
9.5	0.13614616E+00	-0.13422454E-01
10.	0.14416318E+00	0.88278949E-02

A set of 21 noise-free data points was first computed according to

$$y(k) = \theta_1^* \exp(-\theta_2^* t_k),\ k = 0, \ldots, 20, \tag{10}$$

with $t_k = k/2$, $\theta_1^* = 1$ and $\theta_2^* = 0.2$. The data were then generated by

$$y_d(k) = y(k) + \varepsilon(k),\ k = 0, \ldots, 20, \tag{11}$$

where $\varepsilon(k)$ is uniformly distributed between -0.1 and 0.1. The resulting data set is given in Table 1. It will be described by the model $y_m(k, \underline{\theta}) = \theta_1 \exp(-\theta_2 t_k)$, where the prior feasible set for the parameters is given by $\Theta = [0, 5] \times [0, 1]$. Because of the use of a global optimizer, the initial point in the parameter space is not critical and is taken as the center of Θ.

Three different situations are considered to illustrate the behavior of OMNE with and without outliers. In each case, the error is defined by (1).

Correct error bounds

Assume first that $-e_{min}(k) = e_{max}(k) = 0.1$. Since these error bounds are correct, $\underline{\theta}^* \in S$. During the first step of OMNE, a point $\hat{\underline{\theta}}$ is found such that $j(\hat{\underline{\theta}}) = 100\%$. The characterization of S obtained during the second step is given in Figure 1. The corresponding estimated parameter uncertainty intervals satisfy

$$\hat{\theta}_{1min} = 0.952, \qquad \hat{\theta}_{1max} = 1.078, \tag{12}$$

and

$$\hat{\theta}_{2min} = 0.170, \qquad \hat{\theta}_{2max} = 0.228. \tag{13}$$

They contain the true value of the parameters.

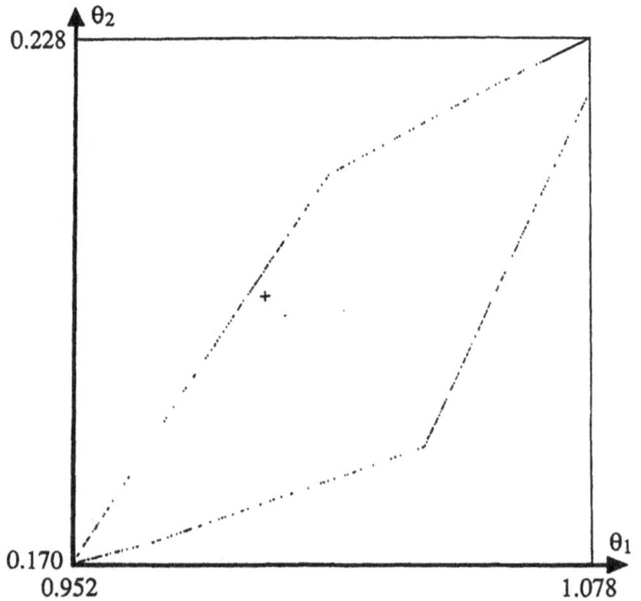

Fig. 1. Estimated membership set with correct error bounds. The cross indicates $\underline{\theta}^*$.

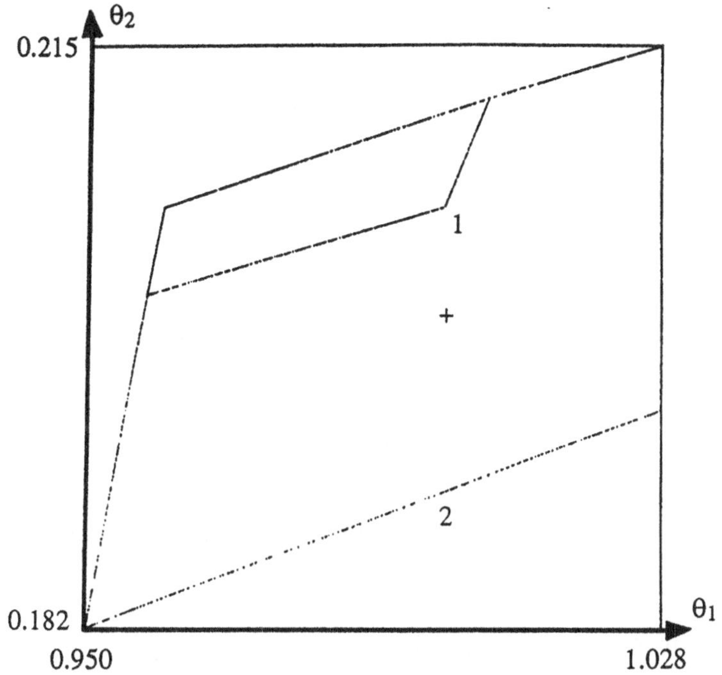

Fig. 2. Estimated membership set with underestimated error. 1: $S^{80.95}$, 2: membership set that would have been obtained if all non detected outliers had been discarded. The cross indicates $\underline{\theta}^*$.

Underestimated error

Assume now that $-e_{min}(k) = e_{max}(k) = 0.05$. From Table 1, we know that this erroneous assumption results in 9 out of the 21 data points becoming outliers, but we are of course not allowed to use this knowledge. During the first step of OMNE, it is no longer possible to find $\hat{\underline{\theta}}$ such that $j(\hat{\underline{\theta}}) = 100\%$, which should warn us that at least one of our hypotheses is erroneous. The best value obtained for j is 80.95%, which corresponds to four data points being (rightly) considered as outliers. Figure 2 gives the membership set at level 80.95. The corresponding estimated parameter uncertainty intervals are given by

$$\hat{\theta}_{1min} = 0.959, \qquad \hat{\theta}_{1max} = 1.005, \tag{14}$$

and

$$\hat{\theta}_{2min} = 0.201, \qquad \hat{\theta}_{2max} = 0.211. \tag{15}$$

They no longer contain the true values for the parameters, which are nevertheless very close, a situation also encountered in more complex examples (Walter and Piet-Lahanier, 1988) and which can be explained as follows. Even if the error bounds are too optimistic, some of the data points not rejected as outliers are still such that

$$e_{min}(k) \leq \varepsilon(k) \leq e_{max}(k). \tag{16}$$

Let S' be the (unknown) membership set associated with these data points. It satisfies $\underline{\theta}^* \in$ S' and $S^{80.95} \subset S'$. Any $\underline{\theta}$ belonging to $S^{80.95}$ therefore satisfies

$$d(\underline{\theta}, \underline{\theta}^*) \leq \text{diam } S', \tag{17}$$

where $d(\underline{\theta}, \underline{\theta}^*)$ is the euclidian distance between $\underline{\theta}$ and $\underline{\theta}^*$ and diam S' is the maximal euclidian distance between two points of S'.

In this simulated example, S' can be computed and is also indicated in Figure 2. Its fairly small size explains why surprisingly good results can be obtained even when the error is grossly underestimated.

Severe outliers

To simulate a situation where serious mistakes have been committed during data collection, 11 out of the 21 data points given in Table 1 have been replaced by totally erroneous values. The corresponding data set is given in Table 2. Assuming that $-e_{min}(k) = e_{max}(k) = 0.1$, we find that 11 data points are rejected as outliers, so that $j(\hat{\underline{\theta}}) = 47.62\%$. Figure 3 gives the estimated membership set at level 47.62. The corresponding estimated parameter uncertainty intervals are given by

$$\hat{\theta}_{1min} = 0.952, \qquad \hat{\theta}_{1max} = 1.469, \tag{18}$$

and

$$\hat{\theta}_{2min} = 0.170, \qquad \hat{\theta}_{2max} = 0.299. \tag{19}$$

Table 2. Data set containing severe outliers

t	y_d	ε
0.	0.31341751E+01	0.21341751E+01
0.5	0.50822043E+01	0.41773667E+01
1.	0.36062460E+01	0.27875152E+01
1.5	0.83734936E+00	0.96531153E-01
2.	0.41763492E+01	0.35060291E+01
2.5	0.69519967E+00	0.88669002E-01
3.	0.39036407E+01	0.33548291E+01
3.5	0.48444059E+00	-0.12144715E-01
4.	0.53270918E+00	0.83380222E-01
4.5	0.44879379E+01	0.408136844E+01
5.	0.57704306E+01	0.54025512E+01
5.5	0.56243811E+01	0.52915101E+01
6.	0.24459681E+00	-0.56597382E-01
6.5	0.23999763E+00	-0.32534152E-01
7.	0.49748559E+01	0.47282591E+01
7.5	0.25536752E+00	0.32237351E-01
8.	0.54020591E+01	0.52001624E+01
8.5	0.12369312E+00	-0.58990397E-01
9.	0.34088013E+01	0.32435024E+01
9.5	0.13614616E+00	0.13422459E-01
10.	0.14416318E+00	0.88278949E-02

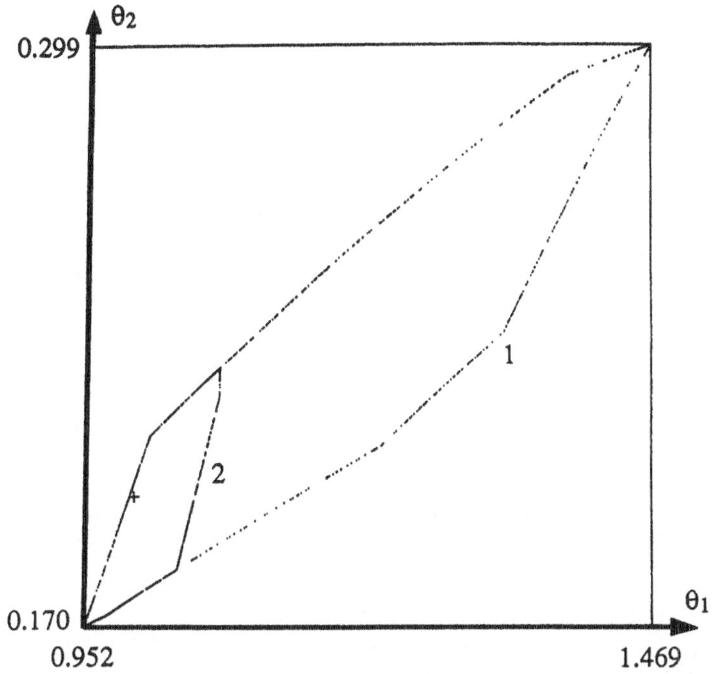

Fig. 3. Estimated membership set with 52.38% of outliers. 1: $S^{47.62}$, 2: membership set of Fig. 1. The cross indicates $\underline{\theta}^*$.

Although the data set now contains a majority of severe outliers, these estimated parameter uncertainty intervals contain the true value for the parameters.

CONCLUSIONS

In the bounded-error context, erroneous hypotheses may result in outliers even if no mistake has been committed during data collection. It is therefore of major importance to use a robust estimator. Most of those developed so far have not been designed to fulfil this requirement. Because data points are either taken into account or totally ignored, OMNE deals very efficiently with severe outliers, which are easily detected and discarded even when their number is larger than that of the regular data points. In the presence of mild outliers, the resulting estimated membership set may not contain the true values of the parameters, unless an appropriate level of protection is chosen. Even when no protection is introduced, the estimated parameter uncertainty intervals turn out, in all examples treated so far, to be close to the true values. More systematic studies of this phenomenon are needed to assess its generality.

REFERENCES

Bekey, G. A., and Masry, S. F., 1983, Random search techniques for optimization of nonlinear systems with many parameters, *Math. Comput. Simulation*, 25:210-213.

Belforte, G., and Milanese, M., 1981, Uncertainty interval evaluation in presence of unknown-but-bounded errors. Nonlinear families of models, *Proc. 1st IASTED Int. Symp. Modeling, Identification, Control*, 75-79.

Fedra, K., van Straten, G., and Beck, M. B., 1981, Uncertainty and arbitrariness in ecosystems modelling: a lake modelling example, *Ecological Modelling*, 13:87-110.
Fogel, E. and Huang Y. F., 1982, On the value of information in system identification - bounded noise case, *Automatica*, 18:229-238.
Lahanier, H., Walter, E., and Gomeni, R., 1987, OMNE: a new robust membership set estimator for the parameters of nonlinear models, *J. Pharmacokin. Biopharm.*, 15:203-219.
Launer, R. L., and Wilkinson, G. N. (Eds.), 1979, "Robustness in Statistics," Academic Press, New York.
Milanese, M., and Belforte, G., 1982, Estimation theory and uncertainty intervals evaluation in presence of unknown but bounded errors: linear families of models and estimators, *IEEE Trans. Autom. Control*, AC-27:408-414.
Norton, J. P., 1986, Problems in identifying the dynamics of biological systems from very short records, *Proc. 25th IEEE Conf. on Decision and Control*, Athens, 286-290.
Norton, J. P., 1987, Identification and application of bounded-parameter models, *Automatica*, 23:497-507.
Piet-Lahanier, H., Walter, E., and Botella, J.-N., 1989, Compensation d'un système de stockage d'informations altimétriques par identification paramétrique directe. *Colloque SMAI "L'automatique pour l'aéronautique et l'espace,"* Paris, to appear.
Pronzato, L., Walter, E., Venot, A., and Lebruchec, J.-F., 1984, A general-purpose global optimizer: implementation and applications, *Math. Comput. Simulation*, 26:412-422.
Richalet, J., Rault, A., and Pouliquen, R., 1971, "Identification des processus par la méthode du modèle," Gordon and Breach, Paris.
Schweppe, F. C., 1968, Recursive state estimation: unknown but bounded errors and system inputs, *IEEE Trans. Autom. Control*, AC-13:22-28.
Schweppe, F. C., 1973, "Uncertain Dynamic Systems," Prentice Hall, Englewood Cliffs.
Smit, M.K., 1983, A novel approach to the solution of indirect measurement problems with minimal error propagation, *Measurement*, 1:181-190.
Walter, E., and Piet-Lahanier, H., 1986, Robust nonlinear estimation in the bounded noise case, *Proc. 25th IEEE Conf. on Decision and Control*, Athens, 1037-1042.
Walter, E., Piet-Lahanier, H., and Happel, J., 1986, Estimation of nonuniquely identifiable parameters via exhaustive modeling and membership set theory, *Math. Comput. Simulation*, 28:479-490.
Walter, E., and Piet-Lahanier, H., 1987, Exact and recursive description of the feasible parameter set for bounded error models, *Proc. 26th IEEE Conf. on Decision and Control*, Los Angeles, 1921-1922.
Walter, E., and Piet-Lahanier, H., 1988, Estimation of the parameter uncertainty resulting from bounded-error data, *Math. Biosci.*, to appear.
Witsenhausen, H. S., 1968, Sets of possible states of linear systems given perturbed observations, *IEEE Trans. Autom. Control*, AC-13:556-558.

2. ROBUST STABILITY AND CONTROL

GENERALIZED NYQUIST TESTS FOR ROBUST STABILITY: FREQUENCY DOMAIN GENERALIZATIONS OF KHARITONOV'S THEOREM

John J. Anagnost, Charles A. Desoer and Robert J. Minnichelli

Department of Electrical Engineering and Computer Science
University of California
Berkeley, CA 94720

0. SUMMARY

This paper presents a simple rigorous development of two major results in robust stability theory: Kharitonov's Theorem for interval polynomials (a previously known result); and a graphical U-stability Nyquist type test for a broad class of parameterized linear time-invariant systems. An example is included for a time delay system with non-linear parameter dependence.

1. INTRODUCTION

This paper presents a simple rigorous development of two major results in robust stability theory. Section 2 presents simplified analytical methods for proving Kharitonov's stability theorem and several extensions, all previously known results. Section 3 presents a generalization of these analytical methods to develop a graphical technique--related to the classical Nyquist criterion--for a much broader class of robust stability problems.

Kharitonov's Theorem states that an *interval class* of polynomials, defined by letting each coefficient vary *independently* in arbitrarily defined intervals, is Hurwitz if and only if *four* special, well-defined polynomials in the class are Hurwitz. The original proof of this theorem was rather complex, but a series of simplifications in the exposition have led up to the simple proof included here; we refer to [Barm. 1], [Yeu. 1], [Das. 1] and [Min. 1] in particular, with additional references included in these. Indeed, the cornerstone of our exposition is the observation that the *image* of the interval class of polynomials, evaluated at any point on the *imaginary axis*, is a level rectangle in $\mathbb{C}$, with corners specified by the four Kharitonov polynomials (Lemma 2.2); this observation is due to Dasgupta [Das. 1]. We consider the motion of this rectangle, using very elementary facts about Hurwitz polynomials, to prove the result without reference to the Hermite-Biehler Theorem.

In Section 3 we apply the analytical methods developed in Section 2 to a much broader class of problems. Instead of the closed right half-plane, we consider arbitrary closed sets U of forbidden zero locations; and instead of an interval class of polynomials--a parallelepiped with edges parallel to the coordinate axes in coefficient space--we consider more general sets: arbitrary polyhedra, convex sets, compact connected sets and even completely arbitrary sets. The resulting test is a graphical technique--first proposed in [Ana. 1]--based on a result sometimes referred to as the 'zero-exclusion

† Research supported by The Aerospace Corporation, El Segundo, CA 90245; Hughes Aircraft Company, El Segundo, CA 90245; and the National Science Foundation Grant ECS 8500993.

principle,' an old idea discernible in Bode's notion of gain and phase margin. Section 3 includes a proof of this result appropriate for the broad class of problems under consideration. Of course, the polyhedral case, with its linear constraints, will have the most numerically efficient solutions. Finally, instead of considering only polynomial functions, we consider a broader class of functions on $\mathbb{C}$; specifically, functions analytic in the region U. This allows us to analyze systems with a variety of infinite-dimensional components: PDE's and time delays being the most important. An example demonstrating the latter is included in Section 3.4.

Related work has been developed by Barmish [Barm. 2,3]; similar graphical tests are proposed, although not exactly of the 'Nyquist' variety used here. The Nyquist type tests, actually plotting the 'nearest point' in the image set, seem to be the most efficient, and the resulting graphical information can be utilized with a traditional Nyquist plot interpretation for the whole family of systems. For the polyhedral case mentioned above (either polynomials or analytic functions), an alternative approach to the Nyquist type tests described here is the root-locus type tests of Bartlett, Hollot and Lin ([Bart. 1], the 'Edge Theorem'). There are even finite algorithms for implementing the Edge Theorem (see [Fu 1] for the special case where U is the right half-plane; [Kra. 1] for the unit circle with low order polynomials; and [Ana. 2] for arbitrary closed U with parameterizable boundary). Even considering these finite implementations, we feel the Nyquist type algorithms will, in general, prove most efficient (see our discussion in [Ana. 2]).

2. STREAMLINED PROOF OF KHARITONOV'S THEOREM

2.1 Statement of the Theorem

We consider a family of *real* polynomials of degree n

$$p(s,a)=\sum_{0}^{n} a_k s^k \qquad 0 < \underline{a}_k \le a_k \le \bar{a}_k \qquad k=0,1,\ldots,n \tag{2.1}$$

where the real numbers $\underline{a}_k$ and $\bar{a}_k$ are given and $a := (a_0, a_1, \ldots, a_n)$. Define

$$A := \{a \in \mathbb{R}^{n+1} \ : \ \underline{a}_k \le a_k \le \bar{a}_k, \quad k=0,1,\ldots,n\}. \tag{2.2}$$

A is a parallelepiped in $\mathbb{R}^{n+1}$ with 2^{n+1} vertices. There is an obvious bijection between the points of A and the polynomials $p(\cdot, a)$, so we consider A as a *family of polynomials*. Using standard set notation we write, for any fixed $s \in \mathbb{C}$,

$$p(s,A) = \{p(s,a) \mid a \in A\} \tag{2.3}$$

Recall that a *polynomial* $q(\cdot)$ (with either real or complex coefficients) is called *Hurwitz* iff all its zeros have *negative* real parts. We say that the *family* A is *Hurwitz* iff all members of A are Hurwitz. We define the four Kharitonov polynomials with respect to A as follows:

$$k_{11}(s) = \underline{a}_0 + \underline{a}_1 s + \bar{a}_2 s^2 + \bar{a}_3 s^3 + \underline{a}_4 s^4 + \underline{a}_5 s^5 + \ldots \tag{2.4}$$

$$k_{12}(s) = \underline{a}_0 + \bar{a}_1 s + \bar{a}_2 s^2 + \underline{a}_3 s^3 + \underline{a}_4 s^4 + \bar{a}_5 s^5 + \ldots \tag{2.5}$$

$$k_{21}(s) = \bar{a}_0 + \underline{a}_1 s + \underline{a}_2 s^2 + \bar{a}_3 s^3 + \bar{a}_4 s^4 + \underline{a}_5 s^5 + \ldots \tag{2.6}$$

$$k_{22}(s) = \bar{a}_0 + \bar{a}_1 s + \underline{a}_2 s^2 + \underline{a}_3 s^3 + \bar{a}_4 s^4 + \bar{a}_5 s^5 + \ldots \tag{2.7}$$

Theorem 2.1 *Kharitonov's Theorem (Real Coefficients)* [Kha. 1]. Consider A, the family of polynomials defined in (2.1) and (2.2). The family A is Hurwitz if and only if the four Kharitonov polynomials $k_{11}(\cdot)$, $k_{12}(\cdot)$, $k_{21}(\cdot)$, $k_{22}(\cdot)$ are Hurwitz.

2.2 Two lemmas

We start with a useful characterization of Hurwitz polynomials. The following analytical tools have been available to the engineering community for a long time; the earliest reference we have found to similar concepts is [Whi. 1, Sec. 6.31, Ex. 2 (1902)]. They are proven here for completeness.

Lemma 2.2 *Characterization of Hurwitz polynomials.* Let

$$q(s) = \sum_{0}^{n} q_k s^k \quad \text{with} \quad q_k \in \mathbb{R}, \forall k, \quad \text{and} \quad q_n > 0. \tag{2.8}$$

i) The polynomial q is Hurwitz if and only if

a) $\arg q(j\omega)$ is well defined $\forall \omega \in \mathbb{R}$, and (2.9)

b) $\lim_{\omega \to \infty} \arg[q(j\omega)] - \arg q(0) = \frac{n\pi}{2}$. (2.10)

ii) If q is Hurwitz then the map $\omega \to \arg q(j\omega)$ is strictly increasing on $\mathbb{R}$.

iii) If q is Hurwitz with $q_n > 0$, then all of its coefficients are positive.

Comment. Geometrically, statements i) and iii) imply that an nth degree real polynomial q with positive coefficients is Hurwitz if and only if the curve traced in $\mathbb{C}$ by $q(j\omega)$, as ω increases from 0 to ∞, starts on the *positive* real axis and rotates around the origin *counterclockwise* by a net change of angle of $n\pi/2$. Statement ii) implies that this rotation is *monotonic*.

Remark. If the coefficients of $q(\cdot)$ in (2.8) are complex with $|q_n| \neq 0$ then statements i) and ii) of Lemma 2.2 remain valid provided (2.10) is replaced by

$$\lim_{\omega \to \infty} [\arg q(+j\omega) - \arg q(-j\omega)] = n\pi. \tag{2.10a}$$

In the proof below we would add $\arg(q_n)$ to the RHS of (2.11) for the complex coefficient case.

Proof. i) $\Rightarrow$. Statement (2.9) holds since q has no zeros on the $j\omega$-axis. Now since $q_n > 0$, denoting the zeros as $z_i = \sigma_i + j\omega_i$, we have

$$\arg[q(j\omega)] = \sum_{1}^{n} \arg(j\omega - z_i). \tag{2.11}$$

Since $\forall i$, $\sigma_i < 0$, for each *real* zero, $\arg(j\omega - z_i)$ increases by $\pi/2$ as ω increases from 0 to ∞; for each pair of complex conjugate zeros, $\arg(j\omega - z_i) + \arg(j\omega - \bar{z}_i)$ increases by π. Hence (2.10) follows.

$\Leftarrow$. Assumption (2.9) implies that q has no $j\omega$-axis zeros. To prove that q is Hurwitz use contraposition. Suppose q has a real zero in the open right-half plane, say $z_1 > 0$. Then $\arg(j\omega - z_1)$ *decreases* by $\pi/2$ as ω increases from 0 to ∞. Since q has *precisely* n zeros, the equality in (2.10) cannot be satisfied. Hence (2.10) rules out open right half plane zeros of q.

ii) If q is Hurwitz then its n zeros are in the open left half plane: hence $\text{Re}\, z_i < 0$, $\forall i$. Now $\arg(j\omega - z_i)$ is a strictly increasing function of ω for all $\omega \in \mathbb{R}$, hence by (2.11) the same holds for $\arg q(j\omega)$.

iii) Since q is a *real* Hurwitz polynomial, its zeros are real or occur in complex conjugate pairs: so $q(s)$ is a product of q_n, monomials $(s - \sigma_i)$ with $\sigma_i < 0$ and binomials $s^2 - 2\sigma_k s + (\sigma_k^2 + \omega_k^2)$ with $\sigma_k < 0$. Since each factor has positive coefficients, their product, $q(\cdot)$, will have positive coefficients. □

We now prove a key property due to Dasgupta.

Lemma 2.3 [Das. 1]. For each fixed $\omega \in \mathbb{R}_+$, $p(j\omega, A)$ is a *rectangle* with edges parallel to the coordinate axes and with vertices determined by the four Kharitonov polynomials $k_{11}(j\omega)$, $k_{12}(j\omega)$, $k_{22}(j\omega)$ and $k_{21}(j\omega)$.

Comment. By (2.1), for any fixed $\omega \in \mathbb{R}$, the map $a \to p(j\omega, a)$ is a *linear* map from $A \subset \mathbb{R}^{n+1}$ into $\mathbb{C}$: since A is a parallelepiped in $\mathbb{R}^{n+1}$, $p(j\omega, A)$ is a *convex polygon* in $\mathbb{C}$. The thrust of Lemma 2.3 is that this polygon is the rectangle with corners $k_{11}(j\omega)$, $k_{12}(j\omega)$, $k_{21}(j\omega)$, and $k_{22}(j\omega)$. (Figure 2.1).

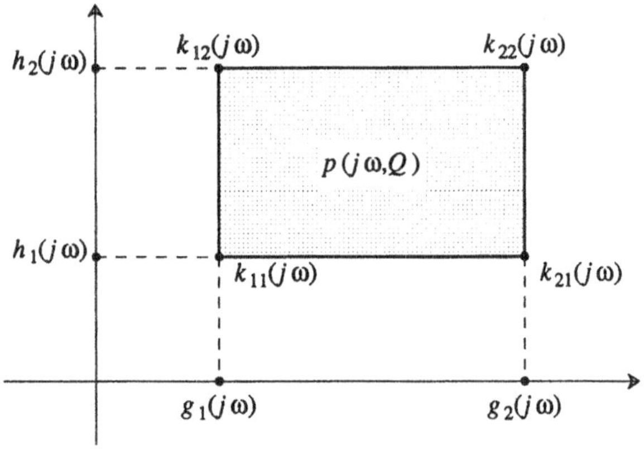

Figure 2.1
Rectangular image $p(j\omega,Q)$ (for $\omega>0$).

Proof. From (2.1) we have, $\forall\omega\in\mathbb{R}$,

$$\underline{a}_0-\bar{a}_2\omega^2+\underline{a}_4\omega^4-\ldots \quad \le \quad \mathrm{Re}\{p(j\omega,a)\} \quad \le \quad \bar{a}_0-\underline{a}_2\omega^2+\bar{a}_4\omega^4-\ldots \tag{2.12}$$

and, $\forall\omega\in\mathbb{R}_+$,

$$\omega(\underline{a}_1-\bar{a}_3\omega^2+\underline{a}_5\omega^4-\ldots) \quad \le \quad \mathrm{Im}\{p(j\omega,a)\} \quad \le \quad \omega(\bar{a}_1-\underline{a}_3\omega^2+\bar{a}_5\omega^4-\ldots). \tag{2.13}$$

Let $g_1(j\omega)$ and $g_2(j\omega)$ be the LHS and RHS of (2.12), and $h_1(j\omega)$ and $h_2(j\omega)$ be j times the LHS and RHS of (2.13). Note that the four polynomials $g_1(s)$, $g_2(s)$, $h_1(s)$ and $h_2(s)$ have real coefficients and that the four Kharitonov polynomials, defined in (2.4)–(2.7), are given by

$$k_{lm}(s)=g_l(s)+h_m(s) \qquad l,m=1,2. \tag{2.14}$$

By (2.12) and (2.13), we see that $p(j\omega,A)$ is the convex hull of the images of the four Kharitonov polynomials:

$$p(j\omega,A)=\mathrm{co}\{k_{11}(j\omega),k_{21}(j\omega),k_{22}(j\omega),k_{12}(j\omega)\} \tag{2.15}$$

Examination of (2.12-2.15) shows that the sides of $p(j\omega,A)$ are parallel to the coordinate axes. □

2.3 Proof of Kharitonov's Theorem

Proof. $\Rightarrow$. If all polynomials of the family A are Hurwitz, then, in particular, k_{11}, k_{12}, k_{21} and k_{22} are Hurwitz.

$\Leftarrow$. By assumption k_{11}, k_{12}, k_{21} and k_{22} are Hurwitz polynomials.

Step 1. Consider the motion of the rectangle $p(j\omega,A)$ as ω increases from 0 to ∞. Clearly, $p(0,A)=[\underline{a}_0,\bar{a}_0]$, a segment of the *positive* real axis since $\underline{a}_0>0$. Since the $k_{lm}(j\omega)$ are polynomials in ω, the rectangle $p(j\omega,A)$ will move continuously in $\mathbb{C}$ as ω increases, keeping at all times its sides parallel to the coordinate axes (Lemma 2.3).

Now k_{21} is Hurwitz and $k_{21}(j\omega)$ is the lower right hand corner of $p(j\omega,A)$; since $\arg k_{21}(j\omega)$ is strictly increasing, $k_{21}(j\omega)$ will push $p(j\omega,A)$ off the real axis into the open first quadrant and then, if $n>1$, will push the *whole rectangle* $p(j\omega,A)$ into the open second quadrant. Now, with $p(j\omega,A)$ in the (open) second quadrant, consider its upper right hand corner $k_{22}(j\omega)$: since arg $k_{22}(j\omega)$ is strictly increasing, if $n>2$, $k_{22}(j\omega)$ will push the whole rectangle $p(j\omega, A)$ into the open third quadrant. Now consider the upper left hand corner $k_{12}(j\omega)$: since arg $k_{12}(j\omega)$ is strictly increasing, if $n>3$, $k_{12}(j\omega)$ will push the whole rectangle into the open fourth quadrant. Now consider the lower left hand corner of $p(j\omega, A)$, namely $k_{11}(j\omega)$: since arg $k_{11}(j\omega)$ is strictly increasing, if $n>4$, $k_{11}(j\omega)$ will push the whole rectangle into the open first quadrant. At this point, we consider a second time $k_{21}(j\omega)$, the lower right hand corner of the rectangle: if $n>5$, $k_{21}(j\omega)$ pushes the rectangle from the open first quadrant into the open second quadrant, as before. This motion--the whole rectangle moving continuously from one open quadrant into the next, never passing through the origin--will go on until the net argument of each corner asymptotically approaches $n\pi/2$, since each corner polynomial is Hurwitz of degree n and (2.10) holds. Thus the whole rectangle $p(j\omega, A)$ starts from the positive real axis and travels continuously through a net angle of $n\pi/2$ as ω increase from zero to infinity.

Step 2. Let $p(\cdot, a)$ be an arbitrary polynomial in A. By (2.12) and (2.13), $\forall \omega \in \mathbb{R}_+$,

$$p(j\omega, a) \in p(j\omega, A) \tag{2.16}$$

By step 1, $\forall \omega \in \mathbb{R}_+$, $p(j\omega, a) \neq 0$, so its argument is a well defined continuous function of ω; furthermore, by step 1 and condition (2.16), condition (2.10) of Lemma 2.2 holds. Hence, by Lemma 2.2, $p(\cdot, a)$ is Hurwitz. □

2.4 Special Cases

Corollary 2.4 ($n=3, 4$ and 5) [And. 1]. Let the notation of (2.1), (2.2) and (2.4)–(2.7) hold.

For $n=3$, the family A is Hurwitz if and only if k_{21} is Hurwitz.

For $n=4$, the family A is Hurwitz if and only if k_{21} and k_{22} are Hurwitz.

For $n=5$, the family A is Hurwitz if and only if k_{21}, k_{22} and k_{12} are Hurwitz.

Proof. We use the ideas of the proof of Sec. 2.3 to prove sufficiency. For $n=3$, the Hurwitzness of k_{21} will move the rectangle $p(j\omega, A)$ from the real axis into the open first quadrant and then into the open second quadrant. As ω increases further, arg $k_{21}(j\omega)$ will increase to become asymptotic to $3\pi/2$. Thus the lower horizontal edge of $p(j\omega, A)$ will enter and remain in the open third quadrant. The top edge will do the same because, for $n=3$,

$$k_{22}(j\omega) = -j\omega^3 \underline{a}_3 - \underline{a}_2\omega^2 + \bar{a}_1 j\omega + \bar{a}_0 \tag{2.17}$$

hence, for ω large, Re$[k_{22}(j\omega)]$ and Im$[k_{22}(j\omega)]$ will eventually become and remain *negative* with arg $k_{22}(j\omega) \to 3\pi/2$. A similar calculation applied to $k_{12}(j\omega)$ leads to the same conclusion. Thus we see that $p(j\omega, A)$ will travel counterclockwise around the origin through a total angle of $3\pi/2$, never intersecting the origin. By step 2 of the proof above, $\forall a \in A$, $p(j\omega, a)$ will do the same, hence the family A is Hurwitz.

The proof for $n=4$ and 5 follows from a similar argument. □

2.5 Complex Coefficients Case

Let A^* be the family of polynomials defined as follows:

$$p(s, a) = (\alpha_n + j\beta_n)s^n + (\alpha_{n-1} + j\beta_{n-1})s^{n-1} + \ldots + (\alpha_0 + j\beta_0) \tag{2.18}$$

where $a_k = \alpha_k + \beta_k$, and $\underline{\alpha}_k \le \alpha_k \le \bar{\alpha}_k$ and $\underline{\beta}_k \le \beta_k \le \bar{\beta}_k$, for $k=0, 1, \ldots, n$; the $\underline{\alpha}_k$'s, $\bar{\alpha}_k$'s, $\underline{\beta}_k$'s and $\bar{\beta}_k$'s are given, and the rectangle $[\underline{\alpha}_n, \bar{\alpha}_n] \times [\underline{\beta}_n \times \bar{\beta}_n]$ is bounded away from zero. Again we visualize A^* as a parallelepiped in $\mathbb{R}^{2n+2}$. Since, $\forall s \in \mathbb{C}$, $a \to p(s, a)$ is a linear map, it maps the convex set A^* into a convex polygon in $\mathbb{C}$.

Since the arguments for the complex case are entirely analogous to those of the real case, we sketch them briefly. There are two important differences: first we must consider two cases $\omega \ge 0$ and $\omega \le 0$; second, $p(0, A^*)$ is now a rectangle in $\mathbb{C}$, namely $[\underline{\alpha}_0, \bar{\alpha}_0] \times [\underline{\beta}_0, \bar{\beta}_0]$.

As in Lemma 2.3, we observe that $\forall a \in A^*$, $\forall \omega \geq 0$

$$g_1^+(j\omega) \leq \mathrm{Re}[p(j\omega, a)] \leq g_2^+(j\omega) \tag{2.19}$$

and

$$\mathrm{Im}[h_1^+(j\omega)] \leq \mathrm{Im}[p(j\omega, a)] \leq \mathrm{Im}[h_2^+(j\omega)] \tag{2.20}$$

where

$$g_1^+(s) := \underline{\alpha}_0 + j\bar{\beta}_1 s + \bar{\alpha}_2 s^2 + j\underline{\beta}_3 s^3 + \underline{\alpha}_4 s^4 + \cdots \tag{2.21}$$

$$g_2^+(s) := \bar{\alpha}_0 + j\underline{\beta}_1 s + \underline{\alpha}_2 s^2 + j\bar{\beta}_3 s^3 + \bar{\alpha}_4 s^4 + \cdots \tag{2.22}$$

$$h_1^+(s) := j\underline{\beta}_0 + \underline{\alpha}_1 s + j\bar{\beta}_2 s^2 + \bar{\alpha}_3 s^3 + j\underline{\beta}_4 s^4 + \cdots \tag{2.23}$$

$$h_2^+(s) := j\bar{\beta}_0 + \bar{\alpha}_1 s + j\underline{\beta}_2 s^2 + \underline{\alpha}_3 s^3 + j\bar{\beta}_4 s^4 + \cdots \tag{2.24}$$

Clearly the four complex polynomials $k_{lm}^+ := g_l^+ + h_m^+$, $l, m = 1, 2$, are in the family A^*. By (2.19) and (2.20) we see that $\forall \omega \geq 0$

$$p(j\omega, A^*) = \mathrm{co}\{k_{11}^+(j\omega), k_{21}^+(j\omega), k_{22}^+(j\omega), k_{12}^+(j\omega)\}. \tag{2.25}$$

Again, $\forall \omega \geq 0$, $p(j\omega, A^*)$ is a rectangle with edges parallel to the coordinate axes.

For $\omega \leq 0$, $\forall a \in A^*$, we obtain again Eqns. (2.19)–(2.24) with g_1^+, g_2^+, h_1^+ and h_2^+ replaced by g_1^-, g_2^-, h_1^-, h_2^-, where g_1^-, g_2^-, h_1^-, h_2^- are defined as in (2.21)–(2.24) except that all the odd power coefficients are interchanged ($\bar{\beta}_1$ is replaced by $\underline{\beta}_1$, etc.). With $k_{lm}^- := g_l^- + h_m^-$, $l, m = 1, 2$ we have $\forall \omega \leq 0$, $\forall a \in A^*$

$$p(j\omega, A^*) = \mathrm{co}\{k_{11}^-(j\omega), k_{12}^-(j\omega), k_{21}^-(j\omega), k_{22}^-(j\omega)\}. \tag{2.26}$$

Thus we have the generalization of Lemma 2.3 for the complex case. Using Lemma 2.2 and Eqns. (2.10a), (2.25) and (2.26), we easily prove the following using arguments analogous to those used for Theorem 2.1 (for the complete proof, see [Min. 1]).

Theorem 2.5 *Kharitonov's Theorem (Complex Coefficients)* [Kha. 2, Bos. 1]. Let A^* be the family of *complex* polynomials defined in (2.18). The family A^* is Hurwitz if and only if the eight complex Kharitonov polynomials $k_{11}^+, k_{11}^-, k_{12}^+, k_{12}^-, k_{21}^+, k_{21}^-, k_{22}^+, k_{22}^-$ are Hurwitz.

3. ROBUST STABILITY FOR LINEAR TIME-INVARIANT SYSTEMS

We propose to generalize the results of Section 2 in two directions: allow for a more flexible definition of stability and allow for less restrictive parameter dependence of the characteristic polynomial coefficients. In Section 2, each of the $n+1$ coefficients of $p(s, a)$ were allowed to vary *independently* inside prescribed intervals. Examples of control systems and circuits show that physical parameters—such as mass, inertia tensor, spring constants, damping factors, resistances, transconductances, inductances, etc.—appear as variables in polynomials that specify the coefficients; usually a parameter appears as a variable in several coefficients, thus the coefficients are no longer independent. (See example in Section 3.4.)

3.1 U-stability

Roughly speaking, we let U be the *closed* set containing all those values of s that are viewed as "undesirable" from a stability point of view. Typically, U includes the closed right-half plane, is symmetric with respect to the real axis, and has a boundary, ∂U, consisting of C^1 curves (hence parameterizable curves). A simple example is

$$U = R_{\sigma_0} := \{s \in \mathbb{C} \mid \mathrm{Re}\{s\} \geq \sigma_0\} \quad \text{for some fixed } \sigma_0 < 0. \tag{3.1}$$

We consider a family of polynomial functions of $s \in \mathbb{C}$ parameterized by $q \in Q \subset \mathbb{R}^m$, $p(s, q)$. Using standard set and functional notation, this family of polynomials is denoted $p(\cdot, Q)$. Note that $p(\cdot, q)$ denotes a particular polynomial in $p(\cdot, Q)$ if $q \in Q$, and $p(s, q) \in \mathbb{C}$ denotes the *value* of that polynomial evaluated as a point $s \in \mathbb{C}$. Finally, $p(s, Q)$ denotes the set of values of all the polynomials $p(\cdot,Q)$ evaluated at s; e.g. $p(s,Q)=\{p(s,q):q\in Q\}$. A polynomial $p(\cdot,q)$ is said to be *U–stable* iff $p(s,q)\neq 0\ \forall s\in U$. A family of polynomials is *U–stable* iff each polynomial $p(\cdot,q)$ is U-stable; i.e. iff $0\notin p(s,Q)\ \forall s\in U$.

3.2 Lumped Linear Time-Invariant Systems

We consider lumped systems with characteristic polynomials of the form

$$p(s,q)=\sum_{0}^{n} a_k(q)\,s^k, \quad q\in Q\subset \mathbb{R}^m \tag{3.2}$$

where the parameterization $p(\cdot,q)$ has been expressed as a parameterization of the polynomial coefficients.

Assumptions:

(A1) The parameter vector $q\in\mathbb{R}^m$ is in a given non-empty set Q, and Q is *connected* and *compact*.

(A2) For $k=0,1,\ldots,n$, the coefficient parameterizations $a_k: Q\to\mathbb{R}$ are *continuous*.

(A3) For all $q\in Q$, $a_n(q)>0$.

For example, Q could be a convex polyhedron in $\mathbb{R}^m$ or a closed ball. (A1) and (A2) imply that $a_k(Q)$ is a compact interval, $k=0,\ldots,n$; then (A3) implies that the interval $a_n(Q)$ is *bounded away* from 0.

We begin the derivation of the main result of this section (Theorem 3.3) by stating two facts. Fact 3.1 is a corollary of [Die. 1, Thm. 9.17.4]; it is a rigorous version of the statement that the zeroes of a polynomial vary *continuously* with respect to its coefficients.[1] Fact 3.2 states that the zeroes of the set of polynomials defined above can be uniformly bounded.

Fact 3.1 Given any *bounded* set $V\subset\mathbb{C}$ and any $q_0\in Q$, if $p(s,q_0)\neq 0,\ \forall s\in\partial V$, then the number of zeros of $p(s,q)$ in V, *counting multiplicities*, is a locally constant function of $q\in Q$ at q_0.

Fact 3.2 Under assumptions (A1)-(A3), there is an $\alpha\in(0,\infty)$ such that for all $q\in Q$, the zeros of $p(s,q)$ belong to the disc $D(0,\alpha)\subset\mathbb{C}$, centered on 0 with radius α.

Proof. Define $\underline{a}_k$, $\bar{a}_k$ by $a_k(Q)=[\underline{a}_k,\bar{a}_k]$. Given any $q\in Q$, suppose z is a zero of $p(\cdot,q)$; i.e. $p(z,q)=0$. Of course, if $z=0$ then $z\in D(0,\alpha)$; so we may assume $z\neq 0$. Then

$$\underline{a}_n|z| \le |a_n(q)z| \le \Big|\sum_{0}^{n-1} a_k(q)z^{k+1-n}\Big| \le \sum_{0}^{n-1}\bar{a}_k\,|z|^{k+1-n}. \tag{3.3}$$

If $|z|\ge 1$, we have

---

[1] We mention an alternative--more formal--approach to characterizing 'continuity' of polynomial zeroes with respect to coefficients. Consider the set of zeroes of a polynomial as an element of the *finite power set* of $\mathbb{C}$, $\mathbf{P}_f(\mathbb{C})$, the set of all nonempty finite subsets of $\mathbb{C}$, equipped with the Hausdorff metric [Mun. 1, Ex. 7, p. 279]. In this metric, two subsets of $\mathbb{C}$ are ε-close if and only if every element of either set is ε-close to some element of the other set. So set ordering and multiplicity are not issues, and two sets can be arbitrarily close to each other even if they don't have the same number of elements. It is not difficult to show that the map from the space of polynomials to the set of polynomial zeroes in $\mathbf{P}_f(\mathbb{C})$ is continuous; indeed, this is implied by Fact 3.1. The proof of Theorem 3.3 then proceeds in a straightforward manner.

This approach to the problem is *mathematically* more powerful, as it produces the result (Theorem 3.3) quite naturally for arbitrary *connected* parameter sets Q. Theorem 3.3 is stated for *compact connected* Q, and in the remark which follows the theorem, it is extended to non-compact *pathwise connected* Q. However, from the engineering perspective of plausible parameter sets, the distinction between connected parameter sets and pathwise connected parameter sets is insignificant.

The approach taken in the text is used because the topological and geometric arguments in the complex plane have a direct conceptual connection to the resulting graphical test; the connection to the Hausdorff topology of $\mathbf{P}_f(\mathbb{C})$ is considerably more abstract.

$$|z| \le \underline{a}_n^{-1} \sum_0^{n-1} \bar{a}_k =: \alpha_1 \tag{3.4}$$

so we choose $\alpha = \max\{1, \alpha_1\}$. □

Theorem 3.3 *U-stability of p(s,Q).* Let the set of polynomials $p(\cdot, Q)$ as defined in (3.2) satisfy assumptions (A1)-(A3), and recall that $U \subset \mathbb{C}$ is closed. Then

1) the set of polynomials $p(\cdot, Q)$ is U–stable (3.5)

if and only if

2) (a) for some $q_0 \in Q$, $p(\cdot, q_0)$ is U–stable, and (3.6)

(b) $\forall s \in \partial U$, $0 \notin p(s, Q)$. (3.7)

Remarks. a) Assumption (A1) can be modified to read:

(A1') The parameter vector $q \in \mathbb{R}^m$ is in a given non-empty set Q, and Q is *pathwise connected.*

So Q is required to be neither closed nor bounded. The simplest way to prove this is to observe that *any* point q' in Q can be connected to the point q_0 of condition 2(a) by a path C in Q; this path is compact. Since $p(s, C) \subset p(s, Q)$, condition 2(b) implies that $0 \notin p(s, C)$ $\forall s \in \partial U$, and Theorem 3.3 (with the original assumption (A1)) implies that $q' \in C$ is U-stable.

b) The theorem can be further extended to arbitrary connected parameter sets Q satisfying (A3) using a different method of proof (see footnote 1); of course, the distinction between connected and pathwise connected parameter sets is not a real engineering concern. In fact, we may even consider completely arbitrary subsets $Q \subset \mathbb{R}^m$ if we require condition 2(a) to hold for some q_0 in *each connected component* of Q.

Comments. a) The choice of U allows for great designer freedom.

b) Note that Q is not required to be convex. The freedom in choosing Q and U allows the engineer to evaluate trade-offs: higher degree of stability versus greater parameter variations.

c) The theorem is a labor saving device: "the set $p(\cdot, Q)$ is U-stable" is equivalent to $0 \notin p(U, Q)$; once condition 2(a) holds, we need only check $0 \notin p(\partial U, Q)$. Condition 2(b) is to be tested on a work station: hence any possibility for obtaining $p(s, Q)$ efficiently should be exploited (see special case below). Note that, $\forall s \in \partial U$, it is not required to actually determine the whole set $p(s, Q)$, we need only check that $0 \notin p(s, Q)$. In case $p(s, Q)$ is convex, we need only a line separating $p(s, Q)$ from the origin, $\forall s \in \partial U$.

Proof. 1⇒2: Suppose $p(\cdot, Q)$ is U-stable. Clearly condition 2(a) is satisfied. We show 2(b) by contradiction. If $s \in \partial U$ and $0 \in p(s, Q)$, then there is some parameter $q^* \in Q$ with $p(s, q^*) = 0$. Thus $p(\cdot, q^*)$ has a zero in $\partial U \subset U$ and is not U-stable, which contradicts the assertion that $p(\cdot, Q)$ is U-stable.

2⇒1: From Fact 2.1 the zeroes of $p(\cdot, q)$ are uniformly bounded for all q in Q, say $|s| < \alpha$ whenever $p(s, q) = 0$ $\forall q \in Q$. Then let $V = U \cap \{s : |s| \le \alpha\}$. Clearly $p(\cdot, q)$ is V-Hurwitz $\Leftrightarrow$ $p(\cdot, q)$ is U-Hurwitz, for all q in Q. Condition 2(b) implies that $p(s, q) \ne 0$ $\forall s \in \partial V$ $\forall q \in Q$, since $s \in \partial V$ implies $s \in \partial U$ or $|s| = \alpha$. Now Fact 3.1 implies that the number of zeroes that $p(\cdot, q)$ has in V is a locally constant function of q on all of Q. Since Q is connected, the number of zeroes that $p(\cdot, q)$ has in V is globally constant on Q [Dug. 1, p. 108], and condition 2(a) guarantees that that number is zero. So $p(\cdot, Q)$ is V-stable, and thus U-stable. □

Special Case: Q is a Convex Polyhedron.

Consider the polynomial $p(s, q)$ given by (3.2), but now replace assumptions (A1)-(A3) by

(A1*) Q is a *convex polyhedron* in $\mathbb{R}^m$ with vertices $\{v_1, v_2, \ldots, v_l\}$.

(A2*) For $k = 0, 1, \ldots, n$, the coefficient parameterization $a_k(\cdot)$ is *affine*; i.e.

$$a_k = \alpha_k + \beta_k^T q \tag{3.8}$$

where $\alpha_k \in \mathbb{R}$ and $\beta_k \in \mathbb{R}^m$ are given and $q \in Q \subset \mathbb{R}^m$.

(A3) For all $q \in Q$, $a_n(q) > 0$.

Assumptions (A1*) and (A2*) imply assumptions (A1) and (A2), so Theorem 3.3 applies. Assumption (A2*) implies that, for any fixed $s \in \mathbb{C}$ the map $q \to p(s, q)$ is *affine*. Hence by (A1*), $p(s, Q)$ is a *convex polygon* in $\mathbb{C}$. In fact

$$p(s, Q) = \text{co}\{p(s, v_1), \ldots, p(s, v_l)\} \tag{3.9}$$

where $\text{co}\{p_1, \ldots, p_m\}$ denotes the *convex hull* of $\{p_1, \ldots, p_m\}$. Usually only a proper subset of the points $p(s, v_i)$ are vertices of the polygon $p(s, Q)$; note that as s varies, that subset may change.

By Theorem 3.3, once it has been verified that for some q_0, $p(\cdot, q_0)$ is U-stable, it remains to check that the *convex polygon* $p(s, Q)$ does not contain the origin $\forall s \in \partial U$. We define the nearest point function, $\text{Nr}(\cdot)$, on closed convex subsets $S \subset \mathbb{C}$ by

$$\text{Nr}(S) := \underset{s \in S}{arg\ min} \{ |s| \}. \tag{3.10}$$

Checking that $p(s, Q)$ does not contain the origin is equivalent to checking that $\text{Nr}(p(s, Q))$ does not equal zero. This can easily be done using Wolfe's nearest point algorithm [Wol. 1, Hau. 1], which computes

$$\text{Nr}(\text{co}\{k_1, \ldots, k_l\}) \tag{3.11}$$

for any finite set $\{k_1, \ldots, k_l\} \subset \mathbb{C}$ in an efficient and finite manner. In our case we wish to compute

$$\text{Nr}(p(s, Q)) = \text{Nr}(\text{co}\{p(s, v_1), p(s, v_2), \ldots, p(s, v_l)\}) \tag{3.12}$$

for various values of $s \in \partial U$. It is easily verified that (3.12) is a *continuous* function from $s \in \partial U$ to $\text{Nr}(p(s, Q)) \in \mathbb{C}$. So, for the typical case where ∂U is composed of a finite number of C^1 curves, we have the following procedure to implement Theorem 3.3:

a) check *any* polynomial in $p(\cdot, Q)$; if it is Hurwitz, condition 2(a) of Theorem 3.3 is satisfied; otherwise $p(\cdot, Q)$ is not U-stable;

b) parameterize the curve(s) ∂U;

c) as s travels along the components of ∂U, plot the point $\text{Nr}(p(s, Q))$;

d) if the resulting curve is bounded away from zero, then condition 2(b) of Theorem 3.3 is satisfied; otherwise, 2(b) is violated and $p(\cdot, Q)$ is not U-stable.

Comments. a) One obviously cannot plot the locus in step c) for *every* value of $s \in \partial U$. Indeed, one would normally partition ∂U, plot those points, and then fill in points as necessary (either manually or 'automatically') until the locus becomes sufficiently smooth to yield a reliable conclusion. The 'filling in' problem is identical to the 'filling in' problem for the conventional Nyquist test.

b) The nearest point calculation in step c) is finite (using the Wolfe algorithm [Wol. 1]). Indeed, in our experience, by using the resulting edge of the polygon containing the nearest point as the starting point for the search at the next value of $s \in \partial U$, we usually required only one or two iterations (mostly one) of the numerical procedure defined in [Wol. 1]. Of course, this cannot be guaranteed; in general, we may need up to l iterations.

Remark. We now consider modifying (A1*) once again to read

(A1**) $Q \subset \mathbb{R}^m$ is *closed* and *convex*

leaving (A2*) and (A3) intact (e.g. Q might be a closed convex set in coefficient space itself, with $a_k(q)$ being simply coordinate projections). The algorithm above still works (that is, the nearest point function is still well-defined), although the nearest point calculation is no longer finite. For this convex case, however, efficient convergent algorithms do exist [Hau. 1]. If we specify *a priori* some acceptable precision for approximating the nearest point, we obtain a finite algorithm for finding Nr($p(s,Q)$).

3.3 Distributed Linear Time-Invariant Systems

Theorem 3.3 is easily generalized to linear time-invariant *distributed* systems. Consider a control system made up of subsystems whose matrix transfer functions have elements in the algebra $\hat{B}(\sigma_0)$, where σ_0 is typically negative [Cal. 1-3, Des. 1, Nett 1; for connections to the semi-group literature, see Cal. 4 and the references therein]. Let R_σ denote the closed right half-plane $\{s \in \mathbb{C} : \text{Re}\{s\} \geq \sigma\}$ and fix $\sigma_0 < 0$. We say that a function $\hat{f}(s) \in \hat{B}(\sigma_0)$ if, for some $\sigma < \sigma_0$:

1. $\hat{f}$ has a finite number of poles in R_σ, and
2. the inverse transform of $\hat{f}$ includes--in addition to the exponentials due to the poles in R_σ--

$$f_a(t) + \sum_{k=0}^{\infty} f_k\, \delta(t-t_k) \tag{3.13}$$

where

$$\int_0^\infty |f_a(t)|\, e^{-\sigma t}\, dt \;+\; \sum_{k=0}^{\infty} |f_k|\, e^{-\sigma t_k} \;<\; \infty \tag{3.14}$$

with $t_0 = 0$ and $t_k > 0 \;\; \forall k$.

So, except for its poles in R_σ, $\hat{f}(s)$ is *analytic* in R_{σ_0} and, except for arbitrarily small neighborhoods of its poles, $\hat{f}(s)$ is *bounded* in R_{σ_0}. In particular, $\hat{f}(s)$ is bounded in R_{σ_0} as $|s|$ goes to infinity. Note that $\hat{f}(s)$ is not necessarily defined on all of $\mathbb{C}$; indeed, there are functions in $\hat{B}(\sigma_0)$ which have no analytic continuation beyond a half-plane R_σ for some $\sigma < \sigma_0$.

The framework above guarantees that the control system matrix transfer functions have coprime matrix factorizations with factors which are *analytic* in s for $s \in R_{\sigma_0}$. In [Cal. 3, Des. 1] it is shown that such a control control system is σ_0–stable[2] if and only if

$$\inf_{\text{Re}\{s\} \geq \sigma_0} |\chi(s)| > 0 \tag{3.15}$$

where the characteristic function $\chi(s)$ is a sum of products of the elements of these matrix factors. Thus we see that the zeroes of a characteristic function of a distributed system have dynamical interpretations similar to zeroes of a characteristic polynomial of a finite dimensional system.

Now suppose that each element of these factorizations depends *continuously* on a parameter $q \in Q \subset \mathbf{R}^m$ with Q *compact* and *connected.* Then the characteristic function becomes $\chi(s,q)$, continuous in q for $q \in Q$ and analytic in s for $s \in R_{\sigma_0}$. We consider 'undesirable' closed sets U of the complex plane which satisfy the assumption:

(A4) $\quad U \subset R_{\sigma_0}$.

Of course, assumption (A4) guarantees that $\chi(s,q)$ will be analytic in s for all $s \in U$. Note that there was no analogous assumption required in the polynomial case, since polynomials are automatically analytic on all of $\mathbb{C}$. We also impose the *well-posedness* assumption:

(A5) $\quad |\chi(s,q)|$ is bounded away from zero as $|s| \to \infty$ in R_{σ_0} for all $q \in Q$.

Assumption (A5) is analogous to assumption (A3) for the polynomial case; indeed, it is equivalent to Fact 3.2, whose proof required (A3). From [Die. 1, Thm. 9.17.4], the zeroes of $\chi(s,q)$ are

2 Here, we say that a control system is σ_0-stable (for $\sigma_0 < 0$) if it is L_p-stable $\forall p \in [1,\infty]$, and, for any input with compact support, the responses are $o(e^{\sigma_0 t})$ as $t \to \infty$.

'continuous' with respect to q; more precisely, Fact 3.1 holds for arbitrary analytic functions, not just for polynomials. Hence the reasoning for Theorem 3.3 applies and we conclude immediately:

Theorem 3.4 For all $q \in Q$, the distributed control system satisfying all the assumptions of the previous paragraph has a characteristic function $\chi(s,q)$ with no zeroes in the closed set $U \subset \mathbb{C}$ if and only if

(a) for some $q_0 \in Q$, $\chi(s,q_0) \neq 0 \quad \forall s \in U$, and

(b) $0 \notin \chi(s,Q)$ for all $s \in \partial U$.

So the graphical algorithms discussed in Section 3.2 apply to distributed systems. In particular, if $\chi(s,q)$ depends *affinely* on $q \in Q$ and $Q \subset \mathbf{R}^m$ is compact and *convex*, then $\chi(s,Q) \subset \mathbb{C}$ is convex for all s in $\mathbb{C}$ and $\mathrm{Nr}(\chi(s,Q))$, $s \in \partial U$, can be computed using the method of Hauser [Hau. 1], as was the case for polynomials. Further, if Q is a *convex polyhedron*, we can apply Wolfe's finite 'nearest point' algorithm as described in Section 3.2.

Remarks. a) The discussion of $\hat{\mathcal{B}}(\sigma_0)$ provides an *a priori* guarantee that factorizations of the open-loop transfer functions exist which are analytic in R_{σ_0}; this implies that the resulting characteristic function is analytic in R_{σ_0}. Combined with assumption (A5), this implies that closed-loop transfer functions are well-defined as elements of $\hat{\mathcal{B}}(\sigma_0)$. Thus the discussion of $\hat{\mathcal{B}}(\sigma_0)$ and assumption (A5) are to be thought of as system theoretic considerations.

b) In many specific examples, the characteristic function is easily obtained and analyticity over certain regions--or all of $\mathbb{C}$--can be verified by inspection (see, e.g., the example of Section 3.4); here we *implicitly* assume that the characteristic function was derived using some appropriate algebraic structure. In these cases, we may consider *arbitrary* closed sets $U \subset \mathbb{C}$ if we modify assumptions (A4) and (A5) to

(A4*) $\chi(s,q)$ is analytic in s for all $s \in U$ and $q \in Q$.

(A5*) $|\chi(s,q)|$ is bounded away from zero as $|s| \to \infty$ in R_{σ_0} for all $q \in Q$.

Now (A5*) is not to be interpreted as a well-posedness condition, nor even as a system theoretic consideration, but simply as an analytic requirement (compare with (A3) and Fact 3.2 in the polynomial case). *Very roughly speaking*, if U and U^c are both unbounded, we may think of the boundary of U as consisting of $\partial U \subset \mathbb{C}$ and a 'point' (or a 'set') at infinity; (A5*) extends condition (b) of Theorem 3.4 to this extra boundary at infinity, so that zeroes cannot enter U neither through ∂U nor through 'infinity.'

3.4 Example: LTI System with Delay

In this section we illustrate the use of Theorem 3.4 by analyzing an LTI plant with a delay. The plant is a regulated motor-inertia system modelled as shown in Figure 3.1. The transfer function is given by

$$\hat{\omega}(s) = \frac{K_m e^{-Ts}}{LJs^2 + (JR + Lb)s + (Rb + K_m^2)} \hat{V}_o(s) \tag{3.16}$$

where ω is the shaft angular velocity and V_0 is the applied voltage to the motor. The *nominal* design parameters are given as

$K_m = 1$ Nm/amp
$L = 1$ H
$R = .01\ \Omega$
$J = 1$ kg m^2
$b = 0$ kg m^2/sec
$T = 0$ sec

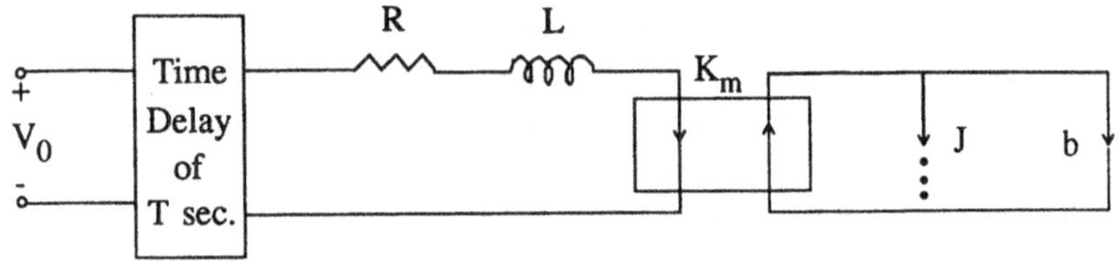

Figure 3.1 Motor-inertia dynamical system with delay

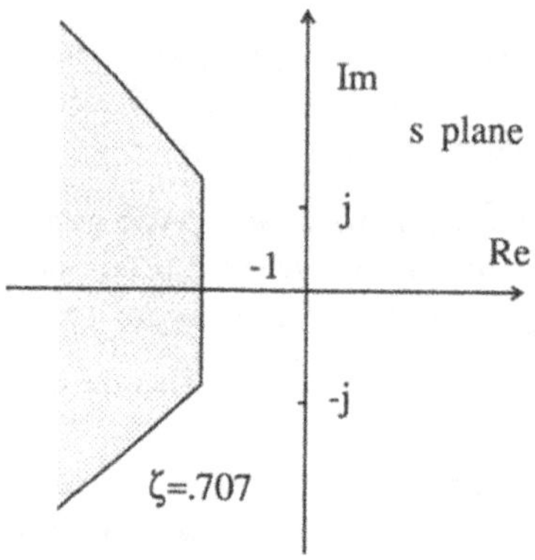

Figure 3.2 Desired region for closed loop poles

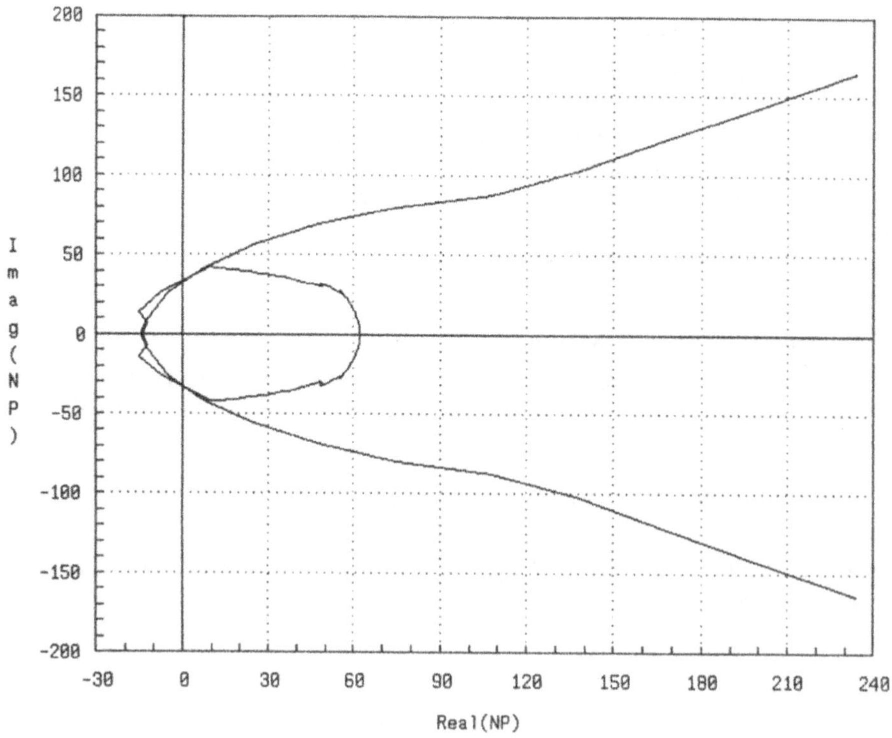

Figure 3.3 Nearest Point Locus with $\tau = 0$

Due to uncertainty, we would like the system to meet specification for parameters in the ranges: $J \in [0.8,1]$, $b \in [0,0.2]$, and $T \in [0,\tau]$. We have not specified τ ahead of time, but instead, we would like to estimate the maximum τ which will work (if any).

The design objective is steady-state regulation of the motor output ω with "good" disturbance rejection. Steady-state regulation is obtained with integral control, while disturbance rejection will be specified in terms of closed-loop pole location according to the region U shown in Figure 3.2 ($\zeta > 0.707$ and $\sigma > 1\ \text{sec}^{-1}$). Specifications were met for the nominal system by using a root-locus design to obtain the following compensator:

$$C_{nom}(s) = \frac{100\,(s^2+2s+2)}{s\,(s+20)}. \tag{3.17}$$

The four closed-loop poles are at $-1.75 \pm j\,1.47$, -2.77 and -13.73. A Nyquist plot of the compensated system shows the nominal system has a 50° phase margin, infinite upper gain margin, and a lower gain margin of -40 dB.

Now we want to find out if the specifications are met for all possible plant perturbations. Using Theorem 3.4, condition (a) is met by the nominal plant, and condition (b) amounts to checking if the characteristic function

$$\chi(s;J,b,T) = 100e^{-Ts}(s^2+2s+2) + [Js^2+(b+0.01J)s+(1+0.01b)](s+20)s \tag{3.18}$$

satisfies $\chi(s_0;J_0,b_0,T_0) = 0$ for some $s_0 \in \partial U$, $J_0 \in [0.8,1]$, $b_0 \in [0,0.2]$ and $T_0 \in [0,0.1]$.

First we discuss the restricted problem of considering variations of $J \in [0.8,1]$ and $b \in [0,0.2]$, fixing $T=0$. In this case, $\chi(s;J,b,0)$ is a polynomial in s whose coefficients are affine functions of J and b. Thus $\chi(s;[0.8,1],[0,0.2],0)$ is a parallelogram in $\mathbb{C}$ for each fixed s. So Theorem 3.3 applies, and, furthermore, the system is one of the 'special cases' discussed after Theorem 3.3. Applying the nearest point algorithm to this parallelogram, we have plotted

$$\text{Nr}\,\{\chi(s;[0.8,1],[0,0.2],0)\} \tag{3.19}$$

in Figure 3.3 for $s \in \partial U$. As s traverses ∂U (see Figure 3.2), the locus circles around the origin without ever intersecting the origin. We conclude that this *restricted* class of perturbed systems ($T \equiv 0$) does robustly meet specifications.

Now we want to consider the whole class $J \in [0.8,1]$, $b \in [0,0.2]$, $T \in [0,\tau]$ using Theorem 3.4 and the extension (for U *not* contained in a right half-plane) in remark (b) following Theorem 3.4. We know by inspection of (3.18), however, that as $T \to 0$ (for J and b fixed), there are infinitely many zeroes of $\chi(s;J,b,T)$ whose real and imaginary parts both go to infinity (in the left half-plane), while the imaginary parts increase in magnitude more rapidly than the real parts (i.e. the ratio is unbounded). Thus 'every' such zero enters the region U of Figure 3.2 for T sufficiently small (but not equal to 0); and for any fixed $T \neq 0$, there are infinitely many zeroes in U, and their magnitudes are not bounded. So we see that Theorem 3.4 does not apply, since the assumption (A5*) is not satisfied: $\chi(s;J,b,T)$ obviously cannot be uniformly (with respect to T) bounded away from zero as $s \to \infty$ in U. (In case one were to apply the test of the 'extended' Theorem 3.3 'blindly' to this problem--i.e. without satisfying assumption (A5*)--there do exist proper finite-dimensional linear controllers which would *seem* to 'guarantee' U-stability for the whole class of systems, a conclusion which is clearly erroneous. This demonstrates the importance of satisfying assumption (A5*)--or (A5) in the case $U \subset R_{\sigma_0}$.)

We repeat the following fact for emphasis: although the zeroes of $\chi(s;J,b,T)$ enter U as $T \to 0$, they also have real parts which tend to $-\infty$. This suggests the following modification of the undesirable region U. We intersect the original region U with the half-plane $\{s : \text{Re}\{s\} \geq -7.5\}$. The modified region U is shown in Figure 3.4. In terms of modal settling times and damping ratios, the modified specifications on the characteristic function zeroes is $\sigma > 1\ \text{sec}^{-1}$, and $\zeta > 0.707$ *for any zero with* $\sigma \leq 7.5\ \text{sec}^{-1}$; zeroes with a corresponding $\sigma > 7.5\ \text{sec}^{-1}$ have no damping margin requirement.

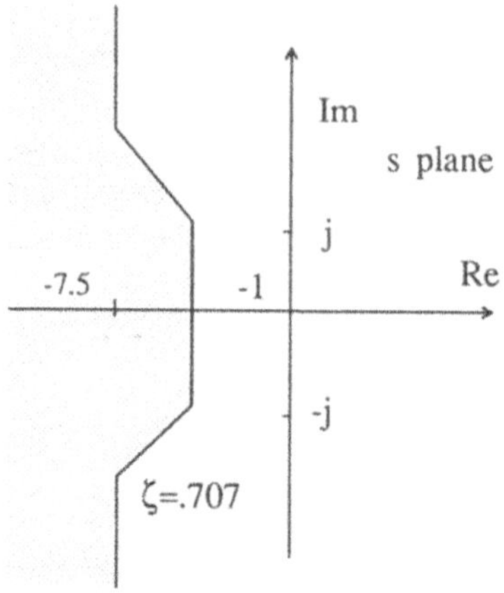

Figure 3.4 Desired region for closed loop poles

With the modified region U, it is clear that assumptions (A4*) and (A5*) are satisfied. In fact, we can give bounds on the zero locations in U if we restrict τ to some arbitrary interval, and we choose $\tau \in [0,.1]$. (If this turns out to be too restrictive--i.e. the whole class meets specification even for $\tau = 0.1$--we can just increase the interval size, or just choose some maximum τ of interest to begin with.) A simple calculation based on Eq. 3.18 shows that $|\chi(s;J,b,T)| > 15$ for all J^*, b^*, $T \in [0,.1]$ and for all s satisfying $\mathrm{Re}\{s\} > -7.5$ and $|s| > 50$. So the zeroes of $|\chi(s;J,b,T)|$ which are in the modified region U must satisfy $|s| < 50$.

Now we apply the test of Theorem 3.4. $\chi(s;[0.8,1],[0,0.2],[0,\tau])$ is *not* a polygon in $\mathbb{C}$, since $\chi(s;J,b,T)$ is not affine in T. We therefore cannot apply Wolfe's nearest point algorithm directly. However, for each *fixed* T^*, we can apply Wolfe's algorithm to find $\mathrm{Nr}\{\chi(s;[0.8,1],[0,0.2],T)\}$. Performing a line search over T^*, we determine $\mathrm{Nr}\{\chi(s;[0.8,1],[0,0.2],[0,\tau]\}$. In Figures 3.5 and 3.6 we have plotted $\mathrm{Nr}\{\chi(s;[0.8,1],[0,0.2],[0,\tau]\}$ for $s \in \partial U$, for $\tau = 0.03$ and $\tau = 0.04$. From the discussion in the previous paragraph, we do not need to plot the image of the whole unbounded boundary ∂U; we need only plot the image of the compact intersection of ∂U with the ball $\{s : |s| \leq 50\}$. Figure 3.5 shows that, for $\tau = 0.03$, the locus remains bounded away from the origin. The shape of the locus is similar to Figure 3.3 at low frequencies, drawing slightly closer to the origin during the 'first pass' around it (probably indicating that the delay does push some of the original poles closer to the boundary of U). Figure 3.6 shows that, for $\tau = 0.04$, the class of characteristic functions (3.18) is *not* U-stable. The low-frequency locus is similar to Figure 3.5, still coming near to, yet remaining bounded away from, the origin as it circles around the origin, and then travels away from the origin. At higher frequencies, indeed, near $s = -5.3 \pm j5.3$, the locus comes back in and *does* intersect the origin. Roughly speaking, we conclude that it is not one of the 'original' zeroes that crosses into the region U, but, instead, one of the (infinitely many) zeroes introduced by the delay.

Figure 3.7 shows a close up near the origin of the locus for $\tau = .025, .030, .035, .040$. Note that once the locus hits the origin for $\tau = .035$, it must intersect the origin for $\tau > .035$. Using additional analysis, we found the limit to be just slightly less than 0.035.

<u>Summary</u>

This example has demonstrated the following:

1) Theorem 3.4 provides a workable test for distributed parameter systems, even when the characteristic function depends nonlinearly on one or more of the unknown parameters. However, the

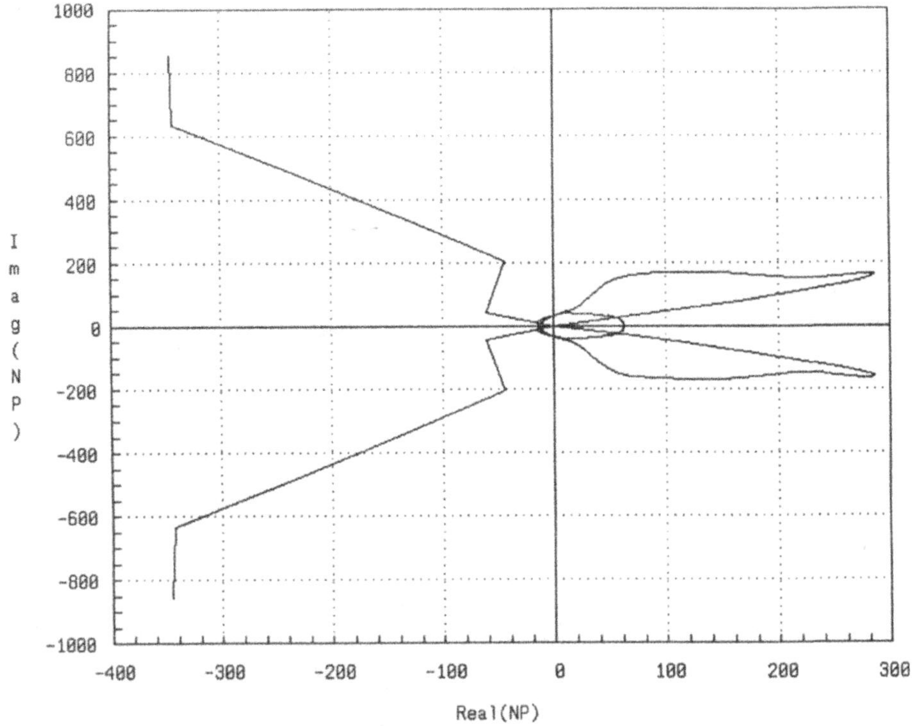

Figure 3.5 Nearest Point Locus for τ = .030

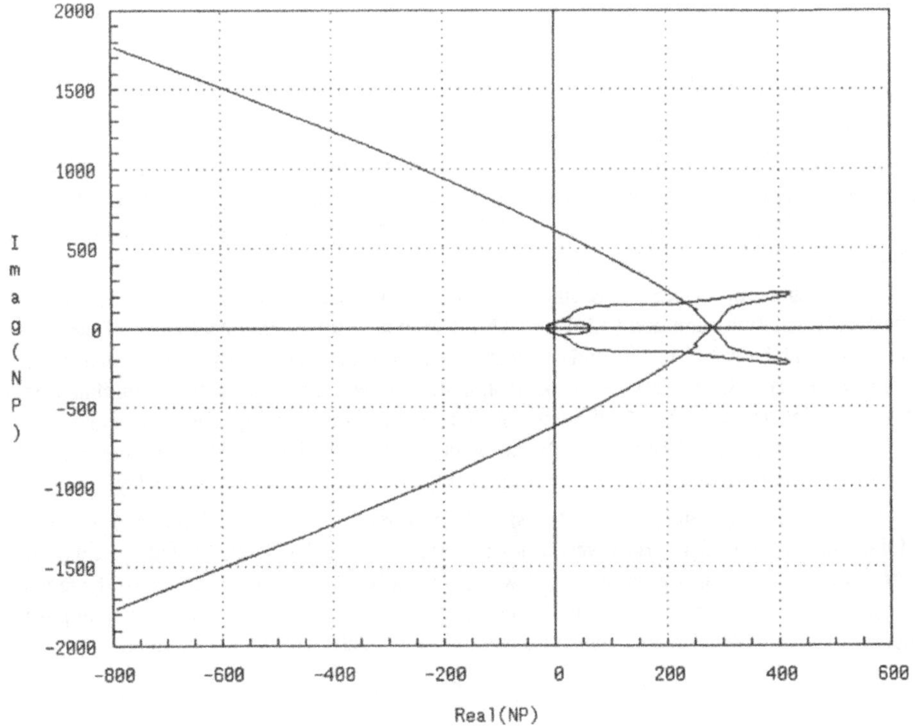

Figure 3.6 Nearest Point Locus for τ = .040

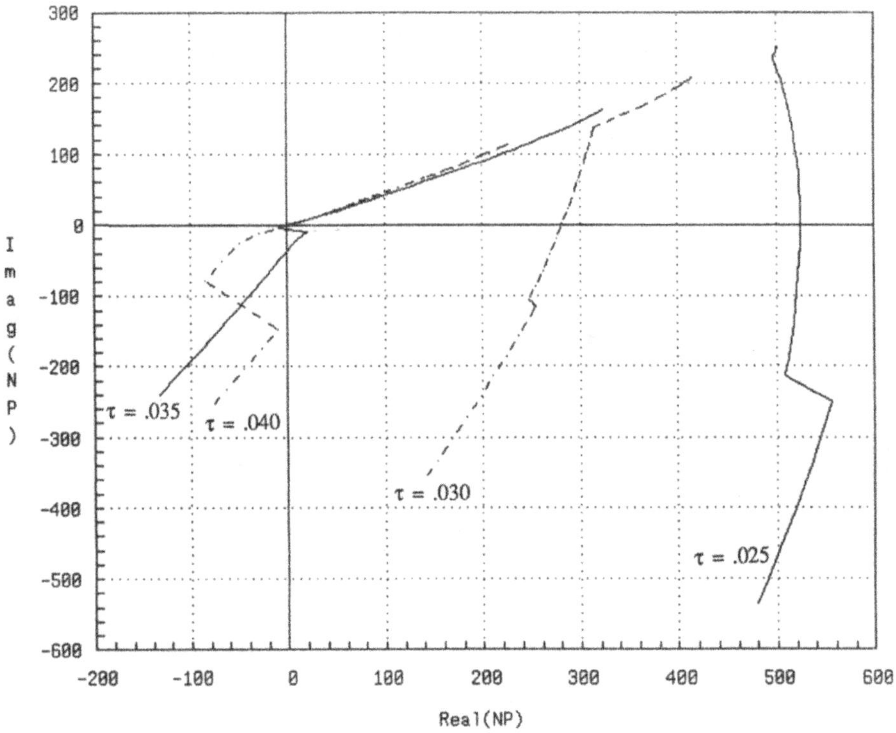

Figure 3.7 Nearest Point Locus for τ = .025, .030, .035, .040

inclusion of nonlinear dependence can severely intensify the numerical calculations. In this example, the nonlinear dependence on T lead to a line search with respect to T^* in the nearest point calculation. Including *several* nonlinear dependencies would mandate more sophisticated minimization algorithms.

2) The role and importance of assumption (A5*). Note that a finite-dimensional system will automatically satisfy assumption (A5*) (or (A5)) if we bound the leading coefficient of the characteristic polynomial away from zero and consider a bounded set of characteristic polynomials (regardless of how the set U is defined). Also note that, in the case where we start with a finite-dimensional system satisfying assumption (A5), if the region U is contained in some right half-plane (assumption (A4)), assumption (A5) will automatically accommodate the addition of unknown time delays. In our example, we had to modify U to fit in a right half-plane when we included the delay.

3) The theory allows assumptions (A4) and (A5) to be replaced by (A4*) and (A5*) (see remark (b) following Theorem 3.4). However, in many common examples of distributed systems, (A5*) will be very difficult to satisfy for regions U which are not bounded on the 'left,' unless the region is very carefully crafted. For our example system (and for any time delay system), a simple positive damping coefficient bound cannot generate a region U for which (A5*) will be satisfied.

4. CONCLUSION

The contributions of this paper should be viewed from the following perspective. Workstations have revolutionized engineering design by their computing power, sophisticated software and graphics. The computing power and the software allow designers to consider much more complicated dynamics as well as more complicated constraints on performance. The combination of computing power, software and graphics allows the study of design trade-offs. Kharitonov's Theorem streamlines the study of the tradeoff between the degree of stability of the nominal system and the size of *coefficient* perturbations that will not destroy stability. Section 3 of this paper develops tools for looking at trade-offs between the degree of stability (choice of region U) for a parameterized class of systems, and the size of that class (choice of the set Q).

5. REFERENCES

[Ana. 1] Anagnost, J. J., Desoer, C. A., and Minnichelli, R. J., "Graphical U-Hurwitz Tests for a Class of Polynomials: A Generalization of Kharitonov's Stability Theorem," Memorandum No. UCB/ERL M87/89, Electronic Research Laboratory, University of California, Berkeley, 1987.

[Ana. 2] Anagnost, J. J., Desoer, C. A., and Minnichelli, R. J., "Graphical Stability Robustness Tests for Linear Time-Invariant Systems: Generalizations of Kharitonov's Stability Theorem," to appear, *Proceedings of the IEEE Conference on Decision and Control*, December, 1988.

[And. 1] Anderson, B. D. O., Jury, E. I., and Mansour, M., "On Robust Hurwitz Polynomials," *IEEE Transactions on Automatic Control*, vol. AC-32, 1987, pp. 909-913.

[Barm. 1] Barmish, B. R., "Invariance of the Strict Hurwitz Property with Perturbed Coefficients," *IEEE Transactions on Automatic Control*, vol. AC-29, 1984, pp. 935-936.

[Barm. 2] Barmish, B. R., "A Generalization of Kharitonov's Four Polynomial Concept for Robust Stability Problems with Linearly Dependent Coefficient Perturbations," Report No. ECE-87-18, Department of Electrical Engineering, University of Wisconsin, Madison, 1987.

[Barm. 3] Barmish, B. R., "New Tools for Robustness Analysis," to appear, IEEE Conference on Decision and Control, December, 1988.

[Bart. 1] Bartlett, A. C., Hollot, C. V. and Lin, L, "Root Locations of an Entire Polytope of Polynomials: It Suffices to Check the Edges," *Proceedings of the American Control Conference* Minneapolis, 1987.

[Cal. 1] Callier, F. M. and Desoer, C. A., "An Algebra of Transfer Functions for Distributed Linear Time-Invariant Systems," *IEEE Transactions on Circuits and Systems*, vol. CAS-25, 1978, pp. 651-663.

[Cal. 2] Callier, F. M. and Desoer, C. A., "Simplifications and Clarifications on the paper 'An Algebra of Transfer Functions for Distributed Linear Time-Invariant Systems,' " *IEEE Transactions on Circuits and Systems*, vol. VAS-27, pp. 320-323, 1980.

[Cal. 3] Callier, F. M. and Desoer, C. A., "Stabilization, Tracking and Disturbance Rejection in Multivariable Convolution Systems," *Annales de la Société Scientifique de Bruxelles*, T. 94, pp. 7-51, 1980

[Cal. 4] Callier, F. M. and Winkin, J., "Distributed System Transfer Functions of Exponential Order," *International Journal of Control*, vol. 43, pp. 1353-1373, 1986.

[Das. 1] Dasgupta, S., *Perspectives on Kharitonov's Theorem: A View from the Imaginary Axis*, Department of Electrical and Computer Engineering, University of Iowa, Iowa City, IA, 52242, 1987.

[Des. 1] Desoer, C. A., Liu, R. W., Murray, J. and Saeks, R., "Feedback System Design: The Fractional Approach to Analysis and Synthesis," *IEEE Transactions on Automatic Control*, vol. AC-25, pp. 399-412, 1980.

[Die. 1] Dieudonné, J., *Foundations of Modern Analysis*, Academic Press, New York, 1969.

[Dug. 1] Dugundji, J., *Topology*, Allyn and Bacon, New York, 1966.

[Fu 1] Fu, M. and Barmish, B. R., "A generalization of Kharitonov's Polynomial Framework to Handle Linearly Dependent Uncertainties," Technical Report ECE-87-9, Department of Electrical and Computer Engineering, University of Wisconsin-Madison, 1987.

[Gil. 1] Gilbert, E. G., "An Iterative Procedure for Computing the Minimum of a Quadratic Form on a Convex Set," *SIAM Journal of Control*, Vol. 4, No. 1, 1966, pp. 61-79.

[Hau. 1] Hauser, J. E., "Proximity Algorithms: Theory and Implementation," Memorandum No. UCB/ERL M86/53, Electronic Research Laboratory, University of California, Berkeley, 1986.

[Kha. 1] Kharitonov, V. L., "Asymptotic Stability of an Equilibrium Position of a Family of Systems of Linear Differential Equations," *Differential Equations*, vol. 14, 1979, pp. 1483-1485.

[Kha. 2] Kharitonov, V. L., "On a Generalization of a Stability Criterion," *Izvestiia Akademii nauk Kazakhskoi SSR, Seria fiziko-matematicheskaia*, vol. 1, pp. 53-57, 1978 (in Russian).

[Kra. 1] Kraus, F., Anderson, B. D. O., Jury, E. I. and Mansour, M., "On Robustness of Low Order Schur Polynomials," *IEEE Transactions on Automatic Control*, vol. AC-35, May 1988, pp. 570-577.

[Min. 1] Minnichelli, R. J., Anagnost, J. J. and Desoer, C. A., "An Elementary Proof of Kharitonov's Theorem with Extensions," Memorandum No. UCB/ERL M87/78, Electronic Research Laboratory, University of California, Berkeley, 1987 (to appear, *IEEE Transactions on Automatic Control*, Aug., 1989).

[Mun. 1] Munkres, J. R., *Topology, a First Course*, Prentice Hall, Englewood Cliffs, N. J., 1975.

[Nett 1] Nett, C. N., Jacobson, C. A. and Balas, M. J., "Fractional Representation Theory: Robustness Results with Applications to Finite Dimensional Control of a Class of Linear Distributed Systems," *Proceedings of the IEEE Conference on Decision and Control*, San Antonio, 1983.

[Whi. 1] Whittaker, E. T. and Watson, G. N., *A Course in Modern Analysis*, 4th Ed., Cambridge University Press, 1946.

[Wol. 1] Wolfe, P., "Finding the Nearest Point in a Polytope," *Mathematical Programming 11*, 1976, pp. 128-149.

[Yeu. 1] Yeung, K. S. and Wang, S. S., "A Simple Proof of Kharitonov's Theorem," *IEEE Transactions on Automatic Control*, vol. AC-32, 1987, pp. 822-823.

EXTENDING KHARITONOV'S THEOREM TO MORE GENERAL SETS OF POLYNOMIALS

Ian R. Petersen

Department of Electrical Engineering
University College, University of New South Wales
Australian Defence Force Academy

INTRODUCTION

In 1978, a significant new result on the stability of families of polynomials was published by V.L. Kharitonov in Russian [1]. When this result became known in the Western literature, there followed an explosion of results related to Kharitonov's Theorem; e.g., see [2]-[15]. One of the reasons for the large amount of interest generated by these results is the fact that they provide powerful tools in the design and analysis of control systems which are robust against parameter uncertainty; e.g., see [15]. Indeed, the family of polynomials under consideration is typically the set of all possible characteristic polynomials for a control system containing uncertain parameters. This family of polynomials is generated by mapping the set of allowable uncertain parameters into the set of allowable polynomials coefficients.

One of the main areas in which research has progressed has been to allow for more general families of polynomials. In Kharitionov's original paper, attention was restricted to families of polynomials which correspond to rectangles in coefficient space. In references [5], [8] and [13]-[15] results have been obtained for the stability of families of polynomials corresponding to convex polytopes in coefficient space. However, as pointed out in [14] and [16] there are numerous situations in practice in which the coefficients of the polynomial will vary as multilinear functions of the uncertain parameters. This will lead to a nonlinear, nonconvex region in coefficient space. In this paper, we present a new result on families of polynomials which correspond to a multilinear mapping between the uncertain parameters and the polynomials coefficients.

FAMILIES OF POLYNOMIALS CORRESPONDING TO MULTILINEAR PARAMETER DEPENDENCE

In this section we introduce a general family of polynomials corresponding to a multilinear mapping between the uncertain parameters and the polynomial coefficients.

Definition 2.1: A mapping $\Psi(\cdot): \mathbf{R}^m \to \mathbf{R}^n$ is said to be a *multilinear mapping* if given any $d \in \mathbf{R}$, any $[\gamma_1 \ \gamma_2 \ \dots \ \gamma_m]' \in \mathbf{R}^m$ and any $\lambda \in \mathbf{R}$, then

$$\Psi(\gamma_1, \gamma_2, \dots, \gamma_{i-1}, \lambda\gamma_i + (1-\lambda)\delta, \gamma_{i+1}, \dots, \gamma_m)$$
$$= \lambda\Psi(\gamma_1, \gamma_2, \dots, \gamma_m) + (1-1)\Psi(\gamma_1, \gamma_2, \dots, \gamma_{i-1}, \delta, \gamma_{i+1}, \dots, \gamma_m)$$

for $i = 1, 2, \dots, m$.

Definition 2.2: Given a multilinear mapping $\Psi(\cdot): \mathbf{R}^m \to \mathbf{R}^n$ and a convex set $\Gamma \subset \mathbf{R}^m$, then the corresponding family of polynomials is defined by

$$F \triangleq \left\{ f(s) = \sum_{i=1}^{n} f_i s^{n-i} : [f_1 \ f_2 \dots f_n]' = \Psi(\gamma) ; \gamma \in \Gamma \right\}. \qquad (2.1)$$

Thus, in coefficient space, we consider the set $\Psi(\Gamma)$. In most applications the set Γ is usually a rectangular region of the form

$$\Gamma = \{\gamma = [\gamma_1 \ \ \gamma_2 \dots \gamma_m]' \in \mathbf{R}^m : \gamma_i^- \le \gamma_i \le \gamma_i^+ \text{ for all } i\}. \qquad (2.2)$$

Associated with this set is the corresponding set of *vertex polynomials*

$$\tilde{\Gamma} \triangleq \left\{\gamma = [\gamma_1 \gamma_2 \cdots \gamma_m]' \in R^m : \gamma_i \in \left\{\gamma_i^-, \gamma_i^+\right\} \text{for all } i\right\}.$$

We now present a result which describes an important property of the set $\Psi(\Gamma)$ for the case in which Γ is of the form (2.2). This result will play an important role in the main result of this paper.

Theorem 2.1: $\Psi(\Gamma) \subset \operatorname{conv}\left\{\Psi(\tilde{\Gamma})\right\}.$

This result is also mentioned in [14] and a similar result is proved in [16]. However, we include the following proof for the sake of completeness.

Proof of Theorem 2.1: Let $f \in \Psi(\Gamma)$ be given and let $\gamma \in \Gamma$ be such that $f = \Psi(\gamma)$. Thus, we can write

$$\gamma_1 = \lambda_1\gamma_1^- + (1-\lambda_1)\gamma_1^+;$$
$$\gamma_2 = \lambda_2\gamma_2^- + (1-\lambda_2)\gamma_2^+;$$
$$\vdots$$
$$\gamma_m = \lambda_m\gamma_m^- + (1-\lambda_m)\gamma_m^+;$$

where $\lambda_i \in [0,1]$ for all i. Hence, using the multilinearity of $\Psi(\cdot)$

$$f = \Psi(\lambda_1\gamma_1^- + (1-\lambda_1)\gamma_1^+, \gamma_2, \ldots, \gamma_m)$$

$$= \lambda_1\Psi(\gamma_1^-, \gamma_2, \ldots, \gamma_m) + (1-\lambda_1)\Psi(\gamma_1^+, \gamma_2, \ldots, \gamma_m)$$

$$= \lambda_1\Psi(\gamma_1^-, \lambda_2\gamma_2^- + (1-\lambda_2)\gamma_2^+, \ldots, \gamma_m) + (1-\lambda_1)\Psi(\gamma_1^+, \lambda_2\gamma_2^- + (1-\lambda_2)\gamma_2^+, \ldots, \gamma_m)$$

$$= \lambda_1\lambda_2\Psi(\gamma_1^-, \gamma_2^-, \ldots, \gamma_m) + \lambda_1(1-\lambda_2)\Psi(\gamma_1^-, \gamma_2^+, \ldots, \gamma_m)$$

$$+ (1-\lambda_1)\lambda_2\Psi(\gamma_1^+, \gamma_2^-, \ldots, \gamma_m) + (1-\lambda_1)(1-\lambda_2)\Psi(\gamma_1^+, \gamma_2^+, \ldots, \gamma_m).$$

Continuing this process, we obtain

$$f = \sum_{i=1}^{2^m}\left(\prod_{j=1}^{m}\tilde{\lambda}_j^i\right)\Psi(g_i)$$

where $g_i \in \tilde{\Gamma}$ is the ith vertex of Γ and

$$\tilde{\lambda}_j^i = \begin{cases} \lambda_j & \text{if the jth component of } g_i \text{ is } \gamma_j^-; \\ (1-\lambda_j) & \text{if the jth component of } g_i \text{ is } \gamma_j^+. \end{cases}$$

Obviously

$$\mu_i \triangleq \prod_{j=1}^{m}\tilde{\lambda}_j^i \geq 0 \text{ for all } i.$$

We now write $\bar{\lambda}_j \triangleq 1-\lambda_j$. However,

$$(\lambda_1 + \bar{\lambda}_1)(\lambda_2 + \bar{\lambda}_2) \ldots (\lambda_m + \bar{\lambda}_m) = \sum_{i=1}^{2^m}\left(\prod_{j=1}^{m}\tilde{\lambda}_j^i\right)$$

and thus we obtain

$$\sum_{i=1}^{2^m}\mu_i = \sum_{i=1}^{2^m}\left(\prod_{j=1}^{m}\tilde{\lambda}_j^i\right) = 1.$$

Furthermore, we have

$$f = \sum_{i=1}^{2^m}\mu_i\Psi(g_i)$$

and hence, we conclude that $f \in \operatorname{conv} \Psi(\tilde{\Gamma})$. This is the required result. ∇∇∇

In order to investigate the stability of the family of polynomials *F*, we now define the *Hurwitz region* in coefficient space.

Definition 2.3: The *Hurwitz Region* $G \subset \mathbf{R}^n$ is defined as

$$G \triangleq \left\{ f = [f_1 f_2 \ldots f_n]' \in R^n : f(s) = \sum_{i=1}^{n} f_i s^{n-i} \text{ is a Hurwitz polynmomial} \right\}.$$

Similarly, if we define an anti-Hurwitz polynomial to be a polynomial which has all of its roots in the open right half plane, then the *Anti-Hurwitz Region* is defined by

$$\tilde{G} \triangleq \left\{ f = [f_1 f_2 \ldots f_n]' \in R^n : f(s) = \sum_{i=1}^{n} f_i s^{n-i} \text{ is an anti-Hurwitz polynmomial} \right\}.$$

A RESULT BASED ON THE NOTION OF CONVEX INTERSECTION SUBSPACES

In reference [13], the notion of Convex Intersection Subspaces was introduced. In this paper, we use the results of [13] together with Theorem 2.1 to derive some new results for a special family of polynomials of the form (2.1) where Γ is of the form (2.2). Indeed, we show that if the mapping $\Psi(\cdot)$ has a certain structure, then $\Psi(\Gamma) \subset G$ if and only if $\Psi(\tilde{\Gamma}) \subset G$. That is, stability is determined purely at the vertex points.

Definition 3.1 (see also [13]): A subspace $S \subset \mathbf{R}^n$ is said to be a *convex intersection subspace* if given any $f \in \mathbf{R}^n$, the set $G \cap \{f + S\}$ is convex.

Lemma 3.1 (see [5] for proof): *The sets*

$$S_e \triangleq \left\{ x = [x_1 x_2 \ldots x_n]' \in R^n : x(s) = \sum_{i=1}^{n} x_i s^{n-i} = h(s^2) \right\}$$
$$S_o \triangleq \left\{ x = [x_1 x_2 \ldots x_n]' \in R^n : x(s) = \sum_{i=1}^{n} x_i s^{n-i} = s g(s^2) \right\}$$

are convex intersection subspaces.

Theorem 3.1: Let $\Psi_1(\cdot): \mathbf{R}^{m1} \to \mathbf{R}^{n1}$ *and* $\Psi_2(\cdot): \mathbf{R}^{m2} \to \mathbf{R}^{n2}$ *be two given multilinear maps. Furthermore, let* $\Gamma_1 \subset \mathbf{R}^{m1}$ *and* $\Gamma_2 \subset \mathbf{R}^{m2}$ *be two given rectangular regions of the form (2.2) and consider the family of polynomials*

$$F \triangleq \left\{ \begin{array}{l} f(s) = h(s^2) + s g(s^2):\ h(s) = \sum_{i=1}^{n_1} h_i s^{n_1 - i};\ g(s) = \sum_{i=1}^{n_1} g_i s^{n_1 - i}; \\ \qquad h = [h_1 h_2 \ldots h_{n_1}]' \in \Psi_1(\Gamma_1);\ g = [g_1 g_2 \ldots g_{n_1}]' \in \Psi_2(\Gamma_2) \end{array} \right\}.$$

This family of polynomials will be stable if and only if the following family of vertex polynomials is stable:

$$\tilde{F} \triangleq \left\{ \begin{array}{l} f(s) = h(s^2) + sg(s^2):\ h(s) = \sum_{i=1}^{n_1} h_i s^{n_1 - i};\ g(s) = \sum_{i=1}^{n_1} g_i s^{n_1 - i}; \\ \qquad h = [h_1 h_2 \ldots h_{n_1}]' \in \Psi_1(\tilde{\Gamma}_1);\ g = [g_1 g_2 \ldots g_{n_1}]' \in \Psi_2(\tilde{\Gamma}_2) \end{array} \right\}.$$

Proof: Given that $\tilde{F} \subset F$, the 'only if ' part of the theorem is obvious. To establish the 'if ' part of the theorem, suppose that the family of vertex polynomials $\tilde{F}$ is stable and let $\hat{f}(s) \in F$ be given. We write

$$\hat{f}(s) = \hat{h}(s^2) + s\hat{g}(s^2)$$

where

$$\hat{h}(s) = \sum_{i=1}^{n_1} \hat{h}_i s^{n_1 - i};\ \hat{g}(s) = \sum_{i=1}^{n_2} \hat{g}_i s^{n_2 - i};$$

$$\hat{h} = [\hat{h}_1 \hat{h}_2 \ldots \hat{h}_{n_1}]' \in \Psi_1(\Gamma_1);\ \hat{g} = [\hat{g}_1 \hat{g}_2 \ldots \hat{g}_{n_2}]' \in \Psi_2(\Gamma_2).$$

We now define a family of polynomials

$$F_e \triangleq \left\{ f(s) = \hat{h}(s^2) + sg(s^2):\ g(s) = \sum_{i=1}^{n_1} g_i s^{n_1 - i};\ g = [g_1 g_2 \ldots g_{n_1}]' \in \Psi_2(\tilde{\Gamma}_2) \right\}.$$

Claim 1: All polynomials in the family F_e are stable.

In order to establish this claim, let $\tilde{f}(s) \in F_e$ be given and write $\tilde{f}(s) = \hat{h}(s^2) + s\tilde{g}(s^2)$ where

$$\tilde{g}(s) = \sum_{i=1}^{n_1} \tilde{g}_i s^{n_1 - i};\ \tilde{g} = [\tilde{g}_1 \tilde{g}_2 \ldots \tilde{g}_{n_1}]' \in \Psi_2(\tilde{\Gamma}_2).$$

Now, the family

$$F_o \triangleq \left\{ f(s) = h(s^2) + s\tilde{g}(s^2):\ h(s) = \sum_{i=1}^{n_1} h_i s^{n_1 - i};\ h = [h_1 h_2 \ldots h_{n_1}]' \in \Psi_1(\tilde{\Gamma}_1) \right\}.$$

is contained in $\tilde{F}$. Hence, all polynomials in F_o must be stable. However, the subspace S_e defined above is a convex intersection subspace. Hence, all polynomials in the family

$$\left\{ f(s) = h(s^2) + s\tilde{g}(s^2):\ h(s) = \sum_{i=1}^{n_1} h_i s^{n_1 - i};\ h = [h_1 h_2 \ldots h_{n_1}]' \in \mathrm{conv}\,\Psi_1(\tilde{\Gamma}_1) \right\}$$

must be stable. Moreover, using Theorem 2.1, it follows that $\hat{h} \in \Psi_1(\Gamma_1) \subset \mathrm{conv}\ \Psi_1(\tilde{\Gamma}_1)$. Therefore, the polynomial $\tilde{f}(s)$ is contained in this family and hence must be stable. This completes the proof of the claim.

Using the above claim and the fact that S_O is a convex intersection subspace, it now follows that all polynomials in the family

$$\left\{ f(s) = \hat{h}(s^2) + sg(s^2) : g(s) = \sum_{i=1}^{n_1} g_i s^{n_1 - i};\ g = [g_1 g_2 \dots g_{n_1}]' \in \operatorname{conv} \Psi_2(\tilde{\Gamma}_2) \right\}$$

are stable. However, using Theorem 2.1, it follows that $\hat{g} \in \Psi_2(\Gamma_2) \subset \operatorname{conv} \Psi_2(\tilde{\Gamma}_2)$. Therefore, the polynomial $\hat{f}(s)$ is contained in this family and hence must be stable. Since, $\hat{f}(s) \in F$ was arbitrary, we conclude that the family F is stable.∇∇∇

We now consider a further class of convex intersection subspaces which were derived in [13].

Lemma 3.2 (see [13] for proof): *Let* $\tilde{w}(s)$ *be a given anti-Hurwitz polynomial. Then the subspaces*

$$S^e_{\tilde{w}} \stackrel{\Delta}{=} \left\{ x = [x_1 x_2 \dots x_n]' \in R^n : x(s) = \sum_{i=1}^{n} x_i s^{n-1} = \tilde{w}(s) h(s^2) \right\}$$

$$S^o_{\tilde{w}} \stackrel{\Delta}{=} \left\{ x = [x_1 x_2 \dots x_n]' \in R^n : x(s) = \sum_{i=1}^{n} x_i s^{n-1} = \tilde{w}(s) s g(s^2) \right\}$$

are convex intersection subspaces.

Note: By combining the results of [15] with the results of [13], this lemma can be extended to the case in which the anti-Hurwitz polynomial $\tilde{w}(s)$ is replaced by a polynomial of the form $\tilde{w}(s)v(s^2)$ where $\tilde{w}(s$ is anti-Hurwitz.

Theorem 3.2: Let $\Psi_{ei}(\cdot): \mathbf{R}^{m_{ei}} \to \mathbf{R}^{n_{ei}}$ *and* $\Psi_{oi}(\cdot): \mathbf{R}^{m_{oi}} \to \mathbf{R}^{n_{oi}}$ *be given multilinear functions for* $i = 1,2, \dots k$. *Furthermore, let* $\Gamma_{ei} \subset \mathbf{R}^{m_{ei}}$ *and* $G_{oi} \subset \mathbf{R}^{m_{oi}}$ *be given rectangular regions of the form* (2.2) *for* $i = 1,2, \dots k$. *Also let* $\{\tilde{w}_i(s)\}_{i=1}^{k}$ *be a given set of anti-Hurwitz polynomials and let* a(s) *be a given polynomial.*

Consider the family of polynomials

$$F \stackrel{\Delta}{=} \left\{ \begin{array}{l} f(s) = a(s) + \sum_{i=1}^{k} \tilde{w}_i(s)\left(h_i(s^2) + s g_i(s^2)\right):\ h_i(s) = \sum_{j=1}^{n_{ei}} h_{ij} s^{n_{ei}-j}; \\ g_i(s) = \sum_{j=1}^{n_{oi}} g_{ij} s^{n_{oi}-j};\ h_i = [h_{i1} h_{i2} \dots h_{in_{ei}}]' \in \Psi_{ei}(\Gamma_{ei}); \\ g_i = [g_{i1} g_{i2} \dots g_{in_{oi}}]' \in \Psi_{oi}(\Gamma_{oi}) \end{array} \right\}$$

Then this family of polynomials will be stable if and only if the family of vertex polynomials

$$\tilde{F} \stackrel{\Delta}{=} \left\{ \begin{array}{l} f(s) = a(s) + \sum_{i=1}^{k} \tilde{w}_i(s)\left(h_i(s^2) + sg_i(s^2)\right):\ h_i(s) = \sum_{j=1}^{n_{ei}} h_{ij} s^{n_{ei}-j}; \\ g_i(s) = \sum_{j=1}^{n_{oi}} g_{ij} s^{n_{oi}-j}; h_i = [h_{i1} h_{i2} \ldots h_{in_{ei}}]' \in \Psi_{ei}(\tilde{\Gamma}_{ei}); \\ g_i = [g_{i1} g_{i2} \ldots g_{in_{oi}}]' \in \Psi_{oi}(\tilde{\Gamma}_{oi}) \end{array} \right\}$$

is stable.

Proof: Given that $\tilde{F} \subset F$, the 'only if ' part of the theorem is obvious. To establish the 'if ' part of the theorem, suppose that all of the vertex polynomials in $\tilde{F}$ are stable and let $\hat{f}(s) \in F$ be given. We can write

$$\hat{f}(s) = a(s) + \sum_{i=1}^{k} \tilde{w}_i(s)\left(\hat{h}_i(s^2) + s\hat{g}_i(s^2)\right)$$

where

$$\hat{h}_i(s) = \sum_{j=1}^{n_{ei}} \hat{h}_{ij} s^{n_{ei}-j};$$

$$\hat{g}_i(s) = \sum_{j=1}^{n_{oi}} \hat{g}_{ij} s^{n_{oi}-j};$$

$$\hat{h}_i = [\, \hat{h}_{i1}\ \hat{h}_{i2} \ldots \hat{h}_{in_{ei}}]' \in \Psi_{ei}(\Gamma_{ei});$$

$$\hat{g}_i = [\, \hat{g}_{i1}\ \hat{g}_{i2} \ldots \hat{g}_{in_{oi}}]' \in \Psi_{oi}(\Gamma_{oi}).$$

We now define a sequence of families of polynomials F^0, F^1, ..., F^k, F^{k+1}, ..., F^{2k}, as follows:

$$F^0 \stackrel{\Delta}{=} \{\hat{f}(s)\};$$

$$F^1 \stackrel{\Delta}{=} a(s) + \left\{ \tilde{w}_1(s) h_1(s^2): h_1(s) = \sum_{j=1}^{n_{e1}} h_{1j} s^{n_{e1}-j};\ h_1 = [h_{11} h_{12} \ldots h_{1n_{e1}}]' \in \Psi_{e1}(\tilde{\Gamma}_{e1}) \right\}$$
$$+ \sum_{i=2}^{k} \tilde{w}_i(s)\hat{h}_i(s^2) + \sum_{i=1}^{k} \tilde{w}_i(s) s\hat{g}_i(s^2);$$

$$F^2 \stackrel{\Delta}{=} a(s) + \left\{ \tilde{w}_1(s) h_1(s^2): h_1(s) = \sum_{j=1}^{n_{e1}} h_{1j} s^{n_{e1}-j};\ h_1 = [h_{11} h_{12} \ldots h_{1n_{e1}}]' \in \Psi_{e1}(\tilde{\Gamma}_{e1}) \right\}$$
$$+ \left\{ \tilde{w}_2(s) h_2(s^2): h_2(s) = \sum_{j=1}^{n_{e2}} h_{2j} s^{n_{e2}-j};\ h_2 = [h_{21} h_{22} \ldots h_{2n_{e2}}]' \in \Psi_{e2}(\tilde{\Gamma}_{e2}) \right\}$$
$$+ \sum_{i=3}^{k} \tilde{w}_i(s)\, \hat{h}_i(s^2) + \sum_{i=1}^{k} \tilde{w}_i(s) s\hat{g}_i(s^2);$$

.
.
.

$$F^{k} \triangleq a(s) + \sum_{i=1}^{k}\left\{ \tilde{w}_i(s)h_i(s^2) : h_i(s) = \sum_{j=1}^{n_{ei}} h_{ij}s^{n_{ei}-j};\ h_i = [h_{i1}h_{i2}\dots h_{in_{ei}}]' \in \Psi_{ei}(\tilde{\Gamma}_{ei})\right\}$$
$$+ \sum_{i=1}^{k}\tilde{w}_i(s)s\hat{g}_i(s^2);$$

.
.
.

$$F^{2k} \triangleq a(s) + \sum_{i=1}^{k}\left\{ \tilde{w}_i(s)h_i(s^2) : h_i(s) = \sum_{j=1}^{n_{ei}} h_{ij}s^{n_{ei}-j};\ h_i = [h_{i1}h_{i2}\dots h_{in_{ei}}]' \in \Psi_{ei}(\tilde{\Gamma}_{ei})\right\}$$
$$+ \sum_{i=1}^{k}\left\{ \tilde{w}_i(s)sg_i(s^2) : g_i(s) = \sum_{j=1}^{n_{oi}} g_{ij}s^{n_{oi}-j};\ g_i = [g_{i1}g_{i2}\dots g_{in_{oi}}]' \in \Psi_{oi}(\tilde{\Gamma}_{oi})\right\}.$$

We first observe that $F^{2k} = \tilde{F}$ and thus all polynomials in the family F^{2k} will be stable. We now establish a claim.

Claim 2 (see also [13]): Let $p \in \{1,2,\dots 2k\}$ be given and suppose that all polynomials in the family F^{p} are stable. Then all polynomials in the family F^{p-1} will be stable.

To establish this claim, suppose that all polynomials in the family F^{p} are stable and let $\tilde{f}(s) \in F^{p-1}$ be given. We will assume that $p \in \{1, 2, \dots, k\}$. (The proof for the case of $p \in \{k+1, k+2, \dots, 2k\}$ is similar.) Hence, $\tilde{f}(s)$ can be written in the form

$$\tilde{f}(s) \triangleq a(s) + \sum_{i=1}^{p-1}\tilde{w}_i(s)\tilde{h}_i(s^2) + \sum_{i=p}^{k}\tilde{w}_i(s)\hat{h}_i(s^2) + \sum_{i=1}^{k}\tilde{w}_i(s)s\hat{g}_i(s^2)$$

where

$$\tilde{h}_i(s) = \sum_{j=1}^{n_{ei}}\tilde{h}_{ij}s^{n_{ei}-j};\ \tilde{h}_i = [\tilde{h}_{i1}\ \tilde{h}_{i2}\dots\tilde{h}_{in_{ei}}]' \in \Psi_{ei}(\tilde{\Gamma}_{ei})$$

for $i = 1, 2, \dots, p-1$. Furthermore, using the fact that the family F^{p} is a family of stable polynomials, it follows that all polynomials in the family

$$\left\{ \begin{array}{l} f(s) \triangleq a(s) + \sum_{i=1}^{p-1}\tilde{w}_i(s)\tilde{h}_i(s^2) + \tilde{w}_p(s)h_p(s^2) + \sum_{i=p+1}^{k}\tilde{w}_i(s)\hat{h}_i(s^2) + \sum_{i=1}^{k}\tilde{w}_i(s)s\hat{g}_i(s^2) : \\ h_p(s) = \sum_{j=1}^{n_{ep}} h_{pj}s^{n_{ei}-j};\ h_p = [h_{p1}h_{p2}\dots h_{pn_{ep}}]' \in \Psi_{ep}(\tilde{\Gamma}_{ep}) \end{array} \right\}$$

will be stable. However, the set $S^{e}_{\tilde{w}_p}$ is a convex intersection subspace. Hence, all polynomials in the family

$$\left\{ \begin{array}{l} f(s) \triangleq a(s) + \sum_{i=1}^{p-1} \tilde{w}_i(s)\tilde{h}_i(s^2) + \tilde{w}_p(s)h_p(s^2) + \sum_{i=p+1}^{k} \tilde{w}_i(s)\hat{h}_i(s^2) + \sum_{i=1}^{k} \tilde{w}_i(s)s\hat{g}_i(s^2): \\ h_p(s) = \sum_{j=1}^{n_{ep}} h_{pj}s^{n_{ei}-j};\ h_p = [h_{p1}h_{p2}\ldots h_{pn_{ep}}]' \in \mathrm{conv}\Psi_{ep}(\tilde{\Gamma}_{ep}) \end{array} \right\}$$

will be stable. Moreover, using Theorem 2.1, we conclude that $\hat{h}_p \in \Psi_{ep}(\Gamma_{ep}) \subset \mathrm{conv}\ \Psi_{ep}(\tilde{\Gamma}_{ep})$. Hence, the polynomial $\tilde{f}(s)$ is contained in this family and therefore, must be stable. Since, $\tilde{f}(s) \in F^{p-1}$ was arbitrary, it follows that the family F^{p-1} is stable. This completes the proof of the claim.

Using the above claim and the fact that the family $F^{2k} = \tilde{F}$ is stable, it now follows that the family $F^0 = \{\hat{f}(s)\}$ is stable. However, $\hat{f}(s) \in F$ was arbitrary. Hence, the family F must be stable. ∇∇∇

EXAMPLE 1

In this section, we consider the stability of a control system containing uncertain parameters. To analyse the stability of this control system, the results of the previous section will be applied. We first consider a dynamical system which consists of an electrical circuit as shown in Figure 1.

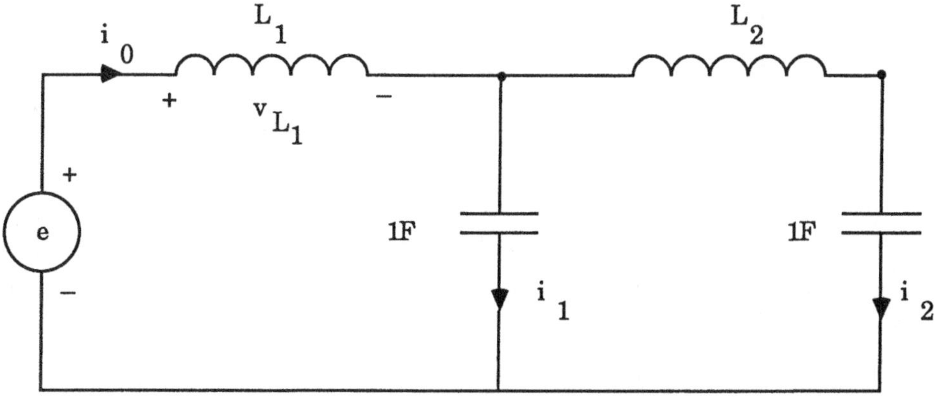

Figure 1.

For this circuit, the inductances L_1 and L_2 represent uncertain parameters. It will be assumed that these uncertain parameters are known to lie within the intervals:

$0.800 \le L_1 \le 1.20;$
$0.833 \le L_2 \le 1.25.$

The dynamical system described by this circuit will have as input the voltage across the independent voltage source e(t). Furthermore, we define the output of the system to be

$$y(t) = i_1(t) - i_2(t) + 3v_{L_1}(t) + 3\phi_2(t) + \int_0^t \phi_2(t)\,dt$$

where $\phi_2(t)$ represents the magnetic flux in the inductor L_2 and $v_{L_1}(t)$ represents the voltage across inductor L_1. For this dynamical system, it is straightforward to verify that the transfer function is given by

$$G(s) = \frac{y(s)}{e(s)} = \frac{s^3 + 3s^2 + 3s + 1}{L_1 s^4 + (2\frac{L_1}{L_2} + 1)s^2 + \frac{1}{L_2}}.$$

Furthermore, if we introduce the notation $\Gamma_2 = 1/L_2$ then we obtain the transfer function

$$G(s) = \frac{s^3 + 3s^2 + 3s + 1}{L_1 s^4 + (2L_1\Gamma_2 + 1)s^2 + \Gamma_2}.$$

When the values of the uncertain parameters are $L_1 = \Gamma_2 = 1$, this system is unstable. However, a feedback controller has been designed to stabilize this system as shown in Figure 2.

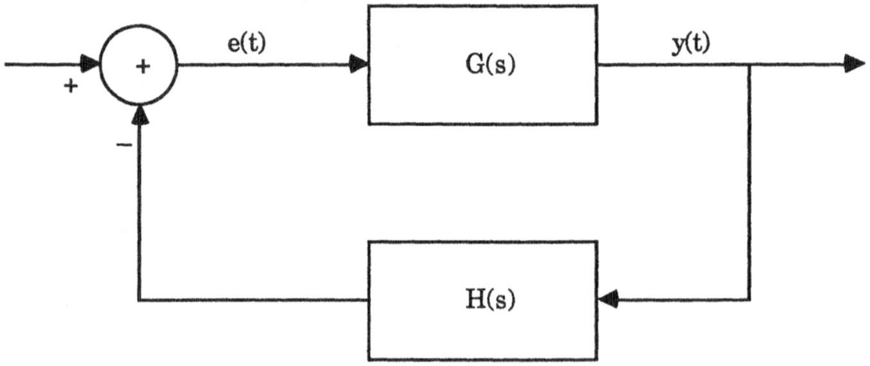

Figure 2.

In this control system, the controller transfer function is given by

$$H(s) = \frac{s + 0.5}{s - 0.1}.$$

It is straightforward to verify that this results in the closed loop transfer function

$$G_{cl}(s) = \frac{(s^3 + 3s^2 + 3s + 1)(s - 0.1)}{s^4 + 3.5s^3 + 4.5s^2 + 2.5s + 0.5 + (s - 0.1)(L_1 s^4 + (2L_1\Gamma_2 + 1)s^2 + \Gamma_2)}.$$

Thus, the closed loop characteristic polynomial will be

contained in the family of polynomials

$$F_{cl} = \left\{ \begin{array}{r} s^4 + 3.5s^3 + 4.5s^2 + 2.5s + 0.5 + (s - 0.1)(L_1 s^4 + (2L_1\Gamma_2 + 1)s^2 + \Gamma_2): \\ 0.8 \le L_1 \le 1.2;\ 0.8 \le \Gamma_2 \le 1.2 \end{array} \right\}$$

This family of polynomials is of the form considered in Theorem 3.2. Therefore, the stability of F_{cl} can be determined from the stability of its four vertex polynomials. That is, the stability of the control system shown in Figure 2 is determined by the following four

$$0.8s^5 + 0.92s^4 + 5.78s^3 + 4.272s^2 + 3.3s + 0.42;$$
$$1.2s^5 + 0.88s^4 + 6.42s^3 + 4.208s^2 + 3.3s + 0.42;$$
$$1.2s^5 + 0.88s^4 + 7.38s^3 + 4.112s^2 + 3.7s + 0.38;$$
$$0.8s^5 + 0.92s^4 + 6.42s^3 + 4.208s^2 + 3.7s + 0.38.$$

Using the Routh-Hurwitz criterion, it is straightforward to verify that each of these polynomials is stable. Hence, using Theorem 3.2, it follows that the control system described above will be stable for all admissible values of the uncertain parameters.

REFERENCES

[1] V.L. Kharitonov, "Asymptotic stability of an equilibrium position of a family of systems of linear differential equations," *Differentail'nye Uraveniya,* Vol. 14, no. 11, pp.1483-1485, 1978.

[2] B.R. Barmish, "Invariance of the strict Hurwitz property for polynomials with perturbed coefficients," *IEEE Transactions on Automatic Control,* Vol. AC-29,

[4] C.V. Hollot and A.C. Bartlett, "Some discrete-time counterparts to Kharitonov's stability criterion for uncertain systems," *IEEE Transactions on Automatic Control,* Vol. AC-31, no. 4, pp. 355-356, 1986.

[5] H.Lin, C.V. Hollot and A. C. Bartlett, "Stability of families of polynomials: Considerations in coefficient space," *International Journal of Control,* Vol. 45, no. 2, pp. 649-660, 1987.

[6] N.K. Bose, "A system-theoretic approach to stability of sets of polynomials," *Contemporary Mathematics,* American Mathematical Society, Vol. 47, pp. 25-34,

[7] S. Bialas and J. Garloff, "Convex combinations of stable polynomials," *Journal of the Franklin Institute,* Vol. 319, no. 3, pp. 373-377, 1985.

[8] A.C. Bartlett, C.V. Hollot and H. Lin, "Root locations of an entire polytope of polynomials: It suffices to check the edges," *Mathematics of Control, Signals , and Systems,* Vol. 1, no. 1, pp. 61-72, 1988.

[9] I.R. Petersen, "A class of stability regions for which a Kharitonov like theorem holds," to appear in the *IEEE Transactions on Automatic Control.*

[10] B.D.O. Anderson, E.I. Jury and M. Mansour, " On robust Hurwitz polynomials," *IEEE Transactions on Automatic Control,* Vol. AC-32, no. 10, pp. 909-912, 1987.

[12] B.D.O Anderson, F.J. Krause, E.I. Jury and M. Mansour, "Robust Schur polynomial stability and Kharitonov's Theorem," *Proceedings of the 26th IEEE Conference on Decision and Control,* pp. 2088-2095, 1987.

[13] I.R. Petersen, "A new extension to Kharitonov's Theorem," *Proceedings of the 26th IEEE Conference on Decision and Control,* pp. 2070-2075, 1987.

[14] B.R. Barmish, "A generalization of Kharitonov's four polynomial concept for robust stability problems with linearly dependent coefficient perturbations," to be

[15] H. Chapellet and S.P. Bhattacharyya, "Geometric conditions for the robust stability of interval

[16] R.R.E. de Gaston and M.G. Safonov, "Exact calculation of the multiloop stability margin," *IEEE Transactions on Automatic Control,* Vol. AC-33, no. 2, pp. 156-171, 1988.

STRONG KHARITONOV THEOREM FOR DISCRETE SYSTEMS

M. Mansour, and F. Kraus

Institute of Automatic Control and Industrial Electronics
Swiss Federal Institute of Technology, Zurich (Switzerland)

B. D. O. Anderson

Australian National University, Canberra (Australia)

Abstract

In [1] robust stability properties of Schur polynomials of the form $f(z) = \sum_{i=0}^{n} a_{n-i} z^i$ were analyzed and a theorem analogous to Kharitonov's weak theorem [2] was derived, where all the corner points of a polyhedron are needed for stability. In this paper the analog of the strong Kharitonov theorem is derived for discrete systems. It is shown that only a relatively small number of corners are needed. The number of corners increases with the system order and can be expressed as a sum of Euler functions.

1. Introduction

Consider the polynomial

$$f(z) = \sum_{i=o}^{n} a_{n-i}\, z^i \tag{1.1}$$

$$a_i \in [\underline{a}_i, \bar{a}_i] \tag{1.2}$$

It is required to find a finite set of conditions such that all the roots of (1.1) lie inside the unit circle. In [1] this problem was solved using the property that f(z) is stable if and only if h(z)/g(z) is discrete lossless positive real, i.e. h(z) and g(z) have simple zeros which lie on $|z| = 1$ and alternate and $|a_n/a_o| < 1$, where h(z) and g(z) are the symmetric and asymmetric parts of f(z) respectively.

$$h(z) = \frac{1}{2}\left[f(z) + z^n f\left(\frac{1}{z}\right)\right] \tag{1.3}$$

$$g(z) = \frac{1}{2}\left[f(z) - z^n f\left(\frac{1}{z}\right)\right] \tag{1.4}$$

Considering the region of the coefficients as given by Fig. (1) for every pair a_i, a_{n-i} it was proved that a necessary and sufficient condition for stability of (1.1) is that all the corner points obtained by every possible combination are stable. Notice that if n is even, $a_{n/2}$ varies in an interval $[\underline{a}_{n/2}, \bar{a}_{n/2}]$.

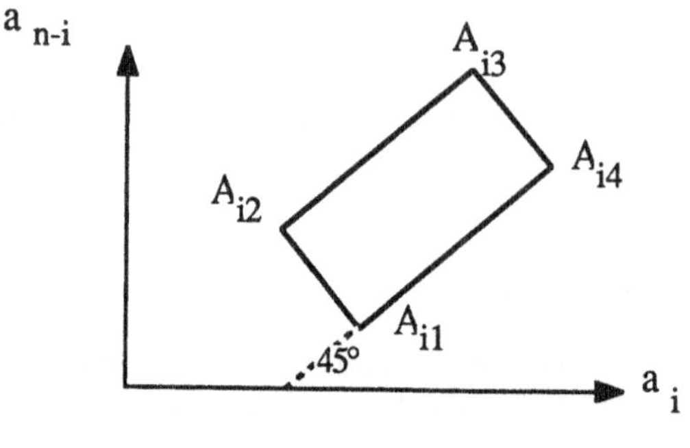

Fig. 1

For the stability of (1.1) subject to (1.2) several necessity and differing sufficiency conditions were derived.

In this paper we use the interlacing property on the unit circle for reducing the number of corner points required. By projecting the zeros of h(z) and g(z) onto the horizontal line [-1,+1] the interlacing property is preserved. Applying Kharitonov-like argumentation we get a result analogous to Kharitonov's strong theorem [2]. In general the number of corners required is four multiplied by a number which increases as the order of the polynomial increases. This number is given by the number of intervals on the line [-1,+1] defined by the projections of the zeros of h(z), g(z) which is in turn given by the roots of some polynomials arrived at through the projection of h(z) and g(z).These polynomials are Chebyshev and Jacobi polynomials. A recursion formula is derived for the number of intervals. Also a method is given to derive the corners the stability of which is necessary and sufficient for stability of (1.1) for the region of coefficients given by Fig. (1). It is also shown that the same result can be easily obtained through frequency domain considerations. For $n<6$ a result analogous to the result in [3] can be obtained where the number of corners is reduced.

2. The projection of h(z) and g(z) on the horizontal line

From (1.3) and (1.4) h(z) and and g(z) are given by

$$\begin{aligned} h(z) &= \frac{a_o+a_n}{2} z^n + \frac{a_1+a_{n-1}}{2} z^{n-1} + \dots + \frac{a_1+a_{n-1}}{2} z + \frac{a_o+a_n}{2} \\ &= \alpha_o z^n + \alpha_1 z^{n-1} + \dots + \alpha_1 z + \alpha_o \end{aligned} \qquad (2.1)$$

$$\begin{aligned} g(z) &= \frac{a_o-a_n}{2} z^n + \frac{a_1-a_{n-1}}{2} z^{n-1} + \dots - \frac{a_1-a_{n-1}}{2} z - \frac{a_o-a_n}{2} \\ &= \beta_o z^n + \beta_1 z^{n-1} + \dots - \beta_1 z - \beta_o \end{aligned} \qquad (2.2)$$

According to the assumption of Fig. (1), α_i and β_i are given as in Fig. (2)

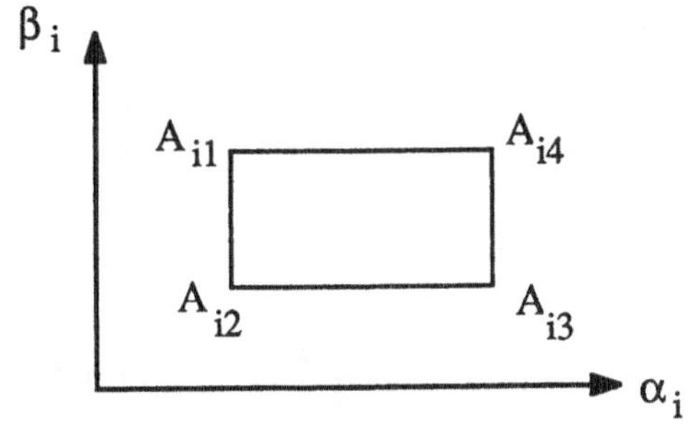

Fig. 2

It is to be noted that according to the necessary condition for stability $|a_n/a_o| < 1$, α_o and β_o can be taken always positive.

For stability, all the zeros of h(z) and g(z) are simple, lie on the unit circle and are interlacing. As two conjugate roots on the unit circle are given by the roots of $z^2 - 2\sigma z + 1$, where σ is the real part of the roots, then we get for n even:

$$h(z) = \alpha_0 \prod_{i=1}^{\nu} (z^2 - 2\sigma_i z + 1) \tag{2.3}$$

$$\text{where } \nu = \frac{n}{2}$$

The "projection" of h(z) on the horizontal line, Fig. (3), gives a polynomial $h'(\lambda)$ of degree $\nu = \frac{n}{2}$

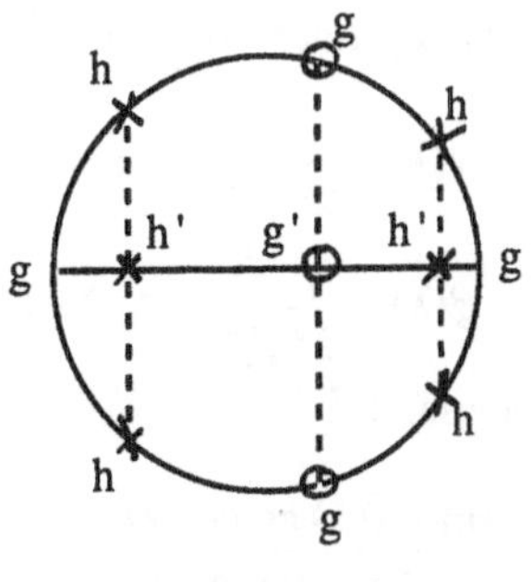

Fig. 3

According to [5],

$$h'(\lambda) = \sum_{i=o}^{\nu} \frac{\alpha_i}{2^i} \sum_{k=0,1,2,\dots} (-1)^k \frac{1}{4^k} \binom{\nu-k-i}{k} \frac{\nu-i}{\nu-k-i} \lambda^{\nu-2k-i} \tag{2.4a}$$

where $\binom{x}{k}$ denotes the binomial coefficient.

$h'(\lambda)$ can be written in the form

$$h'(\lambda) = \frac{1}{2^{\nu-1}}\left[\sum_{i=0}^{\nu-1} \alpha_i T_{\nu-i} + \frac{\alpha_\nu}{2}\right] \tag{2.4b}$$

where T_ν is a Chebyshev polynomial. Also

$$g(z) = \beta_0 (z^2 - 1) \prod_{i=1}^{\nu-1} (z^2 - 2\sigma_i z + 1) \tag{2.5}$$

The "projection" of g(z) on the horizontal line gives a polynomial $g'(\lambda)$ of degree $\frac{n}{2}$ - 1 (here the two roots at +1 and -1 are not considered). From [5] we have

$$g'(\lambda) = \sum_{i=o}^{\nu-1} \frac{\beta_i}{2^i} \sum_{k=0,1,2,\ldots} (-1)^k \frac{1}{4^k} \binom{\nu-k-i-1}{k} \lambda^{\nu-2k-i-1} \tag{2.6a}$$

Now $g'(\lambda)$ can be expressed as a function of Chebyshev polynomial of the second kind U_ν.

$$g'(\lambda) = \frac{1}{2^{\nu-1}} \sum_{i=0}^{\nu-1} \beta_i U_{\nu-1-i} \tag{2.6b}$$

Similarly for n odd:

$$h'(\lambda) = \sum_{i=o}^{\nu} \frac{\alpha_i}{2^i} \sum_{k=0,1,2,\ldots} (-1)^{\left\lceil \frac{k}{2} \right\rceil} \frac{1}{2^k} \binom{\nu - \left\lceil \frac{k}{2} \right\rceil - i}{\left\lfloor \frac{k}{2} \right\rfloor} \lambda^{\nu-k-i} \tag{2.7}$$

and

$$g'(\lambda) = \sum_{i=o}^{\nu} \frac{\beta_i}{2^i} \sum_{k=0,1,2,\ldots} (-1)^{\left\lfloor \frac{k}{2} \right\rfloor} \frac{1}{2^k} \binom{\nu - \left\lceil \frac{k}{2} \right\rceil - i}{\left\lfloor \frac{k}{2} \right\rfloor} \lambda^{\nu-k-i} \tag{2.8}$$

where $\nu = \frac{n-1}{2}$, $\left\lfloor \frac{k}{2} \right\rfloor$ is the lower integer next to $\frac{k}{2}$ and $\left\lceil \frac{k}{2} \right\rceil$ is the higher integer next to $\frac{k}{2}$.

Now $h'(\lambda)$ can be expressed as $\quad h'(\lambda) = \frac{1}{2^\nu} \sum_{i=0}^{\nu} \alpha_i \tau_{\nu-i}$

and $g'(\lambda)$ as $\quad g'(\lambda) = \frac{1}{2^\nu} \sum_{i=0}^{\nu} (2\nu-2i+1)\, \beta_i\, \mu_{\nu-i}$

where τ_ν and μ_ν are Jacobi polynomials [8]

$$\tau_i = \frac{\cos(\overline{i+0.5}) \arccos x)}{\cos(0.5 \arccos x)}, \quad \mu_i = \frac{\sin(\overline{i+0.5}) \arccos x)}{\sin(0.5 \arccos x)}$$

3. The intervals on the line [-1,1]

From the formulas (2.4), (2.6), (2.7) and (2.8) we get table (1) for n = 2 to 10. The term "roots" refers to those values of λ at which one of the polynomials multiplying α_i or β_i changes sign. The number of intervals δ_n on the line [-1,1] is given by one plus the number of different roots γ_n for n even or n odd respectively. i.e.

$$\delta_n = \gamma_n + 1 \tag{3.1}$$

Table 1

		roots
n = 2	$h' = \alpha_0\lambda + \frac{\alpha_1}{2}$ $g' = \beta_0$	0
n = 3	$h' = \alpha_0(\lambda - \frac{1}{2}) + \frac{\alpha_1}{2}$ $g' = \beta_0(\lambda + \frac{1}{2}) + \frac{\beta_1}{2}$	+ 0.5 - 0.5
n = 4	$h' = \alpha_0(\lambda^2 - \frac{1}{2}) + \frac{\alpha_1}{2}\lambda + \frac{\alpha_2}{4}$ $g' = \beta_0\lambda + \frac{\beta_1}{2}$	± 0.707 , 0 0
n = 5	$h' = \alpha_0(\lambda^2 - \frac{\lambda}{2} - \frac{1}{4}) + \frac{\alpha_1}{2}(\lambda - \frac{1}{2}) + \frac{\alpha_2}{4}$ $g' = \beta_0(\lambda^2 + \frac{\lambda}{2} - \frac{1}{4}) + \frac{\beta_1}{2}(\lambda + \frac{1}{2}) + \frac{\beta_2}{4}$	+ 0.5 , + 0.809 , - 0.309 - 0.5 , - 0.809 , + 0.309
n = 6	$h' = \alpha_0(\lambda^3 - \frac{3\lambda}{4}) + \frac{\alpha_1}{2}(\lambda^2 - \frac{1}{2}) + \frac{\alpha_2\lambda}{4} + \frac{\alpha_3}{8}$ $g' = \beta_0(\lambda^2 - \frac{1}{4}) + \frac{\beta_1}{2}\lambda + \frac{\beta_2}{4}$	0 , ± 0.866 , ± 0.707 0 , ± 0.5
n = 7	$h' = \alpha_0(\lambda^3 - \frac{\lambda^2}{2} - \frac{\lambda}{2} + \frac{1}{8}) + \frac{\alpha_1}{2}(\lambda^2 - \frac{\lambda}{2} - \frac{1}{4}) + \frac{\alpha_2}{4}(\lambda - \frac{1}{2}) + \frac{\alpha_3}{8}$ $g' = \beta_0(\lambda^3 + \frac{\lambda^2}{2} - \frac{\lambda}{2} - \frac{1}{8}) + \frac{\beta_1}{2}(\lambda^2 + \frac{\lambda}{2} - \frac{1}{4}) + \frac{\beta_2}{4}(\lambda + \frac{1}{2}) + \frac{\beta_3}{8}$	+ 0.5 , + 0.809 , - 0.309 , - 0.624 , + 0.223 , + 0.901 - 0.5 , - 0.809 , + 0.309 , + 0.624 , - 0.223 , - 0.901
n = 8	$h' = \alpha_0(\lambda^4 - \lambda^2 + \frac{1}{8}) + \frac{\alpha_1}{2}(\lambda^3 - \frac{3\lambda}{4}) + \frac{\alpha_2}{4}(\lambda^2 - \frac{1}{2}) + \frac{\alpha_3}{8}\lambda + \frac{\alpha_4}{16}$ $g' = \beta_0(\lambda^3 - \frac{\lambda}{2}) + \frac{\beta_1}{2}(\lambda^2 - \frac{1}{4}) + \frac{\beta_2}{4}\lambda + \frac{\beta_3}{8}$	0 , ± 0.707 , 0 , ± 0.866 , ± 0.383 , ± 0.924 0 , ± 0.5 , ± 0.707 , 0
n = 9	$h' = \alpha_0(\lambda^4 - \frac{\lambda^3}{2} - \frac{3\lambda^2}{4} + \frac{\lambda}{4} + \frac{1}{16}) + \frac{\alpha_1}{2}(\lambda^3 - \frac{\lambda^2}{2} - \frac{\lambda}{2} + \frac{1}{8})$ $+ \frac{\alpha_2}{4}(\lambda^2 - \frac{\lambda}{2} - \frac{1}{4}) + \frac{\alpha_3}{8}(\lambda - \frac{1}{2}) + \frac{\alpha_4}{16}$ $g' = \beta_0(\lambda^4 + \frac{\lambda^3}{2} - \frac{3\lambda^2}{4} - \frac{\lambda}{4} + \frac{1}{16}) + \frac{\beta_1}{2}(\lambda^3 + \frac{\lambda^2}{2} - \frac{\lambda}{2} - \frac{1}{8})$ $+ \frac{\beta_2}{4}(\lambda^2 + \frac{\lambda}{2} - \frac{1}{4}) + \frac{\beta_3}{8}(\lambda + \frac{1}{2}) + \frac{\beta_4}{16}$	+0.5, +0.809, -0.309, -0.624, +0.223, +0.901, +0.94, -0.174, -0.766, +0.5 -0.5, -0.809, +0.309, +0.624, -0.223, -0.901, -0.94, +0.174, +0.766, -0.5
n = 10	$h' = \alpha_0(\lambda^5 - \frac{5\lambda^3}{4} + \frac{5\lambda}{16}) + \frac{\alpha_1}{2}(\lambda^4 - \lambda^2 + \frac{1}{8}) + \frac{\alpha_2}{4}(\lambda^3 - \frac{3\lambda}{4})$ $+ \frac{\alpha_3}{8}(\lambda^2 - \frac{1}{2}) + \frac{\alpha_4\lambda}{16} + \frac{\alpha_5}{32}$ $g' = \beta_0(\lambda^4 - \frac{3\lambda^2}{4} + \frac{1}{16}) + \frac{\beta_1}{2}(\lambda^3 - \frac{\lambda}{2}) + \frac{\beta_2}{4}(\lambda^2 - \frac{1}{4}) + \frac{\beta_3}{8}\lambda + \frac{\beta_4}{16}$	0 , ± 0.707 , ± 0.866 , ± 0.383 , ± 0.924 , ± 0.588 , ± 0.951 ± 0.309 , ± 0.809 , 0, ± 0.5 , 0 , ± 0.707

It can be seen that as n increases the roots are repeated with different periods of repetition.

For n even: 0 is repeated with a period of 2, while ±0.707 is repeated with a period of 4. ±0.5 and ±0.866 are repeated with a period of 6 while ±0.383, ±0,924 are repeated with a period of 8. ±0.588, ±0.95 are repeated with a period if 10 and so on.

$$\begin{aligned}\gamma_n &= \text{number of different roots}\\ &= \frac{n^2}{4} - \left.\frac{n-2}{2}\right\rfloor \gamma_2 - \left.\frac{n-4}{4}\right\rfloor (\gamma_4 - \gamma_2) - \left.\frac{n-6}{6}\right\rfloor (\gamma_6 - \gamma_4) - \left.\frac{n-8}{8}\right\rfloor (\gamma_8 - \gamma_6) - \left.\frac{n-10}{10}\right\rfloor (\gamma_{10} - \gamma_8) - \dots\\ &= \frac{n^2}{4} - \left.\frac{n-2}{2}\right\rfloor \Phi_2 - \left.\frac{n-4}{4}\right\rfloor \Phi_4 - \left.\frac{n-6}{6}\right\rfloor 2\Phi_6 - \left.\frac{n-8}{8}\right\rfloor \Phi_8 - \left.\frac{n-10}{10}\right\rfloor 2\Phi_{10} - \dots \end{aligned} \tag{3.2}$$

where $\gamma_2 = 1$, Φ_k is the Euler function [8] and $\left.\alpha\right\rfloor$ equals 0 for negative values of α.

For n odd: ± 0.5 is repeated with a period of 6, while ± 0.309 and ± 0.809 are repeated with a period of 10. ± 0.233, ± 0.901, $\pm 0{,}624$ are repeated with a period of 14 while ± 0.940, ± 0.174, ± 0.766 are repeated with a period of 18 and so on. The scheme in (3.3) gives a recursion formula for the number of different roots for n odd. Adding one to this number gives the number of intervals.

$$\begin{aligned}\gamma_n = \text{number of different roots} &= \frac{n^2-1}{4} - \left.\frac{n-3}{6}\right\rfloor \gamma_3 - \left.\frac{n-5}{10}\right\rfloor (\gamma_5 - \gamma_3) - \left.\frac{n-7}{14}\right\rfloor (\gamma_7 - \gamma_5) -\\ &\quad - \left.\frac{n-9}{18}\right\rfloor (\gamma_9 - \gamma_7) - \dots\\ &= \frac{n^2-1}{4} - \left.\frac{n-3}{6}\right\rfloor \Phi_3 - \left.\frac{n-5}{10}\right\rfloor \Phi_5 - \left.\frac{n-7}{14}\right\rfloor \Phi_7 - \left.\frac{n-9}{18}\right\rfloor \Phi_9 - \dots \end{aligned} \tag{3.3}$$

where $\gamma_3 = 2$.

4. Stability of f(z)

Consider the stability of f(z) from (1.1) where a_i and a_{n-i} are given as in Fig. (1) which corresponds to α_i and β_i as shown in Fig. (2). It is clear from section 2 that stability is guaranteed if every $h'(\lambda)$ and $g'(\lambda)$ have interlacing zeros on the line [-1,1]. This property is satisfied if in every interval on [-1,1] the four polynomials corresponding to $(\bar{h}',\bar{g}')$, $(\bar{h}',\underline{g}')$, $(\underline{h}',\bar{g}')$, $(\underline{h}',\underline{g}')$ are stable. Here, $\bar{h}'$ is defined by choosing α_i to equal its greatest or its least value, so that h' is maximized through this choice. Throughout any one interval, the same choice secures the maximization. $\underline{h}'$ is defined so that h' is minimized, and $\bar{g}'$, $\underline{g}'$ are obviously defined. This can be explained as follows for n even and higher than 6:

The sections on the [-1,+1] line corresponding to h' and g' must be interlacing for stability. Fig. (4) gives the transition diagram which shows the situation for n=6

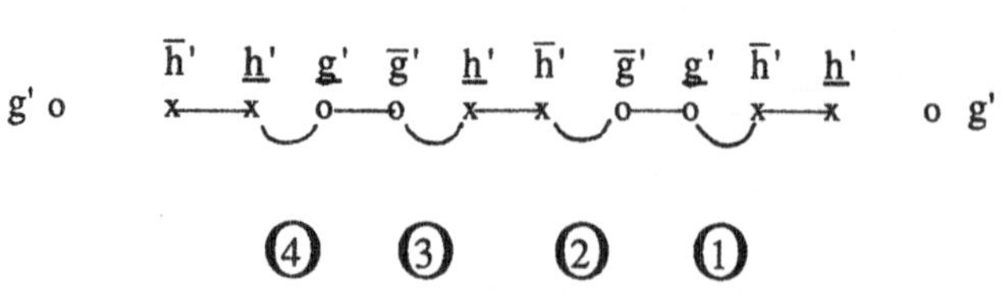

Fig. 4

It is clear that if the transitions between the sections lie in one interval then the stability of the four polynomials given above for every interval guarantees the interlacing property. If the transitions lie in different intervals or between intervals this interlacing property is also guaranteed through the four polynomials in all the intervals.

For n>6 there is a repetition of the transitions so that only four polynomials are sufficient as in Kharitonov's theorem for continuous systems.

Hence the number of corners necessary and sufficient for stability is given by

$$N = 4 * \delta_n \qquad (4.1)$$

where δ_n is the number of intervals on the line [-1,1], (3.1).

For n=10, N = 4 * 20 = 80 corners out of 2^{11} = 2048 corners, i.e. about 4% of the total number of corners are to be checked. For n=30, N = 4 * 144 = 576 out of 2^{31} corners. As n increases the number of corners to consider for stability increases less than quadratically while the total number of corners increases exponentially. Fig. (5) shows the relation for n even and n odd. For n<6 we can reduce the number of corners to be checked as will be shown in section 5.

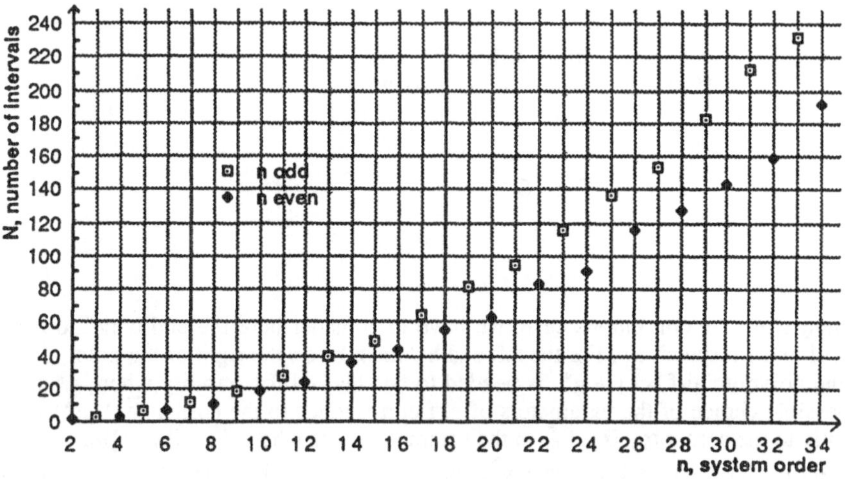

Fig. 5

5. Stability of low order polynomials

In the following n = 2, 3, 4, 5 are considered. As in the continuous case we show that not all the four polynomials are needed for every interval on the line [-1,+1]. In general the number of corners needed is given by:

End conditions + (no. of transitions * no. of intervals)

It is to be noted that the necessary conditions for stability [4] should be checked first.

For n=2:

$$f(z) = a_o z^2 + a_1 z + a_2 \qquad (5.1)$$

necessary conditions for stability: $a_o > 0$

$2a_o < a_1 < 2a_o$

$-a_o < a_2 < a_o$

$$h'(\lambda) = \alpha_o\lambda + \frac{\alpha_1}{2} \qquad (5.2)$$

$$g'(\lambda) = \beta_o \qquad (5.3)$$

The necessary conditions for stability are

$$0 < \alpha_o < a_o$$
$$-2a_o < \alpha_1 = a_1 < 2a_o$$
$$0 < \beta_o < a_o$$

from $h'(\lambda)$ and $g'(\lambda)$ we have one root at $\lambda = 0$.Therefore we have two intervals.

Fig. (6) shows the transition diagram

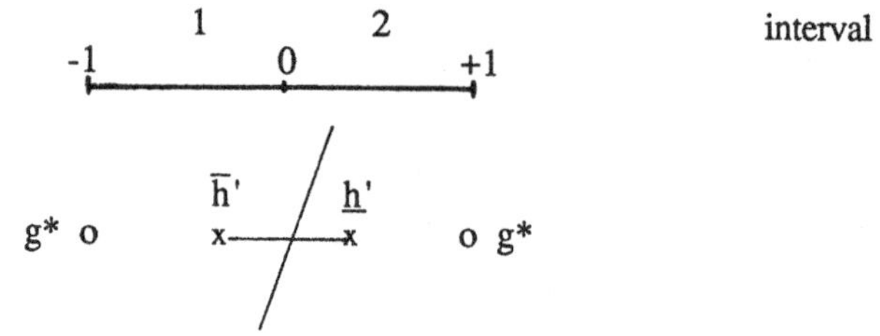

Fig. 6

Different from the continuous case, we have to consider here the end conditions on the points -1 and 1 respectively. For the left end $\bar{h}_1'$ must be on the right of the point -1. Therefore the polynomial $f = \bar{h}_1 + g^*$ is needed to be checked for stability where g^* stays for any possible choice of the parameters of g. f corresponds to the corner $(\bar{h}_1', g^*)$ or more explicitly to the corner $\underline{\alpha}_o, \bar{\alpha}_1, \beta_o^*$ in the parameter space where $\beta_o^* = \bar{\beta}_o$ or $\underline{\beta}_o$.
Similarly for the right end: $f = \underline{h}_2 + g^*$, i.e. corner $\underline{\alpha}_o, \underline{\alpha}_1, \beta_o^*$ is needed to be checked for stability.
From the transition diagram we see that there is no transition and therefore no other polynomial is needed. Therefore for n=2, necessary and sufficient conditions for the stability is that the two corners

$$\underline{\alpha}_o, \bar{\alpha}_1, \beta_o^*$$
$$\underline{\alpha}_o, \underline{\alpha}_1, \beta_o^*$$

are stable.

Special cases:

If $\bar{\alpha}_1 < 0$ only $\underline{\alpha}_o, \underline{\alpha}_1, \beta_o^*$ is needed

If $\underline{\alpha}_1 > 0$ only $\underline{\alpha}_o, \bar{\alpha}_1, \beta_o^*$ is needed

For n=2 we need to check in general $2 + (0 * 2) = 2$ corners.

For n=3:

$$f(z) = a_oz^3 + a_1z^2 + a_2z + a_3 \qquad (5.4)$$

The necessary conditions for stability are

$$0 < a_o$$
$$-3a_o < a_1 < 3a_o$$
$$-a_o < a_2 < 3a_o$$
$$-a_o < a_3 < a_o$$

$$h' = \alpha_0 (\lambda - \frac{1}{2}) + \frac{\alpha_1}{2} \tag{5.5}$$

$$g' = \beta_0 (\lambda + \frac{1}{2}) + \frac{\beta_1}{2} \tag{5.6}$$

The necessary conditions for stability are

$$0 < \alpha_0 < a_0$$
$$-2a_0 < \alpha_1 < 3a_0$$
$$0 < \beta_0 < a_0$$
$$-3a_0 < \beta_1 < 2a_0$$

From h' and g' we have two roots at 0.5 and -0.5, i.e. we have 3 intervals as shown in Fig. (7).

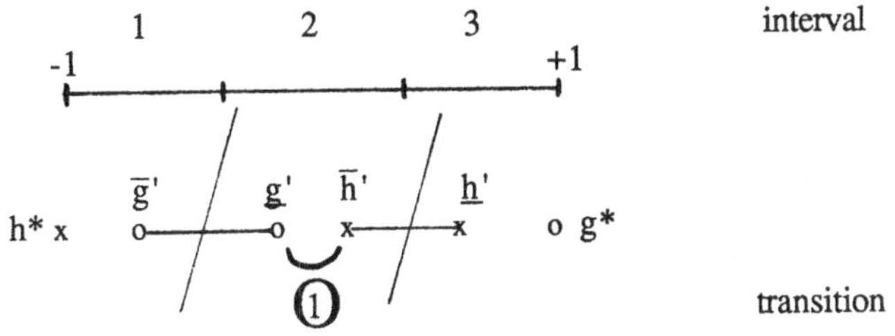

Fig. 7

For the left and for the right end we need the corners given by $(h^*, \bar{g}_1')$ and $(\underline{h}_3', g^*)$ respectively to check for stability. Hence, for both ends we need to check only the corner given by $(\underline{h}_3', \bar{g}_1')$. As we have only one transition and three intervals we need also to check the three corners corresponding to: $(\bar{h}_1', \underline{g}_1')$, $(\bar{h}_2', \underline{g}_2')$ and $(\bar{h}_3', \underline{g}_3')$. Here $h_1' = h_2'$ and $\underline{g}_2' = \underline{g}_3'$. Therefore necessary and sufficient condition for stability of a third order system is the stability of the 4 corners:

$\underline{\alpha}_0, \underline{\alpha}_1, \underline{\beta}_0, \bar{\beta}_1$

$\underline{\alpha}_0, \bar{\alpha}_1, \bar{\beta}_0, \underline{\beta}_1$

$\underline{\alpha}_0, \bar{\alpha}_1, \underline{\beta}_0, \underline{\beta}_1$

$\bar{\alpha}_0, \bar{\alpha}_0, \underline{\beta}_0, \underline{\beta}_1$

out of $2^4 = 16$ corners.

Special cases:

i) If $\bar{\alpha}_1 > 0, \underline{\beta}_1 > 0$ it is easy to show that only $(\bar{h}_1', \underline{g}_1')$ is needed for the transition i.e. the stability of the two corners

$\underline{\alpha}_0, \underline{\alpha}_1, \underline{\beta}_0, \bar{\beta}_1$

$\underline{\alpha}_0, \bar{\alpha}_1, \bar{\beta}_0, \underline{\beta}_1$

is necessary and sufficient for stability.

ii) If $\bar{\alpha}_1 > 0$, $\underline{\beta}_1 < 0$ it is easy to show that only $(\bar{h}_1', \underline{g}_2')$ is needed for the transition i.e. we need only the two corners

$\underline{\alpha}_0, \underline{\alpha}_1, \underline{\beta}_0, \bar{\beta}_1$

$\underline{\alpha}_0, \bar{\alpha}_1, \underline{\beta}_0, \underline{\beta}_1$

iii) If $\bar{\alpha}_1 < 0$, $\beta_1 > 0$ no corner is needed for the transition. In this case the stability of one corner namely

$$\underline{\alpha}_o, \underline{\alpha}_1, \underline{\beta}_o, \bar{\beta}_1$$

is necessary and sufficient for stability.

Summarizing for n=3 we need to check in general $1 + (1 * 3) = 4$ corners.

For n=4:

$$f(z) = a_o z^4 + a_1 z^3 + a_2 z^2 + a_3 z + a_4 \tag{5.7}$$

necessary conditions for stability

$$\begin{array}{rcl} a_o &>& 0 \\ -4a_o < & a_1 & < 4a_o \\ -2a_o < & a_2 & < 6a_o \\ -4a_o < & a_3 & < 4a_o \\ -a_o < & a_4 & < a_o \end{array}$$

$$h'(\lambda) = \alpha_o(\lambda^2 - \frac{1}{2}) + \frac{\alpha_1}{2}\lambda + \frac{\alpha_2}{4} \tag{5.8}$$

$$g'(\lambda) = \beta_o\lambda + \frac{\beta_1}{2} \tag{5.9}$$

The necessary conditions for stability are

$$\begin{array}{rcl} 0 < & \alpha_o & < a_o \\ -4a_o < & \alpha_1 & < 4a_o \\ -2a_o < & \alpha_2 & < 6a_o \\ 0 < & \beta_o & < a_o \\ -4a_o < & \beta_1 & < 4a_o \end{array}$$

from $h'(\lambda)$, $g'(\lambda)$ we have the roots $\lambda = 0, \pm\frac{\sqrt{2}}{2}$, i.e. we get 4 intervals.

Fig. (8) shows the transition diagram where we have two transitions $(\bar{h}', \underline{g}')$ and $(\bar{h}', \bar{g}')$.

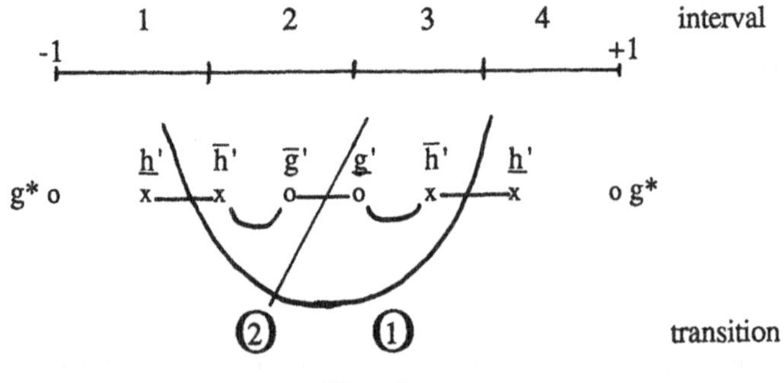

Fig. 8

For the left and for the right end we need to check the corner corresponding to $(\underline{h}_1', g^*)$ and $(\underline{h}_4', g^*)$ respectively.

For the two transitions we need to check the corners corresponding to

$(\bar{h}_1', \underline{g}_1')$, $(\bar{h}_2', \underline{g}_2')$, $(\bar{h}_3', \underline{g}_3')$, $(\bar{h}_4', \underline{g}_4')$,

$(\bar{h}_1', \bar{g}_1')$, $(\bar{h}_2', \bar{g}_2')$, $(\bar{h}_3', \bar{g}_3')$, $(\bar{h}_4', \bar{g}_4')$.

Therefore necessary and sufficient condition for stability of a fourth order system is the stability of the 10 corners:

(1) $\underline{\alpha}_0, \bar{\alpha}_1, \underline{\alpha}_2, \beta_0^*, \beta_1^*$

(2) $\underline{\alpha}_0, \underline{\alpha}_1, \underline{\alpha}_2, \beta_0^*, \beta_1^*$

(3) $\bar{\alpha}_0, \underline{\alpha}_1, \bar{\alpha}_2, \bar{\beta}_0, \underline{\beta}_1$

(4) $\underline{\alpha}_0, \underline{\alpha}_1, \bar{\alpha}_2, \bar{\beta}_0, \underline{\beta}_1$

(5) $\underline{\alpha}_0, \bar{\alpha}_1, \bar{\alpha}_2, \underline{\beta}_0, \underline{\beta}_1$

(6) $\bar{\alpha}_0, \bar{\alpha}_1, \bar{\alpha}_2, \underline{\beta}_0, \underline{\beta}_1$

(7) $\bar{\alpha}_0, \underline{\alpha}_1, \bar{\alpha}_2, \underline{\beta}_0, \bar{\beta}_1$

(8) $\underline{\alpha}_0, \underline{\alpha}_1, \bar{\alpha}_2, \underline{\beta}_0, \bar{\beta}_1$

(9) $\underline{\alpha}_0, \bar{\alpha}_1, \bar{\alpha}_2, \bar{\beta}_0, \bar{\beta}_1$

(10) $\bar{\alpha}_0, \underline{\alpha}_1, \bar{\alpha}_2, \bar{\beta}_0, \bar{\beta}_1$

Special cases:

- If $\underline{\beta}_1 > 0$ we need only the corners (1),(2),(3),(4),(7),(8)
- If $\underline{\beta}_1 < 0, \bar{\beta}_1 > 0$ we need the corners (1),(2),(5),(6),(9),(10)
- If $\bar{\beta}_1 < 0$ we need the corners (1),(2),(5),(6),(7),(8)

In general we need $2 + (2 * 4) = 10$ corners.

For n=5:

$$f(z) = a_0 z^5 + a_1 z^4 + a_2 z^3 + a_3 z^2 + a_4 z + a_5, \quad a_0 > 0 \tag{5.10}$$

necessary conditions for stability

$$\begin{aligned} -5a_0 &< a_1 < 5a_0 \\ -2a_0 &< a_2 < 10a_0 \\ -10a_0 &< a_3 < 10a_0 \\ -3a_0 &< a_4 < 5a_0 \\ -a_0 &< a_5 < a_0 \end{aligned}$$

$$h'(\lambda) = \alpha_0 \left(\lambda^2 - \frac{\lambda}{2} - \frac{1}{4}\right) + \frac{\alpha_1}{2}\left(\lambda - \frac{1}{2}\right) + \frac{\alpha_2}{4} \tag{5.11}$$

$$g'(\lambda) = \beta_0 \left(\lambda^2 + \frac{\lambda}{2} - \frac{1}{4}\right) + \frac{\beta_1}{2}\left(\lambda + \frac{1}{2}\right) + \frac{\beta_2}{4} \tag{5.12}$$

necessary conditions for stability

$$\begin{aligned} 0 &< \alpha_0 < a_0 \\ -4a_0 &< \alpha_1 < 5a_0 \\ -6a_0 &< \alpha_2 < 10a_0 \\ -0 &< \beta_0 < a_0 \\ -5a_0 &< \beta_1 < 4a_0 \\ -6a_0 &< \beta_2 < 10a_0 \end{aligned}$$

From $h'(\lambda)$ and $g'(\lambda)$ we have the roots $\lambda = \pm 0.5, \pm 0.309, \pm 0.809$; i.e. we have 7 intervals. Fig. (9) shows the transition diagram where we have 3 transitions:

$(\bar{h}', \underline{g}'), (\bar{h}', \bar{g}'), (\underline{h}', \bar{g}')$.

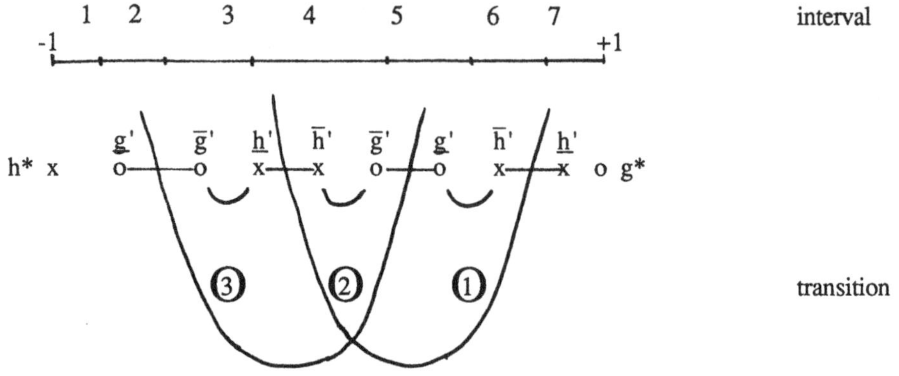

Fig. 9

For the left and for the right end we consider the corners corresponding to $(h^*, \underline{g}_1')$ and $(\underline{h}_7', g^*)$. Therefore for both ends only the corner given by $(\underline{h}_7', \underline{g}_1')$ has to be checked for stability. As we have three transitions and seven intervals we need to check 21 corners in addition. These are given by:

$$(\bar{h}_i', \underline{g}_i'),\ (\bar{h}_i', \bar{g}_i'),\ (\underline{h}_i', \bar{g}_i') \qquad \text{for } i= 1,2,\ldots\ldots,7$$

Therefore the necessary and sufficient condition for stability is the stability of the following corners:

$\underline{\alpha}_o, \underline{\alpha}_1, \underline{\alpha}_2, \underline{\beta}_o, \bar{\beta}'_1, \underline{\beta}_2$

$\bar{\alpha}_o, \underline{\alpha}_1, \bar{\alpha}_2, \beta_o, \bar{\beta}_1, \beta_2$

$\bar{\alpha}_o, \underline{\alpha}_1, \bar{\alpha}_2, \bar{\beta}_o, \bar{\beta}_1, \underline{\beta}_2$

$\bar{\alpha}_o, \underline{\alpha}_1, \bar{\alpha}_2, \bar{\beta}_o, \underline{\beta}_1, \underline{\beta}_2$

$\underline{\alpha}_o, \underline{\alpha}_1, \bar{\alpha}_2, \bar{\beta}_o, \underline{\beta}_1, \underline{\beta}_2$

$\underline{\alpha}_1, \underline{\alpha}_2, \bar{\alpha}_2, \underline{\beta}_o, \underline{\beta}_1, \underline{\beta}_2$

$\underline{\alpha}_o, \bar{\alpha}_1, \bar{\alpha}_2, \underline{\beta}_o, \underline{\beta}_1, \underline{\beta}_2$

$\bar{\alpha}_o, \bar{\alpha}_1, \bar{\alpha}_2, \underline{\beta}_o, \underline{\beta}_1, \underline{\beta}_2$

$\bar{\alpha}_o, \underline{\alpha}_1, \bar{\alpha}_2, \bar{\beta}_o, \underline{\beta}_1, \bar{\beta}_2$	$\underline{\alpha}_o, \bar{\alpha}_1, \underline{\alpha}_2, \bar{\beta}_o, \underline{\beta}_1, \bar{\beta}_2$
$\bar{\alpha}_o, \underline{\alpha}_1, \bar{\alpha}_2, \underline{\beta}_o, \underline{\beta}_1, \bar{\beta}_2$	$\underline{\alpha}_o, \bar{\alpha}_1, \underline{\alpha}_2, \underline{\beta}_o, \underline{\beta}_1, \bar{\beta}_2$
$\bar{\alpha}_o, \underline{\alpha}_1, \bar{\alpha}_2, \underline{\beta}_o, \bar{\beta}_1, \bar{\beta}_2$	$\underline{\alpha}_o, \bar{\alpha}_1, \underline{\alpha}_2, \underline{\beta}_o, \bar{\beta}_1, \bar{\beta}_2$
$\underline{\alpha}_o, \underline{\alpha}_1, \bar{\alpha}_2, \underline{\beta}_o, \bar{\beta}_1, \bar{\beta}_2$	$\bar{\alpha}_o, \bar{\alpha}_1, \underline{\alpha}_2, \underline{\beta}_o, \bar{\beta}_1, \bar{\beta}_2$
$\underline{\alpha}_1, \underline{\alpha}_2, \bar{\alpha}_2, \bar{\beta}_o, \bar{\beta}_1, \bar{\beta}_2$	$\bar{\alpha}_o, \bar{\alpha}_1, \underline{\alpha}_2, \bar{\beta}_o, \bar{\beta}_1, \bar{\beta}_2$
$\underline{\alpha}_o, \bar{\alpha}_1, \bar{\alpha}_2, \bar{\beta}_o, \bar{\beta}_1, \bar{\beta}_2$	$\bar{\alpha}_o, \underline{\alpha}_1, \underline{\alpha}_2, \bar{\beta}_o, \bar{\beta}_1, \bar{\beta}_2$
$\bar{\alpha}_o, \bar{\alpha}_1, \bar{\alpha}_2, \bar{\beta}_o, \bar{\beta}_1, \bar{\beta}_2$	$\underline{\alpha}_o, \underline{\alpha}_1, \underline{\alpha}_2, \bar{\beta}_o, \bar{\beta}_1, \bar{\beta}_2$

Total number of corners to be checked = $1 + (3 * 7) = 22$

For $n \geq 6$ the number of transitions is four and no end conditions are needed because they are included in the transitions. (3.1) with (3.2) and (3.3) give the number of intervals for n even and n odd. The number of corners to be checked is given by 4 * number of intervals. Fig. (5) shows the number of intervals as a function of n. Appendix 1 gives the corners to be checked for different n.

6. Stability of f(z) using Frequency domain Ideas

Analogously to the result in [7] one can derive the strong Kharitonov result for discrete systems using the frequency domain approach. We follow the argument in [6].

Substituting $z = e^{j\Theta}$ in (2.1) & (2.2) we get for n even ($n = 2\nu$)

$$h(e^{j\theta})=2e^{j\frac{n}{2}\theta}\left[\alpha_0\cos\nu\theta + \alpha_1\cos(\nu-1)\theta + ... + \alpha_{\nu-1}\cos\theta + \frac{1}{2}\alpha_\nu\right] \tag{6.1}$$

$$g(e^{j\theta})=2e^{j\frac{n}{2}\theta}\left[\beta_0\sin\nu\theta + \beta_1\sin(\nu-1)\theta + ... + \beta_{\nu-1}\sin\theta\right] \tag{6.2}$$

For n odd ($n = 2\nu - 1$) we get

$$h(e^{j\theta}) = 2e^{j\frac{n}{2}\theta}\left[\alpha_0\cos(\nu-0.5)\theta + \alpha_1\cos(\nu-1.5)\theta + ... + \alpha_{\nu-1}\cos\frac{\theta}{2}\right] \tag{6.3}$$

$$g(e^{j\theta}) = 2e^{j\frac{n}{2}\theta}\left[\beta_0\sin(\nu-0.5)\theta + \beta_1\sin(\nu-1.5)\theta + ... + \beta_{\nu-1}\sin\frac{\theta}{2}\right] \tag{6.4}$$

$$f(e^{j\Theta}) = 2e^{j\frac{n}{2}\Theta}\,[h^*(\Theta) + jg^*(\Theta)]$$

where $h^*(\Theta)$ and $g^*(\Theta)$ are the terms in brackets in equations (6.3) and (6.4). For a fixed value $\hat{\Theta}$ we get a rectangular box R* in the complex plane as shown in Fig. (10).

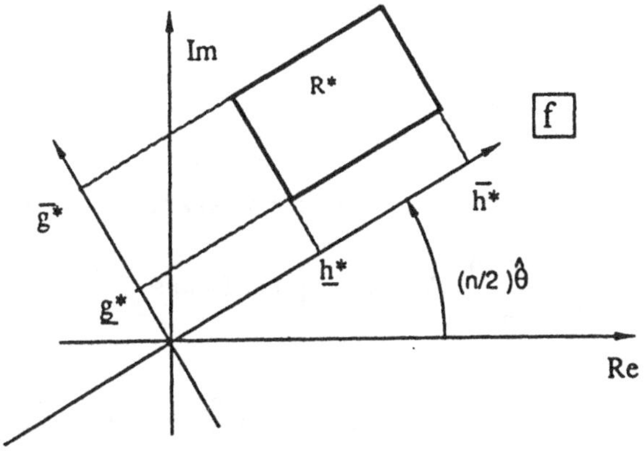

Fig. 10

With respect to a rotating coordinate frame the box is parallel to the axes. The corners of the box are:

$\bar{h}^*$ & $\underline{g}^*$ $\Rightarrow f_1$

$\bar{h}^*$ & $\bar{g}^*$ $\Rightarrow f_2$

$\underline{h}^*$ & $\bar{g}^*$ $\Rightarrow f_3$

$\underline{h}^*$ & $\underline{g}^*$ $\Rightarrow f_4$

Applying the Cremer-Leonhard-Michailow criterion, the function $f(e^{j\Theta})$ should have a change of argument of $n\pi$ for stability if Θ varies from 0 to π. For the function

$$f^*(e^{j\Theta}) = \frac{1}{2}e^{-j\frac{n}{2}\Theta}f(z) = h^*(\Theta) + j\,g^*(\Theta) \tag{6.5}$$

the change of argument reduces to $\frac{n}{2}\pi$. We therefore get a box parallel to the axes and we have the same situation as in the continuous case [7]. Therefore the stability conditions include only polynomials of the corner points of R*, i.e. dependent on $\bar{h}^*$, $\underline{h}^*$, $\bar{g}^*$, $\underline{g}^*$. These are in their turn dependent on Θ. The maxima and minima of h* and g* with respect to α_k and β_k depend on the sign of the cosine and sine terms in (6.3) and (6.4). The change of these signs determines the bounds of the intervals where the four corners of the box R* remain unchanged. Fig. (11) shows the Θ-intervals where $\bar{\alpha}_k$, $\bar{\beta}_k$ maximizes h* & g* respectively.

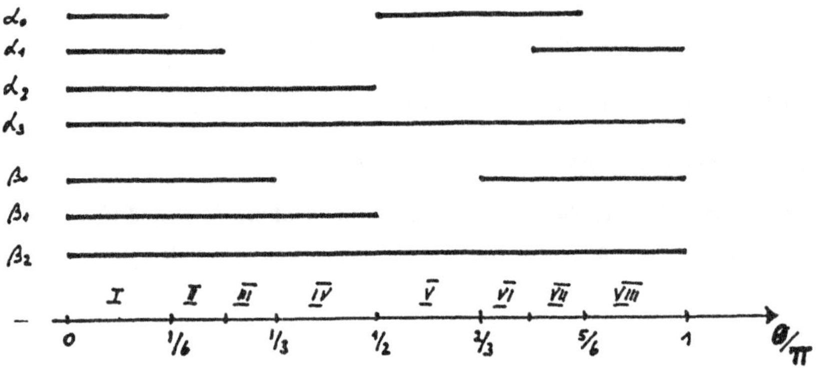

Fig. 11

A recursion formula for the number of intervals can be obtained as follows:

Let $\frac{n}{2} = p_1^{k_1} p_2^{k_2} \dots p_\eta^{k_\eta}$ for n even
$n = p_1^{k_1} p_2^{k_2} \dots p_\eta^{k_\eta}$ for n odd
where p_i are prime factors

Then $N_n = N_{n-2} + n - 1 - \Delta$ (6.6)

where n-1 is the number of new roots of $\cos\frac{n}{2}\Theta$ and $\sin\frac{n}{2}\Theta$ on $\Theta \in [0,\pi]$ and Δ is the number of different multiples of p_i which are already considered. For n=8 is for example $\Delta=3$. Using the formula (6.6) we get the following table for n even and n odd:

n	2	4	6	8	10	12	14	16	18	20
N_n	2	4	8	12	20	24	36	44	56	64

n	3	5	7	9	11	13	15	17	19	21
N_n	3	7	13	19	29	41	49	65	83	95

Using Euler functions the number of intervals for n odd is given by

$$\text{for } n \geq 3 \qquad N_n = 1 + \sum_{k=3,5,7,\dots} \phi(k) \tag{6.7}$$

$$\text{and for } n \geq 2 \qquad N_n = 1 + \sum_{k=4,8,12,\dots} \phi(k) + 2 \sum_{k=6,10,14,\dots} \phi(k) \tag{6.8}$$

For every interval one needs four corner polynomials. For $n \leq 6$ one needs less than four corner polynomials for every interval as shown before. It can be easily shown that the formulas for $h^*(\Theta)$ and $g^*(\Theta)$ give directly the Chebyshev and Jacobi polynomials obtained in section 2.

Conclusions

Necessary and sufficient conditions for the stability of discrete systems with parameters in a certain domain of the parameter space are derived. The result is the analog of Kharitonov's strong theorem. Two methods are used to arrive at this result, one by projecting the roots of the symmetric and the asymmetric part of the polynomial f(z) on the [-1, +1] line. The resulting Chebyshev and Jacobi polynomials give certain intervals on the [-1, +1] line. In each interval we need to check the four corner polynomials corresponding to Kharitonov's strong theorem for continuous systems. The number of intervals increases with n. The other method is the frequency domain method where the intervals are easily obtained through the roots of trigonometric functions. A recursion formula is derived and the number of intervals is shown to be a sum of Euler functions.

References

[1] F. Kraus, B.D.O. Anderson, and M. Mansour: Robust Schur Polynomial Stability and Kharitonov's Theorem. Proceedings of the IEEE Control and Decision Conference, Los Angeles (1987), pp. 2088 -2095

[2] V.L. Kharitonov: Asymptotic stability of an equilibrium position of a family of systems of linear differential equations. Differential Equations 14 (1979), pp. 1483 - 1485

[3] B.D.O. Anderson, E.I. Jury, and M. Mansour: On robust Hurwitz polynomials. IEEE Trans. Autom. Control, AC-32 (1987), pp.

[4] M. Mansour: Instability Criteria of Linear Discrete Systems. Automatica, 2 (1965), pp. 167 - 178

[5] M. Mansour and F. Kraus: On Robust Stability of Schur Polynomials. Report No. 87-05, Institut für Automatik und Industrielle Elektronik, ETH Zürich, Switzerland

[6] F. Kraus and M. Mansour: Robuste Stabilität im Frequenzgang, Report No 87-06, Institut für Automatik und Industrielle Elektronik, ETH Zürich, Switzerland

[7] R. J. Minnichelli, J. J. Anagnost and C. A. Desoer: An Elementary Proof of Kharitonov's Stability Theorem with Extensions. Memorandom No. UCB/ERL M87/78, Berkeley, 1987

[8] M. Abramowitz, I. A. Stegun: Handbook of mathematical functions, Dover

Appendix 1

Corners to be checked for different n

here (-) denotes minimum, (+) denotes maximum and (±) denotes maximum or minimum.

n = 2	α_0:	- -
	α_1:	+ -
	β_0:	± ±
n = 3	α_0:	- - - +
	α_1:	- + + +
	β_0:	- + - -
	β_1:	+ - - -

n = 4	α_o:	- - + - - + + - - +
	α_1:	+ - - - + + - - + +
	α_2:	- - + + + + + + + +
	β_o:	± ± + + - - - - + +
	β_1:	± ± - - - - + + + +
n = 5	α_o:	- - - - + + + - + + + - - - + + + + - - - +
	α_1:	- + + + + + - - - - - - - + + - - - - - + +
	α_2:	- - - - - - - - + + + + + + + + + + + + + +
	β_o:	- + - - - + + + - + + + - - - + - - - + + +
	β_1:	+ - - + + + + + + + - - - - - - - + + + + +
	β_2:	- + + + + + + + - - - - - - - + + + + + + +

For $n \geq 6$ all the 4 combinations $(\bar{h}',\bar{g}')$, $(\bar{h}',\underline{g}')$, $(\underline{h}',\bar{g}')$ and $(\underline{h}',\underline{g}')$ are considered . Here $\bar{h}'$ and $\bar{g}'$ are given. $\underline{h}'$ and $\underline{g}'$ are their inverse i.e. (+) and (-) are interchanged.

n = 6 $\bar{h}'$
- + + + - - - +
+ + - - - - + +
- - - - + + + +
+ + + + + + + +

$\bar{g}'$
+ + + - - + + +
- - - - + + + +
+ + + + + + + +

n = 7 $\bar{h}'$
- - - + + + + - - - - - +
+ + + + + - - - - - - + +
- - - - - - - - - + + + +
+ + + + + + + + + + + + +

$\bar{g}'$
- + + + + + - - - - + + +
+ + - - - - - - + + + + +
- - - - + + + + + + + + +
+ + + + + + + + + + + + +

n = 8 $\bar{h}'$
+ - - - - + + - - - - +
- - + + + + - - - - + +
+ + + - - - - - - + + +
- - - - - - + + + + + +
+ + + + + + + + + + + +

$\bar{g}'$
- - - + + + - - - + + +
+ + + + - - - - + + + +
- - - - - - + + + + + +
+ + + + + + + + + + + +

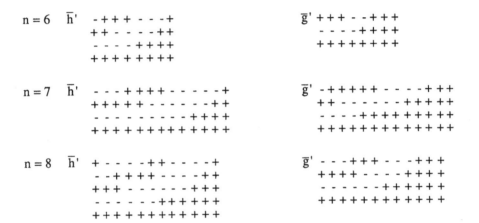

POLYTOPES OF POLYNOMIALS WITH ZEROS IN A PRESCRIBED REGION: NEW CRITERIA AND ALGORITHMS

Minyue Fu

Department of Electrical and Computer Engineering
Wayne State University
Detroit, Michigan 48202

Abstract. This paper is concerned with the robust stability problem of families of polynomials. Our main focus is on a general polytope of polynomials described by

$$\mathcal{P}^\varepsilon \doteq \{p(s,\mathbf{q}) = p_0(s) + \sum_{i=0}^{n} a_i(\mathbf{q})s^i : \mathbf{q} \in \varepsilon Q \subset \mathbf{R}^m\}$$

where $p_0(s)$ is the nominal polynomial of n-th order, $\mathbf{q} = [q_1, q_2, \cdots, q_m]'$ is a vector of perturbation parameters, $a_i(\mathbf{q})$ are linear functions of $\mathbf{q}$, Q is a prescribed polytope in $\mathbf{R}^m$ containing the origin, and $\varepsilon \geq 0$ is a parameter which controls the size of Q. Given an open set D in the complex plane, our objective is to provide simple methods for determining the maximal ε, call it $\varepsilon_{\max}$, such that $\mathcal{P}^\varepsilon$ is D-stable (i.e., every polynomial in $\mathcal{P}^\varepsilon$ has all zeros interior to D) for all $\varepsilon < \varepsilon_{\max}$. This maximal size can be compared against any given *varepsilon*, the size of $\mathcal{P}^\varepsilon$, to obtain the so-called *robustness measure* of $\mathcal{P}^\varepsilon$. Our first result provides a closed-form description of $\varepsilon_{\max}$ using a "zero exclusion approach". Then we give a simple computing algorithm for calculating $\varepsilon_{\max}$ which works effectively when the number of vertices of the $\mathcal{P}^\varepsilon$ is not too large. Our special attention then is paid to an important class of polytopes, called parallelotopes, of polynomials for which the set Q is a hyper-rectangle in $\mathbf{R}^m$. For a parallelotope of polynomials, a highly efficient algorithm is proposed. The computation is further reduced for the Hurwitz stability of a special polytope of polynomials which has a Kharitonov-like structure. Finally, extension of our main results is made to solving nonlinear coefficient perturbation problems, and some sufficient conditions are obtained.

The methods we develop in this paper have several other advantages. Namely, the polytope of polynomials is allowed to contain polynomials with different orders; the assumptions on the set D are rather weak; the polynomials can be complex; and some technical tools developed here may be suggestive to handling nonlinear coefficient perturbation problems. The results in the paper can also be readily extended to time-delay systems and multivariate polynomials.

1 INTRODUCTION

Robust stability of a control system has become a great interest of control researchers and engineers in recent years. The general problem can be motivated by considering the characteristic polynomial (real or complex) of a linear system with uncertain parameters

$$p(s,\mathbf{q}) = p_0(s) + \sum_{i=0}^{n} a_i(\mathbf{q})s^i$$

where $p_0(s)$ is the *nominal characteristic polynomial* of n-th order, $\mathbf{q} = [r_1, r_2, \cdots, q_m]'$ is a set of *perturbation parameters* which belongs to some prescribed region $Q \subset \mathbf{R}^m$ containing the origin, and the coefficients $a_i(\cdot)$ are linear or nonlinear functions of $\mathbf{q}$ with $a_i(0) = 0$. The objective is to determine the robust stability of $p(s,\mathbf{q})$ for all admissible $\mathbf{q} \in Q$; i.e., to check the robust stability of the family of polynomials

$$\mathcal{P} \doteq \{p_0(s) + \sum_{i=0}^{n} a_i(\mathbf{q})s^i : \mathbf{q} \in Q\}. \tag{1.1}$$

The first important result on this problem was given by Kharitonov [1] which shows that an interval polynomial $\mathcal{P}_I$ (a family of polynomials with each coefficient lying in an interval) is Hurwitz stable (i.e., the roots of every member of $\mathcal{P}_I$ stay in the open left half plane) if and only if four specially chosen vertex polynomials of $\mathcal{P}_I$ are Hurwitz stable. This result was later extended by Kharitonov [2] to complex interval polynomials (where each coefficient lies in a rectangle in the complex plane) and eight vertices are shown to be necessary and sufficient. Kharitonov's Theorems, however, are limited by the assumptions that the coefficients of the polynomials are independent and that the stability region is restricted to the open left half plane. A considerable body of research has been made to relax these assumptions so that more general robust stability problems can be handled; see [3]–[25] and their bibliographies. An important breakthrough was made by Bartlett, Hollot and Lin [4] where a polytope of polynomials (see Section 2 for definition) and a general stability region were considered. The polytopic structure of $\mathcal{P}$ can be motivated by assuming that the polynomial coefficients $a_j(\cdot)$ are linear functions of $\mathbf{q}$ and that each perturbation parameter r_i lies in a bounded interval given by $[\underline{q}_i, \bar{q}_i]$ with $\underline{q}_i < 0$ and $\bar{q}_i > 0$; i.e., Q is a hyper-rectangle. Consequently, $\mathcal{P}$ becomes

$$\mathcal{P}_L \doteq \{p_0(s) + \sum_{i=1}^{m} q_i \delta p_i(s) : q_i \in [\underline{q}_i, \bar{q}_i], i = 1, 2, \cdots, m\} \tag{1.2}$$

where for every $i = 1, 2, \cdots, m$, $\delta p_i(s)$ is obtained from $p(s,\mathbf{q}) - p_0(s)$ by setting $q_i = 1$ and $q_j = 0$ for all $j \neq i$. We call $\delta p_i(s)$ the *perturbation polynomials.* Note that $\mathcal{P}_L$ is a polytope of polynomials. If $\delta p_i(s)$ are linearly independent, then this polytope is called a *parallelotope* [26]. In particular, $\mathcal{P}_L$ is a line segment if $m = 1$, or a parallelogram if $m = 2$. If $m = 3$, then $\mathcal{P}_L$ becomes a parallelepiped. Also note that an interval polynomial is a special parallelotope of polynomials. There seems no standard mathematical terminology for a degenerate parallelotope for which $\delta p_i(s)$ are linearly dependent. For notational convenience, we also call this class of polytopes parallelotopes although it may be an abuse of terminology. General polytopes of polynomials can be obtained by considering the situation when the uncertain parameters $\mathbf{q}$ lie in a polytope in $\mathbf{R}^m$.

It was shown in Bartlett, Hollot and Lin [4] that a polytope of n-th order real polynomials $\mathcal{P}$ (i.e., every member of $\mathcal{P}$ is n-th order) is so-called D-stable (i.e., the roots of every member of $\mathcal{P}$ stay in D) for a simply connected set D in the complex plane if and only if all the edges of $\mathcal{P}$ are D-stable. This result, often referred to as the Edge Theorem, allows linear dependence of the polynomial coefficients and D regions other than the open left half plane. In particular, it applies to the stability of discrete-time systems where the set D is the open unit disk. Since the requirement of simple connectedness on D may not hold in many applications (for example, dominant pole assignment), Fu and Barmish [5] extended this Edge Theorem to include disconnected D sets. Further generalization of the results in [4] and [5] is made by Fu, Olbrot and Polis [18] to handle robust stability problem of time-delay systems: similar Edge Theorem for the D-stability of a polytope of quasipolynomials was established and graphical tests were given for checking the edges. For the special case where D is the open left plane and the polytope consists of linear combinations of interval polynomials, Chapellat and Bhattacharyya [17] showed that the number of edges of $\mathcal{P}$ necessary to check can be reduced.

Although the Edge results provide good computational reduction, it should be noted that the number of possible edges of a polytope may increase dramatically with respect to the number of vertices. This phenomenon is referred to as the "combinatoric explosion" [7]. Another problem associated with Edge results is that they are not reducible to the Kharitonov's results when $\mathcal{P}$ becomes an interval polynomial and D, the open left half plane. To overcome these weaknesses, Barmish [7] developed a new method using a zero exclusion approach. Consequently, a robust stability testing function $H(d)$ was generated for every $d \in \partial D$ and it was shown that the D-stability of $\mathcal{P}$ can be verified by checking the positivity of $H(d)$ for all $d \in \partial D$ (the boundary of D). The construction of this testing function is roughly as follows: First, an auxiliary path $\partial\Gamma$ in the complex plane is selected which encircles the origin. Then, for every $d \in \partial D$ and $\gamma \in \partial\Gamma$, a function $h(d,\gamma)$ is created using all the vertices of $\mathcal{P}$. Finally, $H(d)$ is calculated by maximizing $h(d,\gamma)$ over all γ on the auxiliary path. Compared with the Edge Theorems, this approach greatly reduces the computation when the number of vertices is large. Furthermore, for the special case when $\mathcal{P}$ is an interval polynomial and D is the open left half plane, "the Kharitonov polynomials 'fall out' immediately" from $H(d)$ [7]. The results of [7] have also been extended by Barmish and Khargonekar [8] to include unmodelled dynamics.

In many application examples, we may not only be interested in determining the robust stability of a family of polynomials with a fixed size, but also want to know the "maximal bound" of the coefficient perturbations for which the D-stability is preserved. In other words, given a polytope of polynomials

$$\mathcal{P}^{\varepsilon} \doteq \{p_0(s) + \sum_{i=0}^{n} a_i(\mathbf{q})s^i : \mathbf{q} \in \varepsilon Q\} \tag{1.3}$$

where $\varepsilon \geq 0$ is used to control the size of the polytope of polynomials, we want to determine the maximal ε, call it $\varepsilon_{\max}$, for which $\mathcal{P}^{\varepsilon}$ is D-stable for all $\varepsilon < \varepsilon_{\max}$. Such a maximal bound will be called the *maximal D-stability bound.* Note that if Q is a hyper-rectangle, i.e., if $\underline{q}_i \leq q_i \leq \bar{q}_i, i = 1,2,\cdots,m$, then $\mathcal{P}^\varepsilon$ becomes a parallelotope of polynomials

$$\mathcal{P}_L^\varepsilon \doteq \{p_0(s) + \sum_{i=1}^{m} q_i\delta p_i(s) : q_i \in [\varepsilon\underline{q}_i, \varepsilon\bar{q}_i], i = 1,2,\cdots,m\}. \tag{1.4}$$

In Barmish [19] and Bialas and Garloff [20], Khartionov's Theorem [1] was used to obtain the maximal Hurwitz stability bound for an interval polynomial by an iterative process. The closed form representation of this maximal Hurwitz stability bound was obtained recently by Fu and Barmish [24]. In Soh, Berger and Baker [21], L_2-norm was used for measuring perturbations, and maximal stability bounds were obtained for both continuous-time and discrete-time systems. The calculations of these bounds were simplified by Chapellat and Bhattacharyya [23] and Fu [22]. However, the coefficient perturbations of the polynomial have to be independent in the papers cited above. For linearly dependent coefficient perturbations, Fu and Barmish [24] provided a method for calculating the maximal stability bounds when there is only one perturbation parameter. This method, however, is not extendable to multi-parameter perturbation problems, and the stability region is restricted to the open left half plane (or open unit disk using bilinear transformation). For a polytope of polynomials and a general D set, $\varepsilon_{\max}$ can certainly be solved by iteratively applying the Edge Theorems or the test in [7] on $\mathcal{P}^\varepsilon$ for different values of ε until the minimal ε is found for which $\mathcal{P}^\varepsilon$ is no longer D-stable. This, however, introduces an additional dimension of searching.

The main objective of this paper is to provide simple criteria and computing algorithms for calculating the maximal D-stability bound $\varepsilon_{\max}$ for a polytope of polynomials $\mathcal{P}^\varepsilon$ as in (1.3). A fundamental idea in this paper is inspired by the work of Barmish [7] where a zero exclusion approach is used for determining the D-stability of a polytope of polynomials. Given a family of polynomials $\mathcal{P}$ with a nominal polynomial $p_0(s)$ and an open set D in the complex plane, we consider

$$\delta\mathcal{P} \doteq \{p(s) - p_0(s) : p(s) \in \mathcal{P}\}$$

and use the "normalized" value set

$$V(\delta\mathcal{P}, d) \doteq \{\delta p(d)/p_0(d) : \delta p(s) \in \delta\mathcal{P}\}$$

for various $d \in \partial D$ to determine the D-stability of $\mathcal{P}$. Its formal description will be given in Theorem 3.1. This result, which will be called the Boundary Theorem, basically claims that $\mathcal{P}$ is D-stable if and only if $-1 \notin V(\delta\mathcal{P}, d)$ for all $d \in \partial D$, provided that the nominal polynomial $p_0(s)$ is D-stable.

By applying the Boundary Theorem to $\mathcal{P}^\varepsilon$, we obtained our first main result — Minimum Intersection Theorem. This theorem gives a simple closed form description of $\varepsilon_{\max}$ in terms of the minimum intersection of $V(\delta\mathcal{P}, d)$ with the real axis for all $d \in \partial D$, where $\delta\mathcal{P}$ is the shorthand for $\delta\mathcal{P}^\varepsilon, \varepsilon = 1$. Using the fact that $V(\delta\mathcal{P}, d)$ is a convex polygon in the complex plane, its minimum intersection with the real axis must happen on either a vertex or an edge. The problem now boils down to determining the vertices and edges of $V(\delta\mathcal{P}, d)$. We then obtained a simple algorithm for calculating the minimum intersection which works effectively when the number of vertices of $V(\delta\mathcal{P}, d)$ is not too large. For a parallelotope of polynomials $\mathcal{P}_L^\varepsilon$ as in (1.4), we found surprisingly that $V(\delta\mathcal{P}_L, d)$ has at most $2m$ vertices and thus $2m$ edges![1] Based on this discovery, another computing algorithm was established. It turns out that this algorithm needs to construct at most $[(m+3)/2]$ of these $2m$ vertices for determining the minimum intersection value mentioned above. To illustrate the simplicity, let us consider the case when $\mathcal{P}^L$ has 10 perturbation parameters, i.e., $m = 10$. The Edge Theorems need to check 5120 edges and the Method in Barmish [7] needs to use 1024 vertices and an auxiliary path at each $d \in \partial D$.[2] Using our method, however, at most 6 vertices of $V(\delta\mathcal{P}_L, d)$ need to be constructed at each $d \in \partial D$.

Once the maximal robust stability bound $\varepsilon_{\max}$ is found, the *robustness measure* of $\mathcal{P}^\varepsilon$ for any given *varepsilon* can be defined as $1 - \varepsilon/\varepsilon_{\max}$ or as $20\log(\varepsilon_{\max}/\varepsilon)$ in dB. This robustness measure serves as an indication of how robust stable $\mathcal{P}^\varepsilon$ is in a relative sense and it can be used as a design consideration of a robust controller.

We then consider the Hurwitz stability of the following special polytope of polynomials

$$\mathcal{P}_S \doteq \{p(s) = \sum_{i=1}^{\ell} p_i(s) f_i(s) : p_i(s) \in \mathcal{P}_i, i = 1, 2, \cdots, \ell\} \tag{1.5}$$

where $f_i(s)$ are fixed polynomials and $\mathcal{P}_i$ are interval polynomials of n-th order; see Section 5 and [23] for motivations of this class of perturbations. Using the Kharitonov's polynomials of every $\mathcal{P}_i$, we show that the number of vertices of $V(\mathcal{P}_S, d)$ needed to check can be reduced to at most $[(2\ell+3)/2]$ although $\mathcal{P}_S$ may have up to $2^{(n+1)\ell}$ vertices and many more edges.

Stimulated by the effectiveness of the Minimum Intersection Theorem in solving the D-stability of polytopes of polynomials, we extend this result to general families of polynomials. A sufficient condition is given which converts the D-stability problem to a nonlinear minimization problem. This sufficient condition is also necessary for a class of families of polynomials. Two interesting corollaries of the sufficient condition are provided, and one of them turns out to be a well known fact which shows that the Hurwitz stability (or Schur stability) of a nominal polynomial $p_0(s)$ carries over to $p_0(s) + \delta p(s)$ if the H_∞ norm of $\delta p(s)/p_0(s)$ is less than the unity.

Some other generalities of the results in this paper are also worth of mentioning. Namely, the members in a family of polynomials can have different orders, the assumptions on the set D are rather week, and the polynomials are allowed to be complex. Furthermore, the results can be extended to time-delay systems and multivariate polynomials.

This paper is organized as follows: Section 2 to follow gives notation, definitions and assumptions. Section 3 provides two preliminary results: Boundary Theorem and a result on vertex reduction. Section 4 establishes the main results: Minimum Intersection Theorem and the associated computing algorithms for the robust stability of

[1] This fact has also been pointed out in a recent paper by Djaferis and Hollot [25] in a slightly different way but we provide a simple analytic form for the vertices and edges.

[2] It can be shown that an m-parameter parallelotope has at most 2^m vertices and $m2^{m-1}$ edges.

general polytopes and parallelotopes of polynomials. Section 5 is focused on the Hurwitz stability of the parallelotopes of polynomials in the form of (1.5). Extension of the Minimum Intersection Theorem is made in Section 7 to general families of polynomials. A numerical example is shown in Section 8 and the conclusion is drawn in Section 9. Appendix A gives the proof of Theorem 3.3.

2 NOTATION, DEFINITIONS, AND ASSUMPTIONS

Given a set X in the complex plane $\mathcal{C}$, we use ∂X and X^c to denote the boundary and the complement of X, respectively. The integer part of a non-negative real number a is denoted by $[a]$.

Let $\mathcal{P}$ be a family of polynomials with real or complex coefficients and $p_0(s)$ be a *nominal polynomial* in $\mathcal{P}$, we define *a family of perturbation polynomials*

$$\delta\mathcal{P} \doteq \{\delta p(s) = p(s) - p_0(s) : p(s) \in \mathcal{P}\}. \tag{2.1}$$

If $\mathcal{P}$ is a polytope of polynomials and $p^i(s), i = 1, 2, \cdots, r$ are its vertices, then $\mathcal{P}$ is the collection of all convex combinations of $p^i(s)$, i.e.,

$$\mathcal{P} = \text{conv}\{p^1(s), p^2(s), \cdots, p^r(s)\}. \tag{2.2}$$

Given any $d \in \mathcal{C}$ such that $p_0(d) \neq 0$, we define the value set

$$V(\delta\mathcal{P}, d) \doteq \{\delta p(d)/p_0(d) : \delta p(s) \in \delta\mathcal{P}\}. \tag{2.3}$$

Note that if $\mathcal{P}$ is a polytope of polynomials given as above, then $V(\delta\mathcal{P}, d)$ is a convex polygon in the complex plane and it is given by

$$V(\delta\mathcal{P}, d) = \text{conv}\{\rho^1(d), \rho^2(d), \cdots, \rho^r(d)\} \tag{2.4}$$

where

$$\rho^i(s) \doteq (p^i(s) - p_0(s))/p_0(s). \tag{2.5}$$

That is, the set of vertices of $V(\delta\mathcal{P}, d)$ is either $\{\rho^1(d), \rho^2(d), \cdots, \rho^r(d)\}$ or a subset of it. For a parallelotope of polynomials $\mathcal{P}_L$ as in (1.2), we have

$$V(\delta\mathcal{P}_L, d) = \{\sum_{i=1}^{m} q_i\rho_i(d) : q_i \in [\underline{q}_i, \bar{q}_i], i = 1, 2, \cdots, m\} \tag{2.6}$$

where

$$\rho_i(s) \doteq \delta p_i(s)/p_0(s). \tag{2.7}$$

A family of polynomials $\mathcal{P}_I$ is called a (real) *interval polynomial* if

$$\mathcal{P}_I \doteq \{p(s) = a_0 + a_1 s + a_2 s^2 + \cdots + a_n s^n : a_i \in [\alpha_i, \beta_i], i = 0, 1, \cdots, n\} \tag{2.8}$$

for some non-negative integer n and some $\alpha_i, \beta_i \in \mathbf{R}, i = 0, 1, \cdots, n$. The four Kharitonov polynomials of $\mathcal{P}_I$ are given by

$$\begin{aligned} p^1(s) &\doteq h_1(s^2) + s g_1(s^2); \\ p^2(s) &\doteq h_2(s^2) + s g_1(s^2); \\ p^3(s) &\doteq h_2(s^2) + s g_2(s^2); \\ p^4(s) &\doteq h_1(s^2) + s g_2(s^2) \end{aligned} \tag{2.9}$$

where

$$\begin{aligned} h_1(s) &\doteq \alpha_0 + \beta_2 s^2 + \alpha_4 s^4 + \beta_6 s^6 + \cdots; \\ h_2(s) &\doteq \beta_0 + \alpha_2 s^2 + \beta_4 s^4 + \alpha_6 s^6 + \cdots; \\ g_1(s) &\doteq \alpha_1 s + \beta_3 s^3 + \alpha_5 s^5 + \beta_7 s^7 + \cdots; \\ g_2(s) &\doteq \beta_1 s + \alpha_3 s^3 + \beta_5 s^5 + \alpha_7 s^7 + \cdots \end{aligned} \tag{2.10}$$

It is straightforward to verify that [7], for every $\omega \geq 0$,

$$\{p(j\omega) : p(s) \in \mathcal{P}_I\} = \text{conv}\{p^1(j\omega), p^2(j\omega), p^3(j\omega), p^4(j\omega)\}. \tag{2.11}$$

Defining the nominal polynomial

$$p_0(s) \doteq (p^1(s) + p^2(s) + p^3(s) + p^4(s))/4, \tag{2.12}$$

and the perturbation polynomials

$$\begin{aligned} \delta p_1(s) &\doteq (h_2(s) - h_1(s))/2; \\ \delta p_2(s) &\doteq (g_2(s) - g_1(s))/2. \end{aligned} \tag{2.13}$$

Then, we have

$$V(\delta\mathcal{P}_I, j\omega) = \{q_1\rho_1(j\omega) + q_2\rho_2(j\omega) : q_1, q_2 \in [-1, 1]\} \tag{2.14}$$

where $\rho_1(s)$ and $\rho_2(s)$ are given by (2.7).

Definition 2.1 Given a region $D \subset \mathcal{C}$, a polynomial $p(s)$ is called *D-stable* if $p(d) \neq 0$ for all $d \in D^c$. In particular, if D is the open left half plane (resp. open unit disk) and $p(s)$ is D-stable, then $p(s)$ is called *strictly Hurwitz* or *Hurwitz stable* (resp. *strictly Schur* or *Schur stable*). A family of polynomials $\mathcal{P}$ is called *D-stable* if every member of $\mathcal{P}$ is D-stable.

The following assumptions are required for the results in this paper:

Assumption 2.2 D is an open set, D^c is nonempty, and ∂D is the union of a finite number of continuous paths in the complex plane.

Assumption 2.3 The nominal polynomial $p_0(s) \in \mathcal{P}$ is D-stable.

3 PRELIMINARY RESULTS: BOUNDARY THEOREM AND VERTEX REDUCTION

In this section, we provide two important preliminary theorems. The first one, called Boundary Theorem, claims that the D-stability of a family of polynomials can be verified by using all $V(\delta\mathcal{P}, d), d \in \partial D$. Several forms similar to this theorem have appeared in the literature; see Fam and Meditch [12], Fu and Barmish [13], Argoun [14], Hertz, Jury and Zeheb [16], Gaston and Safonov [15], and Barmish [7]. However, our theorem requires rather weak assumptions, and a simple proof of the theorem is provided. The second theorem, Theorem 3.3, shows that the number of possible vertices of $V(\delta\mathcal{P}_L, d)$ corresponding to a parallelotope of polynomials $\mathcal{P}_L^\epsilon$ as in (1.4) can be dramatically reduced from 2^m to $2m$. Thus, significant computational reduction can be achieved. The proof of Theorem 3.3 is given in Appendix A.

Theorem 3.1 (Boundary Theorem) *Consider a family of polynomials $\mathcal{P}$ and a region $D \subset C$ satisfying Assumptions 2.2-2.3. Suppose $\mathcal{P}$ is connected. Then, $\mathcal{P}$ is D-stable if and only if $-1 \notin V(\delta\mathcal{P}, d)$ for all $d \in \partial D$.*

Proof: The necessity is self-evident because $\partial D \subset D^c$. Consequently, $\mathcal{P}$ is D-stable implies that $p(d) \neq 0$ or $(p(d) - p_0(d))/p_0(d) \neq -1$ for all $p(s) \in \mathcal{P}$ for all $d \in \partial D$, i.e., $-1 \notin V(\delta\mathcal{P}, d)$. In order to establish the sufficiency, we first define, for any polynomial $p(s)$ and any set $X \subset C$,

$$M(p, X) \doteq \{p(x) : x \in X\}.$$

Using this definition, a polynomial $p(s)$ is D-stable if and only if $0 \notin M(p, D^c)$. Therefore, $p_0(s)$ being D-stable implies that $0 \notin M(p_0, D^c)$. Suppose, on the contrary, that there exists some $p_1(s) \in \mathcal{P}$ such that $p_1(s)$ is not D-stable, i.e., $0 \in M(p_1, D^c)$. We need to show that there exists $d \in D^c$ such that $-1 \in V(\delta\mathcal{P}, d)$, or equivalently, to show there exists some $p_\lambda(s) \in \mathcal{P}$ such that $0 \in M(p_\lambda, \partial D)$. Indeed, let

$$\Gamma \doteq \{\gamma(t) : t \in [0, 1]\}$$

with $\gamma(0) = p_0(s)$ and $\gamma(1) = p_1(s)$ be any continuous path in $\mathcal{P}$ connecting $p_0(s)$ and $p_1(s)$. For every $p_t(s) \in \Gamma$, we define a "distance function"

$$d(p_t) \doteq \begin{cases} \min\{|m| : m \in M(p_t, D^c)\} & \text{if } 0 \notin M(p_t, D^c) \\ -\min\{|m| : m \in M(p_t, D^c)\} & \text{if } 0 \in M(p_t, D^c) \end{cases}$$

Note that $d(p_t) = 0$ if and only if $0 \in \partial M(p_t, D^c)$. Using the continuity of Γ and the minimum function with respect to t, we know that $d(\cdot)$ is a continuous function on Γ. Since $d(p_0) > 0$ and $d(p_1) \leq 0$, we conclude that there must exist at least one $t \in (0, 1]$ such that $d(p_t) = 0$. Let

$$\lambda \doteq \min\{t : d(p_t) = 0; t \in (0, 1]\}.$$

It follows that $0 \in \partial M(p_\lambda, D^c)$. Since the mapping $M(p_\lambda, \cdot) : \mathcal{C} \to \mathcal{C}$ is a linear mapping, we claim that there must exist some $d \in \partial D$ such that $p_\lambda(d) = 0$. Indeed, if the mapping is one to one, then the image of any point on $\partial M(p_\lambda, D^c)$ must be on the boundary of D^c (i.e., ∂D) and we are done. If the kernel of the mapping is at least one-dimensional, then the kernel must intersect ∂D and again, our claim holds. Therefore, $0 \in M(p_\lambda, \partial D)$. □

Remark 3.2 If $\mathcal{P}$ consists of only real polynomials and D is symmetric with respect to the real axis, then the points on ∂D with negative imaginary parts are not necessary to check. In other words, ∂D in the Boundary Theorem can be reduced to

$$\partial D_+ \doteq \{d : d \in \partial D, \mathrm{Im}(d) \geq 0\}.$$

This simplification is also applicable to other results in this paper.

Theorem 3.3 *Consider a convex polygon $V \subset \mathcal{C}$ given by*

$$V \doteq \{\sum_{i=1}^{m} q_i \rho_i : q_i \in [\underline{q}_i, \bar{q}_i]\} \tag{3.1}$$

where $\rho_i \in \mathcal{C}$ are nonzero numbers satisfying

$$0 \leq \angle(\rho_1) \leq \angle(\rho_2) \leq \cdots \leq \angle(\rho_m) < 180°, \tag{3.2}$$

$\underline{q}_i < 0$ and $\bar{q}_i > 0$ for all $i = 1, 2, \cdots, m$. Then, V has at most $2m$ vertices which are given by

$$\begin{aligned}
v_1 &= \underline{q}_1\rho_1 + \underline{q}_2\rho_2 + \cdots + \underline{q}_m\rho_m \\
v_2 &= \underline{q}_1\rho_1 + \underline{q}_2\rho_2 + \cdots + \underline{q}_{m-1}\rho_{m-1} + \bar{q}_m\rho_m \\
v_3 &= \underline{q}_1\rho_1 + \underline{q}_2\rho_2 + \cdots + \underline{q}_{m-2}\rho_{m-2} + \bar{q}_{m-1}\rho_{m-1} + \bar{q}_m\rho_m \\
&\cdots\cdots \\
v_m &= \underline{q}_1\rho_1 + \bar{q}_2\rho_2 + \cdots + \bar{q}_m\rho_m \\
v_{m+1} &= \bar{q}_1\rho_1 + \bar{q}_2\rho_2 + \cdots + +\bar{q}_m\rho_m \\
v_{m+2} &= \bar{q}_1\rho_1 + \bar{q}_2\rho_2 + \cdots + +\bar{q}_{m-1}\rho_{m-1} + \underline{q}_m\rho_m \\
v_{m+3} &= \bar{q}_1\rho_1 + \bar{q}_2\rho_2 + \cdots + \bar{q}_{m-2}\rho_{m-2} + \underline{q}_{m-1}\rho_{m-1} + \underline{q}_m\rho_m \\
&\cdots\cdots \\
v_{2m} &= \bar{q}_1\rho_1 + \underline{q}_2\rho_2 + \cdots + \underline{q}_m\rho_m
\end{aligned} \tag{3.3}$$

and at most $2m$ edges, which are given by $\mathrm{conv}\{v_i, v_{i+1}\}$, *$i = 1, 2, \cdots, 2m-1$, and* $\mathrm{conv}\{v_{2m}, v_1\}$. *Furthermore, $\angle(v_1) \leq 0$, $\angle(v_{m+1}) \geq 0$, and v_1, $v_2, \cdots, v_{2m}, v_1$ traverse in the clockwise direction.*

Example 3.4: To demonstrate the results in Theorem 3.3, the vertices and edges of the following example is given in Figure 1:

$$V \doteq \{q_1(1+j0) + q_2(1+j) + q_3(-1+j) + q_4(-2+j) : q_i \in [-1,1], i = 1,2,3,4\}.$$

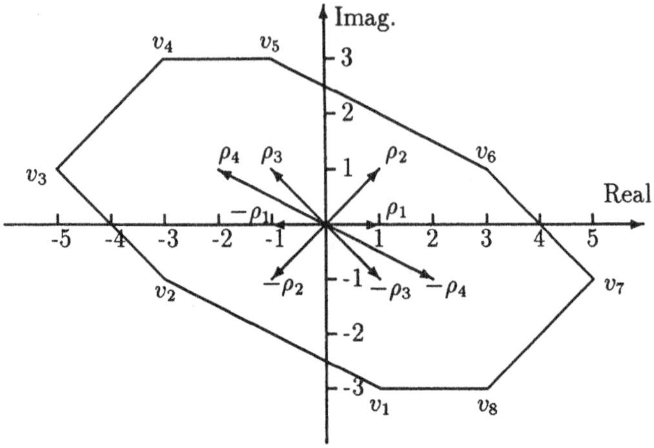

Figure 1. The Convex Polygon of V in Example 3.4

4 MINIMUM INTERSECTION THEOREM AND COMPUTING ALGORITHMS

In this section, the main results of this paper are presented.

Consider a polytope of polynomials $\mathcal{P}^\varepsilon$ as in (1.3) and a given set $D \subset \mathcal{C}$, our purpose is to determine the maximal ε, $\varepsilon_{\max}$, such that $\mathcal{P}^\varepsilon$ is D-stable for all $0 < \varepsilon < \varepsilon_{\max}$.

Suppose Assumptions 2.2- 2.3 are satisfied. Using Theorem 3.1, we know that $\mathcal{P}^\varepsilon$ is D-stable if and only if $-1 \notin V(\delta\mathcal{P}^\varepsilon, d)$, or, equivalently, $-1/\varepsilon \notin V(\delta\mathcal{P}, d)$, where $\delta\mathcal{P}$ is the shorthand for $\delta\mathcal{P}^\varepsilon, \varepsilon = 1$. That is, $\mathcal{P}^\varepsilon$ is D-stable if and only if for every $d \in \partial D$, the minimum intersection of $V(\delta\mathcal{P}, d)$ with the real axis, call it $I(d)$, is greater than $-1/\varepsilon$. Hence, $\varepsilon_{\max}$ is given by

$$\varepsilon_{\max} = \frac{1}{|\inf\{I(d) : d \in \partial D\}|} .$$

This is summarized in the following theorem:

Theorem 4.1 (Minimum Intersection Theorem) *Consider a polytope of polynomials as in* (1.3) *and a set $D \subset C$ satisfying Assumptions* 2.2-2.3. *For every $d \in \partial D$, let $I(d)$ be the minimum intersection of $V(\delta\mathcal{P}, d)$ with the real axis. Then, $\mathcal{P}^\varepsilon$ is D-stable if and only if $I(d) \geq -1/\varepsilon$ for all $d \in \partial D$. Consequently, the maximal ε, $\varepsilon_{\max}$, which guarantees the D-stability of $\mathcal{P}^\varepsilon$ for all $0 \leq \varepsilon < \varepsilon_{\max}$ is given by*

$$\varepsilon_{\max} = \frac{1}{|\inf\{I(d) : d \in \partial D\}|}. \tag{4.1}$$

Now, we want to provide an simple but general algorithm for calculating $I(d)$. Let $V_+(\delta\mathcal{P}, d)$ (resp. $V_-(\delta\mathcal{P}, d)$, $V_0(\delta\mathcal{P}, d)$) contains all vertices $\rho^i(d)$ having positive (resp. negative, zero) imaginary parts. Then, the minimum intersection of $V(\delta\mathcal{P},d)$ is achieved either by a vertex in $V_0(\delta\mathcal{P},d)$ or on a line segment formed by a vertex in $V_+(\delta\mathcal{P},d)$ and another in $V_-(\delta\mathcal{P},d)$. Notice that the intersection with the real axis of the line segment formed by $\rho^i(d) \in V_+(\delta\mathcal{P},d)$ and $\rho^j(d) \in V_-(\delta\mathcal{P},d)$ is given by

$$I_{ij}(d) \doteq \frac{\mathrm{Im}(\rho^i(d))\mathrm{Re}(\rho^j(d)) - \mathrm{Im}(\rho^j(d))\mathrm{Re}(\rho^i(d))}{\mathrm{Im}(\rho^i(d)) - \mathrm{Im}(\rho^j(d))}. \tag{4.2}$$

Therefore, we have

$$I(d) = \min\{I_{ij}(d), \rho_k(d) : \rho_i(d) \in V_+(\delta\mathcal{P},d), \rho_j(d) \in V_-(\delta\mathcal{P},d), \rho_k(d) \in V_0(\delta\mathcal{P},d)\}. \tag{4.3}$$

This is summarized in the following algorithm:

Computing Algorithm 4.2

Step 1: Divide $V(\delta\mathcal{P},d)$ into $V_+(\delta\mathcal{P},d)$, $V_-(\delta\mathcal{P},d)$ and $V_0(\delta\mathcal{P},d)$;

Step 2: For every $\rho^i(d) \in V_+(\delta\mathcal{P},d)$ and $\rho^j(d) \in V_-(\delta\mathcal{P},d)$, calculate $I_{ij}(d)$ using (4.2);

Step 3: Calculate $I(d)$ using (4.3).

Remark 4.3 Notice that Step 1 above requires r real comparisons and Steps 2-3 can be shown to require at most $r^2/4$ calculations of $I_{ij}(d)$ and that number of real comparisons. Therefore, the algorithm above works effectively when r is not too big. Note, however, for a parallelotope of polynomials with m parameters, the number of vertices r is equal to 2^m, which increases exponentially with respect to m. For this reason, we apply Theorem 3.3 to obtain the algorithm below which will completely solve the "combinatoric explosion" problem.

Computing Algorithm 4.4 Given any $d \in \partial D$, the minimum intersection of $V(\delta\mathcal{P}_L,d)$ with the real axis can be calculated using the following procedure:

Step 1: Eliminate zero $\rho_i(d)$'s and reduce m accordingly;

Step 2: For each i, if $\mathrm{Im}(\rho_i(d)) < 0$ or $\mathrm{Im}(\rho_i(d)) = 0$ but $\mathrm{Re}(\rho_i(d)) < 0$, then replace $\rho_i(d)$, $\underline{q}_i$ and $\bar{q}_i$ by $-\rho_i(d)$, $-\bar{q}_i$ and $-\underline{q}_i$, respectively;

Step 3: Reorder $\rho_i(d)$ and the associated $\underline{q}_i$ and $\bar{q}_i$ such that

$$0 \leq \angle(\rho_1(d)) \leq \angle(\rho_2(d)) \leq \cdots \leq \angle(\rho_m(d)) < 180°.$$

If $\angle(\rho_m(d)) = 0$, then

$$I(d) = \sum_{i=1}^{m} \underline{q}_i \rho_i(d) \tag{4.4}$$

and we are done; Else,

Step 4: Let $t = [m/2] + 1$ and use (3.3) to calculate v_t. If $\text{Im}(v_t) = 0$, then set $k = t$ and go to Step 5. Else, if $\text{Im}(v_t) < 0$, then calculate $v_{t+1}, v_{t+2}, \cdots$ until v_k such that either $\text{Im}(v_k) = 0$ or $\text{Im}(v_{k-1}) < 0$ but $\text{Im}(v_k) > 0$. If $\text{Im}(v_t) > 0$, then calculate $v_{t-1}, v_{t-2}, \cdots$ until v_k such that $\text{Im}(v_k) = 0$ or until v_{k-1} such that $\text{Im}(v_{k-1}) < 0$ but $\text{Im}(v_k) > 0$.

Step 5: If $\text{Im}(v_k) = 0$, then $I(d) = v_k$. Else,

$$I(d) = \frac{\text{Im}(v_k)\text{Re}(v_{k-1}) - \text{Im}(v_{k-1})\text{Re}(v_k)}{\text{Im}(v_k) - \text{Im}(v_{k-1})}. \tag{4.5}$$

Remark 4.5 It is not difficult to see that there are at most $[(m+3)/2]$ number of vertices needed to calculate in Step 4 above. This is due to the fact that the process in Step 4 has to stop either at v_1 or v_{m+1} because $\text{Im}(v_1) < 0$ and $\text{Im}(v_{m+1}) > 0$ when $\angle(\rho_m) > 0$.

Proof of Computing Algorithm 4.4: Steps 1–3 are used to reorganize $V(\delta\mathcal{P}_L, d)$ so that Theorem 3.3 can be applied. If $\angle(\rho_m(d)) = 0$ (after reordering), then $V(\delta\mathcal{P}, d)$ must lie on the real axis. In this case, it is obvious that the minimum intersection $I(d)$ is given by (4.4). If $\angle(\rho_m) > 0$ (after reordering), then $V(\delta\mathcal{P}, d)$ does not lie on the axis because we have now $\text{Im}(v_1) < 0$ and $\text{Im}(v_{m+1}) > 0$. The minimum intersection then happens on either a vertex v_k or a line segment $\text{conv}\{v_{k-1}, v_k\}$ for some $1 < k \leq m$. This vertex or line segment is searched in Step 4 using the fact that $v_1, v_2, \cdots$ traverse in the clockwise direction. Step 5 gives the value of the intersecting vertex or the intersection of this line segment with the real axis. □

Remark 4.6 (Discontinuity of $I(d)$) It is found that $I(d)$ may be discontinuous with respect to d. In fact, $I(d)$ may have "sparks" at some points; see the example in Section 7. This problem makes the sweeping of ∂D a little difficult because the infimum of $I(d)$ may not be approximated using a fine but arbitrary discretization of ∂D. Fortunately, the discontinuity happens only when $V(\delta\mathcal{P}, d)$ lies on the real axis. This requires that all $\rho_i(d)$ have zero imaginary parts. In order to "capture" the "sparks", we suggest that the imaginary parts of $\rho_i(d)$ be set to zero when their absolute values become sufficiently small. With this modification, the minimum intersection value at a discontinuous point d can be approximated by using the points in a sufficiently small neighborhood of d.

5 HURWITZ STABILITY OF A SPECIAL CLASS OF POLYTOPES OF POLYNOMIALS

In this section, we consider the Hurwitz stability of the following polytope of polynomials in (1.5). For notational simplicity, we assume in this section that every polynomial is real. The results can be extended to the complex polynomial case simply by replacing the Kharitonov polynomials for real interval polynomials with those for complex interval polynomials given in [2]. Our goal is to reduce the number of possible vertices and edges of $V(\delta\mathcal{P}_S, j\omega)$ needed by the test criteria in Section 4 for checking the Hurwitz stability of $\mathcal{P}_S$.

The problem above for $\ell = 2$ can be motivated by the robust stability of the

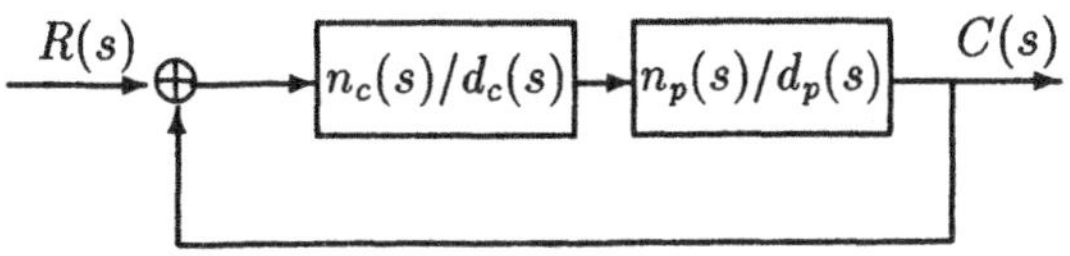

Figure 2. A Feedback Control System

feedback control system shown in Figure 2, where the numerator $n_p(s)$ (resp. the denominator $d_p(s)$) of the plant belongs to some interval polynomial $\mathcal{P}_n$ (resp. $\mathcal{P}_d$) and the compensator $n_c(s)/d_c(s)$ is fixed. We want to know the stability of the characteristic polynomial $n_p(s)n_c(s) + d_p(s)d_c(s)$ for all $n_p(s) \in \mathcal{P}_n$ and $d_p(s) \in \mathcal{P}_d$. The problem for $\ell > 2$ can be similarly related to the robust stability problem of multi-input-single-output or single-input-multi-output systems [17].

Let $p_{0,i}(s), \delta p_{1,i}(s)$ and $\delta p_{2,i}(s)$ be the nominal polynomial and the perturbation polynomials of $\mathcal{P}_i$, respectively, as defined in (2.12) and (2.13). We can define the nominal polynomial of $\mathcal{P}_S$ as

$$p_0(s) = \sum_{i=1}^{\ell} p_{0,i}(s)f_i(s) \tag{5.1}$$

and let

$$\rho_{1,i}(s) = \delta p_{1,i}(s)f_i(s)/p_0(s), \quad \rho_{2,i}(s) = \delta p_{2,i}(s)f_i(s)/p_0(s). \tag{5.2}$$

Using (2.14), it is clear that, for every $\omega \geq 0$,

$$V(\delta\mathcal{P}_S, j\omega) = \{\sum_{i=1}^{\ell} q_{1,i}\rho_{1,i}(j\omega) + \sum_{i=1}^{\ell} q_{2,i}\rho_{2,i}(j\omega) : q_{1,i}, q_{2,i} \in [-1,1], i = 1,2,\cdots,\ell\}. \tag{5.3}$$

Therefore, we have the following result:

Theorem 5.1 *Consider a polytope of polynomials $\mathcal{P}_S$ given by* (1.5). *Then, $\mathcal{P}_S$ is Hurwitz stable if and only if the following polytope of polynomials is Hurwitz stable:*

$$\begin{aligned}\tilde{\mathcal{P}}_S \doteq \{p_0(s) \;&+\; \sum_{i=1}^{\ell} r_{1,i}\delta p_{1,i}(s)f_i(s) + \sum_{i=1}^{\ell} r_{2,i}\delta p_{2,i}(s)f_i(s) : \\ & r_{1,i}, r_{2,i} \in [-1,1], i = 1,2,\cdots,\ell\}\end{aligned} \tag{5.4}$$

where $p_0(s)$ is given by (5.1) *and $\delta p_{1,i}(s)$ and $\delta p_{2,i}(s)$ are defined using* (2.13).

Using Theorem 4.1, we conclude that $\mathcal{P}_S$ is Hurwitz stable if and only if the minimum intersection of $V(\delta\tilde{\mathcal{P}}_S, j\omega)$ with the real axis is greater than -1 for all $\omega \geq 0$. By applying the Computing Algorithm 4.4 to $\tilde{\mathcal{P}}_S$, the number of vertices of $V(\delta\tilde{\mathcal{P}}_S, j\omega)$ needed to check at each $\omega \geq 0$ is now reduced to at most $[(2\ell+3)/2]$.

6 EXTENSION: D-STABILITY OF GENERAL FAMILIES OF POLYNOMIALS

This section provides an extension of the Minimum Intersection Theorem for handling general families of polynomials. Consequently, some sufficient conditions are generated.

Theorem 6.1 *Consider a family of polynomials $\mathcal{P}$ as in* (1.1) *and a region $D \subset C$ satisfying Assumptions* 2.2-2.3. *Suppose $\mathcal{P}$ is connected. Then, $\mathcal{P}$ is D-stable if for every $d \in \partial D$,*

$$I(d) \doteq \min\{\mathrm{Re}(\rho(d)) : \mathrm{Im}(\rho(d)) = 0; \rho(d) \in V(\delta\mathcal{P}, d)\} > -1. \tag{6.1}$$

In addition, if the set

$$V(\delta\mathcal{P}, d) \cap (-\infty, 0] \tag{6.2}$$

is connected for all $d \in \partial D$, then the condition in (6.1) *becomes also necessary for the D-stability of $\mathcal{P}$.*

Proof: Using Theorem 3.1, we know that $\mathcal{P}$ is D-stable if and only if for every $d \in \partial D$, $-1 \notin V(\delta\mathcal{P}, d)$, which is equivalent to $-1 \notin V(\delta\mathcal{P}, d) \cap (-\infty, 0]$. Therefore, the sufficiency of (6.1) is evident. If the set in (6.2) is connected, then the necessity of (6.1) is also obvious because $V(\delta\mathcal{P}, d)$ contains the origin for every $d \in \partial D$. □

Since the minimization problem in (6.1) may be difficult to solve in general, we provide two simple sufficient conditions (6.3) and (6.4) in the corollary to follow. The first sufficient condition is obtained by removing the constrain $\mathrm{Im}(\rho(d)) = 0$ in (6.1) while the second one, a well known fact, is derived by substituting the minimum with H_∞-norm. The proof is obvious and therefore omitted.

Corollary 6.2 *Consider a family of polynomials $\mathcal{P}$ as in* (1.1) *and a region $D \subset C$ satisfying Assumptions* 2.2-2.3. *Suppose $\mathcal{P}$ is connected. Then, $\mathcal{P}$ is D-stable if*

$$\inf\{\mathrm{Re}(\delta p(d)/p_0(d)) : d \in \partial D; \delta p(s) \in \delta\mathcal{P}\} > -1 \tag{6.3}$$

where $\delta\mathcal{P}$ is defined in (2.1). *In particular, $\mathcal{P}$ is strictly Hurwitz (resp. strictly Schur) if*

$$\sup\{\|\delta p(s)/p_0(s)\|_\infty : \delta p(s) \in \delta\mathcal{P}\} < 1 \tag{6.4}$$

where $\|\cdot\|_\infty$ denotes the H_∞ norm, given by

$$\|F(s)\|_\infty \doteq \sup\{|F(j\omega)| : \omega \in \mathbf{R}\}$$

(resp.

$$\|F(s)\|_\infty \doteq \sup\{|F(e^{j\theta})| : \theta \in [-\pi, \pi]\}\ ).$$

7 A NUMERICAL EXAMPLE

To illustrate the results in Section 4, we consider the following parallelotope of polynomials:

$$\mathcal{P}_L^\varepsilon = \{p_0(s) + \sum_{i=1}^{4} q_i \delta p_i(s) : q_i \in [-\varepsilon, \varepsilon], i = 1,2,3,4\}$$

where

$$\begin{aligned} p_0(s) &= s^4 + 12s^3 + 47s^2 + 70s + 50; \\ \delta p_1(s) &= s^3 + 10.75s^2 + 32.5s + 18.75; \\ \delta p_2(s) &= 0.75s^2 + 7.5s + 18.75; \\ \delta p_3(s) &= s^3 + 7s^2 + 12s + 10; \\ \delta p_4(s) &= 0.25s^2 + 0.5s + 0.5. \end{aligned}$$

The roots of the nominal polynomial $p_0(s)$ are calculated to be $-5, -5, -1+j$ and $-1-j$. The D set is given by

$$D \doteq D_1 \cup D_2 \cup D_3$$

where

$$\begin{aligned} D_1 &\doteq \{d : |d - (-1+j)| < 0.25\}; \\ D_2 &\doteq \{d : |d - (-1-j)| < 0.25\}; \\ D_3 &\doteq \{d : |d - (-5)| < 1\}. \end{aligned}$$

The objective is to determine the maximal ε, $\varepsilon_{\max}$, such that $\mathcal{P}^\varepsilon$ remains D-stable for all $\varepsilon < \varepsilon_{\max}$. Using Remark 3.2, we can replace ∂D in Theorem 4.1 by ∂D_+, which is given by the union of

$$\partial D_1 = \{-1 + j + 0.25e^{j\pi\theta} : \theta \in [0,2]\}$$

and

$$\partial D_{3,+} = \{-5 + e^{j\pi\theta} : \theta \in [0,1]\}.$$

By applying the Computing Algorithm 4.3, we obtain the curves of $I(d)$ (i.e., $I(d(\theta))$) on ∂D_1 and $\partial D_{3,+}$ in Figures 3 and 4, respectively. In Figure 3, the minimum of $I(d)$ is found to be approximately -3.4 at $\theta = 1.25$. Similarly, the minimum of $I(d)$ in Figure 4 is found to be approximately -1.65 at $\theta = 0$ (Note that this corresponds to a discontinuous point). Using (4.1), we conclude that $\varepsilon_{\max} \approx 1/3.4 \approx 0.29$. Consequently, the robustness measure of $\mathcal{P}^\varepsilon$ is $1 - \varepsilon/0.29$ or $20\log(0.29/\varepsilon)$ in dB.

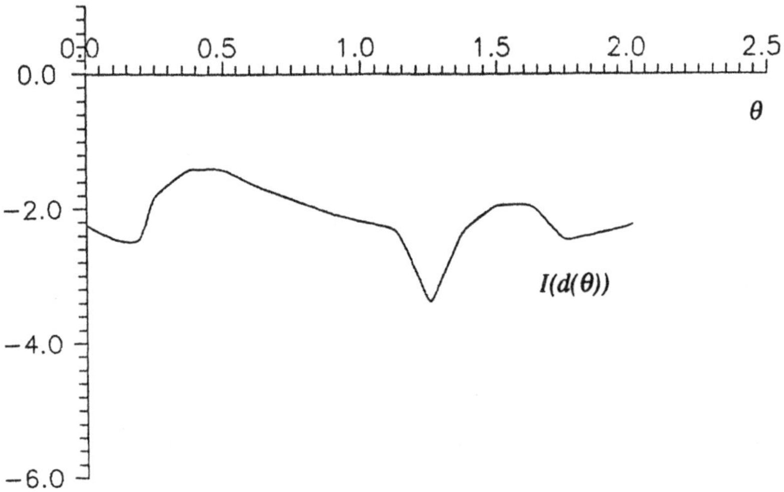

Figure 3. $I(d)$ on ∂D_1

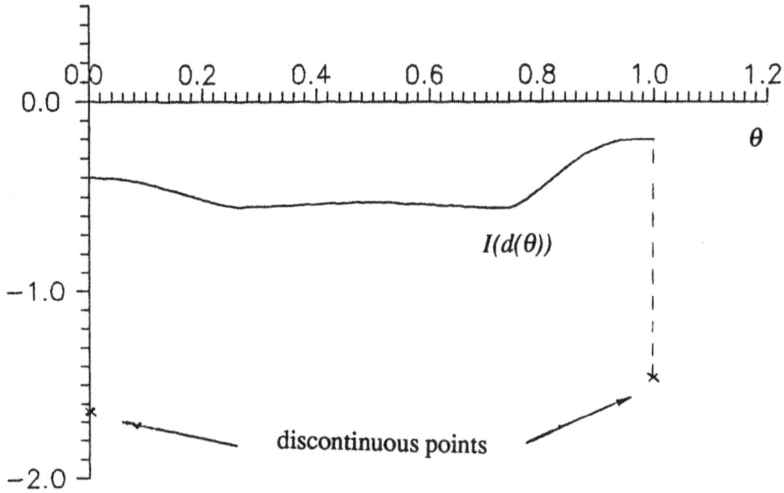

Figure 4. $I(d)$ on $\partial D_{3,+}$

8 CONCLUSION

The robust stability problem of families of polynomials has been considered and a number of new criteria and computing algorithms have been provided. For a polytope of polynomials $\mathcal{P}^\varepsilon$ in (1.3), a closed form description has been given for the maximal D-stability bound $\varepsilon_{\max}$ for which the D-stability of $\mathcal{P}^\varepsilon$ is preserved for all $\varepsilon < \varepsilon_{\max}$. By comparing this maximal size against the size of a given polytope of polynomials, we have obtained the so-called ***robustness measure*** of that given polytope of polynomials. A simple algorithm has been given for calculating this maximal bound which works effectively when the number of vertices of $\mathcal{P}^\varepsilon$ is not too large. For a parallelotope of polynomials $\mathcal{P}_L^\varepsilon$ as in (1.4) with m parameters, we have provided another algorithm which allows us to determine this maximal bound by calculating no more than $[(m+3)/2]$ vertices of the value set $V(\delta\mathcal{P}_L, d)$ at each $d \in \partial D$, where $V(\delta\mathcal{P}_L, d)$ is defined in (2.3). No auxiliary sweeping parameter is required in the calculation. Thus, the "combinatoric explosion" problem is completely solved. Extension of the results on the polytopes of polynomials has been made to nonlinear coefficient perturbation problems and some sufficient conditions have been obtained.

It should be realized that the polytopic structure of polynomials describes only a small class of perturbations in the real systems. It is straightforward to show by examples that the coefficients of the characteristic polynomials of a system are nonlinear with respect to perturbation parameters in general even for the case when the perturbations in the system matrices are linear; see, for example, [27]. Consequently, the results on the robust stability of polytopes of polynomials may not be applicable. It is hoped that some ideas given in Section 8 may be suggestive in attacking the nonlinear coefficient perturbation problems.

Appendix A

Proof of Theorem 3.3: Unfortunately, the proof is a bit lengthy.

Let V be a convex polygon in the form of (3.1). First, it is trivial that $\angle(v_1) \le 0$ and $\angle(v_{m+1}) \ge 0$ because $\mathrm{Im}(\rho_i) \ge 0$ for all $i = 1, 2, \cdots, m$. We now want to show that $v_1, v_2, \cdots, v_{2m}, v_1$ traverse in the clockwise direction. To demonstrate this, it is sufficient to prove that

$$\angle(v_2 - v_1) \ge \angle(v_3 - v2) \ge \cdots \ge \angle(v_{2m} - v_{2m-1}) \ge \angle(v_1 - v_{2m}). \quad \text{(A.1)}$$

Indeed, using (3.3) we have

$$\begin{aligned}
v_2 - v_1 &= (\bar{q}_m - \underline{q}_m)\rho_m \\
v_3 - v_2 &= (\bar{q}_{m-1} - \underline{q}_{m-1})\rho_{m-1} \\
&\cdots \\
v_{m+1} - v_m &= (\bar{q}_1 - \underline{q}_1)\rho_1 \\
v_{m+2} - v_{m+1} &= (\underline{q}_m - \bar{q}_m)\rho_m \\
v_{m+3} - v_{m+2} &= (\underline{q}_{m-1} - \bar{q}_{m-1})\rho_{m-1} \\
&\cdots \\
v_{2m} - v_{2m-1} &= (\underline{q}_2 - \bar{q}_2)\rho_2 \\
v_1 - v_{2m} &= (\underline{q}_1 - \bar{q}_1)\rho_1.
\end{aligned}$$

Therefore, (A.1) follows from (3.2).

Secondly, we claim that every v_i is a boundary point of V (if not a vertex). To verify this, we define

$$\sigma_i \doteq \rho_i e^{-j\pi/2} = \mathrm{Im}(\rho_i) - j\mathrm{Re}(\rho_i) \tag{A.2}$$

for every $1 \le i \le m$. Then the projection of an arbitrary point

$$\rho = \sum_{k=1}^{m} q_k \rho_k \in V$$

on σ_i can be written as

$$\begin{aligned} P(\rho, \sigma_i) &\doteq \left(\mathrm{Re}(\sum_{k=1}^{m-1} q_k\rho_k)\mathrm{Im}(\rho_i) - \mathrm{Im}(\sum_{k=1}^{m-1} q_k\rho_k)\mathrm{Re}(\rho_i)\right) / |\rho_i| \\ &= \sum_{k=1}^{m-1} q_k(\mathrm{Re}(\rho_k)\mathrm{Im}(\rho_i) - \mathrm{Im}(\rho_k)\mathrm{Re}(\rho_i))/|\rho_i|. \end{aligned} \tag{A.3}$$

Obviously, the projection of ρ_k on σ_i is non-negative for $1 \le k \le i$ and nonpositive for $i+1 \le k \le m$, i.e.,

$$\mathrm{Re}(\rho_k)\mathrm{Im}(\rho_i) - \mathrm{Im}(\rho_k)\mathrm{Re}(\rho_i) \ge 0, \quad 1 \le k \le i;$$

$$\mathrm{Re}(\rho_k)\mathrm{Im}(\rho_i) - \mathrm{Im}(\rho_k)\mathrm{Re}(\rho_i) \le 0, \quad i+1 \le k \le m.$$

Therefore, the minimum (resp. the maximum) of (A.3) is achieved by setting $q_k = \underline{q}_k$ (resp. $q_k = \bar{q}_k$) for $1 \le k \le i$ and $q_k = \bar{q}_k$ (resp. $q_k = \underline{q}_k$) for $i+1 \le k \le m$. That is, the minimum and the maximum of (A.3) are reached by v_{m-i+1} and v_{2m-i+1}, respectively. Hence, all v_i's are boundary points.

Now we want to show inductively that the v_i's given by (3.3) include all vertices of V. This holds obviously for the cases $m = 1$ and $m = 2$. Now we assume $m > 2$ and that the following convex polygon

$$V^* \doteq \{\sum_{i=1}^{m-1} q_i\rho_i : q_i \in [\underline{q}_i, \bar{q}_i], i = 1, 2, \cdots, m-1\}$$

has at most $2(m-1)$ vertices which are given by

$$\begin{aligned} v_1^* &= \underline{q}_1\rho_1 + \underline{q}_2\rho_2 + \cdots + \underline{q}_{m-1}\rho_{m-1} \\ v_2^* &= \underline{q}_1\rho_1 + \underline{q}_2\rho_2 + \cdots + \underline{q}_{m-2}\rho_{m-2} + \bar{q}_{m-1}\rho_{m-1} \\ &\cdots\cdots \\ v_{m-1}^* &= \underline{q}_1\rho_1 + \bar{q}_2\rho_2 + \cdots + \bar{q}_{m-1}\rho_{m-1} \\ v_m^* &= \bar{q}_1\rho_1 + \bar{q}_2\rho_2 + \cdots + +\bar{q}_{m-1}\rho_{m-1} \\ v_{m+1}^* &= \bar{q}_1\rho_1 + \bar{q}_2\rho_2 + \cdots + +\bar{q}_{m-2}\rho_{m-2} + \underline{q}_{m-1}\rho_{m-1} \\ &\cdots\cdots \\ v_{2(m-1)}^* &= \bar{q}_1\rho_1 + \underline{q}_2\rho_2 + \cdots + \underline{q}_{m-1}\rho_{m-1}\,. \end{aligned} \tag{A.4}$$

Using V^*, V can be expressed as

$$V = \{\rho^* + q_m\rho_m : \rho^* \in V^*, q_m \in [\underline{q}_m, \bar{q}_m]\}.$$

Obviously, the possible vertices of V are given by

$$\begin{aligned} v_i' &= v_i^* + \underline{q}_m\rho_m, \\ v_i'' &= v_i^* + \bar{q}_m\rho_m, \quad i = 1, 2, \cdots, 2(m-1). \end{aligned} \tag{A.5}$$

Comparing (A.4) and (A.5) with (3.3), we find that $v_1 = v_1'$, $v_2 = v_1''$, $v_3 = v_2''$, $v_4 = v_3''$, $\cdots$, $v_m = v_{m-1}''$, $v_{m+1} = v_m''$, $v_{m+2} = v_m'$, $v_{m+3} = v_{m+1}'$, $\cdots$, $v_{2m} = v_{2(m-1)}'$. Therefore, we only need to show that $v_2', \cdots, v_{m-1}', v_{m+1}'', \cdots, v_{2(m-1)}''$ can be expressed as convex combinations of other v_k' and v_k''. This implies that only v_1^* and v_m^* can possibly create new vertices when $q_m\rho_m$ is added to V^*. For this purpose, we let σ_m be given by (A.2). A similar analysis as before can demonstrate that the minimum and the maximum of the projection of V^* on σ_m are achieved by v_1^* and v_m^*, respectively. It follows that for every $1 \le k \le 2(m-1)$, the projection of every vertex v_k^* on σ_m can be expressed as a convex combination of $P(v_1^*, \sigma_m)$ and $P(v_m^*, \sigma_m)$; i.e., there exists some $0 \le \lambda_k \le 1$ such that

$$P(v_k^*, \sigma_m) = \lambda_k P(v_1^*, \sigma_m) + (1 - \lambda_k) P(v_m^*, \sigma_m). \tag{A.6}$$

Let

$$\nu_k \doteq \lambda_k v_1^* + (1 - \lambda_k) v_m^*.$$

Then equation (A.6) implies that $v_k^* - \nu_k$ is parallel to ρ_m. Using the facts that v_i^* traverse in the clockwise direction when i increases and that $\angle(v_1^*) \le 0$ and $\angle(v_m^*) \le \angle(\rho_m)$, the direction of $v_k^* - \nu_k$ (if $v_k^* - \nu_k \neq 0$) must be the same as the direction of ρ_m if $1 < k < m-1$ or the opposite of that of ρ_m when $m - 1 < k < 2(m-1)$. For $1 < k < m-1$, the conclusion above implies that there exists $\gamma_k \ge 0$ such that $v_k^* - \nu_k = \gamma_k \rho_m$. Assuming $1 < k < m$, we claim that v_k' can be expressed as the convex combination of v_k'' and $\nu_k + \underline{q}_m\rho_m$. Indeed, it is straightforward to verify that the solution of

$$v_k' = \eta v_k'' + (1 - \eta)(\nu_k + \underline{q}_m\rho_m)$$

is given by

$$\eta = \frac{v_k^* - \nu_k}{v_k^* - \nu_k + (\bar{q}_m - \underline{q}_m)\rho_m} = \frac{\gamma_k}{\gamma_k + \bar{q}_m - \underline{q}_m}.$$

Consequently, $0 \le \eta \le 1$. Therefore, v_k' is a convex combination of v_k'' and $\nu_k + \underline{q}_m\rho_m$. Since ν_k is a convex combination of v_1^* and v_m^*, $\nu_k + \underline{q}_m\rho_m$ is a convex combination of v_1' and v_m'. It follows that for any $1 < k < m-1$, v_k' is a convex combination of v_k'', v_1' and v_m', thus can be eliminated from the set of vertices of V. Similar argument can be given to show that v_k'' is a convex combination of v_k', v_1'' and v_m'' if $m-1 < k < 2(m-1)$. Hence, only $v_1, v_2, \cdots, v_{2m}$ are possible vertices of V. In other words, the set of vertices of V must be either $\{v_1, v_2, \cdots, v_{2m}\}$ or a subset of it.

Finally, it is straightforward to see that $\mathrm{conv}\{v_i, v_1\}, i = 1, 2, \cdots, 2m-1$ and $\mathrm{conv}\{v_{2m}, v_1\}$ form the boundary (i.e., the set of edges) of V because v_i traverse in the clockwise direction and they are all boundary points. □

References

[1] V. L. Kharitonov, "Asymptotic Stability of an Equilibrium Position of a Family of Systems of Linear Differential Equations," *Differentsial, Uravnen.*, vol. 14, no. 11, pp. 2086-2088, 1978.

[2] V. L. Kharitonov, "On a Generalization of a Stability Criterion," *Izv. Akad. Nauk. Kazakh. SSR Ser. Fiz. Mat.*, vol. 1, pp. 53-57, 1978 (in Russian).

[3] S. Bialas and J. Garloff, "Convex Combinations of Stable Polynomials," *Journal of the Franklin Institute*, vol. 319, no. 3, pp. 373-377, 1985.

[4] A. C. Bartlett, C. V. Hollot and H. Lin, "Root Locations of an Entire Polytope of Polynomials: It suffices to Check the Edges," *Mathematics of Control Signals and Systems*, vol. 1, pp. 61-71, 1987.

[5] M. Fu and B. R. Barmish, "Polytopes of Polynomials with Zeros in a Prescribed Region," *Proceedings of American Control Conference*, pp. 2461-2464, Atlanta, Georgia, June 1988, also to appear in *IEEE Transactions on Automatic Control.*

[6] S. Bialas, "A Necessary and Sufficient Condition for the Stability of Convex Combinations of Stable Polynomials and Matrices," *Bulletin of Polish Academy of Sciences, Technical Sciences*, vol. 33, no. 9-10, pp. 473-480, 1985.

[7] B. R. Barmish,"A Generalization of Kharitonov's Four Polynomial Concept for Robust Stability Problems with Linearly Dependent Coefficient Perturbations," *Proceedings of the 1988 American Control Conference*, Atlanta, Georgia, June 1988.

[8] B. R. Barmish, and P. P. Khargonekar, "Robust stability of Feedback Control Systems with Uncertain Parameters and Unmodelled Dynamics," *Proceedings of the 1988 American Control Conference*, Atlanta, Georgia, June 1988.

[9] C. V. Hollot, D. P. Looze, and A. C. Bartlett, "Unmodeled Dynamics: Performance and Stability via Parameter Space Methods," *Proceedings of the 26th Conference on Decision and Control*, pp. 2076-2081, Los Angeles, CA, December 1987.

[10] I. R. Petersen,"A New Extension to Kharitonov's Theorem," *Proceedings of the 26th Conference on Decision and Control*, pp. 2070-2075, Los Angeles, CA, December 1987.

[11] I. R. Petersen,"A Class of Stability Regions for which a Kharitonov Like Theorem Holds," *Proceedings of the 26th Conference on Decision and Control*, pp. 440-444, Los Angeles, CA, December 1987.

[12] A. T. Fam and J. S. Meditch, "A Canonical Parameter Space for Linear Systems," *IEEE Transactions on Automatic Control*, vol. AC-23, no. 3, pp. 454-458, 1978.

[13] M. Fu and B. R. Barmish, "Stability of Convex and Linear Combinations of Polynomials and Matrices Arising in Robustness Problems," *Proceedings of Conference on Information Science and Systems*, John Hopkins University, Baltimore, 1987.

[14] M. B. Argoun, "Stability of Hurwitz Polynomials under Coefficient Perturbations: Necessary and Sufficient Conditions," *International Journal of Control*, vol. 45, no. 2, pp. 739-744, 1987.

[15] R. R. E. de Gaston and M. G. Safonov,"Exact Calculation of Multiloop Stability Margin," *IEEE Transactions on Automatic Control*, vol. 33, no. 2, pp. 156-171, 1988.

[16] D. Hertz, E. I. Jury and E. Zeheb, "Root Exclusion from Complex Polynomials and Some of its Applications," *Automatica*, vo. 23, no. 3, pp. 399-404, 1987.

[17] H. Chapellat and S. P. Bhattacharyya, "A Generalization of Kharitonov's Theorem for Robust Stability of Interval Plants," to appear.

[18] M. Fu, A. W. Olbrot and M. P. Polis, "Robust Stability for Time-Delay Systems: the Edge Theorem and Graphical Tests," to appear.

[19] B. R. Barmish, "Invariance of the Strict Hurwitz Property for Polynomials with Perturbations," *IEEE Transactions on Automatic Control*, vol. AC-29, no. 10, pp. 935–936, 1984.

[20] S. Bialas and J. Garloff, "Stability of Polynomials Under Coefficient Perturbations," *IEEE Transactions on Automatic Control*, vol. AC-30, no. 3, 1985.

[21] C. B. Soh, C. S. Berger, and K. P. Dabke, "On the Stability Properties of Polynomials with Perturbed Coefficients," *IEEE Transactions on Automatic Control*, vol. AC-30, no. 10, pp. 1033-1036, 1985.

[22] M. Fu, "Robustness Bounds of Hurwitz and Schur Polynomials," to appear in *Journal of Optimization Theory and Applications.*

[23] H. Chapellat and S. P. Bhattacharyya, "Exact Calculation of Stability Margin with Respect to Transfer Function Coefficients," to appear.

[24] M. Fu and B. R. Barmish, "Maximal Unidirectional Perturbation Bounds for Stability of Polynomials and Matrices," *Systems and Control Letters*, vol. 11, pp. 173-179, 1988.

[25] T. E. Djaferis, and C. V. Hollot, "Parameter Partitioning via Shaping Conditions for the Stability of Families of Polynomials," *Proceedings of 1988 American Control Conference*, Atlanta, Georgia, June 1988.

[26] S. R. Lay, *Convex Sets and their Applications*, John Wiley and Sons, Inc., New York, 1982.

[27] B. R. Barmish, M. Fu and S. Saleh, "Stability of a Polytope of Matrices: Counterexamples," *IEEE Transactions on Automatic Control*, vol. 33, no. 6, pp. 569-572, June 1988.

ROBUSTNESS BOUNDS FOR CLASSES OF STRUCTURED PERTURBATIONS

A. Vicino and A. Tesi

Dipartimento di Sistemi e Informatica
Universitá di Firenze
Via di Santa Marta, 3
50139 Firenze (Italy)
E-mail: vicino@itopoli.bitnet
vicino@ifiidg.bitnet

ABSTRACT

In this paper two methods for robust pole location (generalized stability) analysis of linear dynamical systems with structured real parametric uncertainties are proposed. The first approach solves the problem of computing maximal polytopic domains in parameter space for fairly general regions of pole location, when families of polynomials with coefficients affine in a set of real parameters are considered. This approach is based on the fact that certain sets bounding the regions of interest in parameter space are linear manifolds for each fixed value of a parameterizing scalar variable. The solution of the maximal polytope problem allows to solve also other problems of interest in stability robustness analysis of uncertain control systems.

The second approach, based on algebraic matrix properties, deals with state space models where system matrix entries are perturbed by polynomial functions of a set of physical uncertain parameters. A method of analysis converting the generalized stability problem in the nonsingularity analysis of a suitable matrix is proposed. The proposed method requires to check positivity of a multinomial form over a hyperrectangular domain in parameter space. This problem, which can be reduced to finding the real solutions of a system of polynomial equations, simplifies considerably when considering cases with one or two uncertain parameters. For these cases, necessary and sufficient conditions for stability are given in terms of the solution of suitable real eigenvalue problems.

1. INTRODUCTION

The growing interest in robust control literature for the study of dynamical behavior of systems with unknown but bounded parametric uncertainties has been greatly stimulated by the fundamental work of Kharitonov [1]. Of main importance are also [2,3] which among first posed and started the analysis of the problem. Numerous papers have been devoted to robust stability analysis of dynamical feedback control systems subject to bounded parametric uncertainties of the plant or of the controller. Most of the proposed approaches study system generalized stability in terms of the roots of its characteristic polynomial with coefficients assumed subject to certain classes of perturbations ([4]-[20]); in particular, [11,12] contain extensive lists of references on the subject. Other approaches, which in principle are more general, assume the system given in state space with uncertain parameters entering model matrices. These methods (see e.g.,[21,22]), although more realistic, often provide conservative results for stability problems. An interesting approach providing an algorithm for nonconservative multiloop stability margin computation, suitable for dealing with perturbed matrices, has been proposed in [24,25]; this algorithm seems to work satisfactorily when the problem involves a limited number of uncertain parameters.

In this paper we present two methods for investigating system behavior when certain classes of structured parameter perturbations are considered. In a first geometric approach we deal with classes of polynomials with coefficients affine in a set of parameters belonging to a polytopic uncertainty set. We observe that a solution to the problem of root location of polytopes of polynomials in coefficient space has been given in [10]. This result, stating that the root location region of an entire polytopic family in coefficient space is determined by that relative to the exposed edges of the polytope, becomes of difficult application with increasing problem dimensionality. The approach presented in this paper is in the spirit of [6,13,17] and is based on the following ideas. Given a *nominal* parameter vector p^o, a class of *admissible* perturbations in parameter space and a region of pole location Λ in the complex plane, we look for maximal regions around p^o, such that polynomial roots remain in Λ (assuming of course that p^o generates a *nominal* polynomial with roots in Λ). This means finding the distance, according to a suitable norm, from p^o to the surfaces in parameter space corresponding to polynomials having at least one root on the boundary of Λ (this distance is also frequently called in robust control contexts *stability margin* of the perturbed system). These surfaces partition the parameter space in a number of regions and the location of p^o determines the only region we are interested in. When the relation between polynomial coefficients and parameters is (affine) linear, this problem, which can be formulated in general as a nonlinear programming problem, can be solved as a one parameter optimization search. This fact has been used in [6] to find maximal stability spheres in polynomial coefficient space, in [12] to compute maximal stability ellipsoids in parameter space for polynomials with linearly dependent coefficients and in [17,19] to compute maximal box type regions in coefficient space for stability of discrete time systems and for more general pole location regions. In this paper we solve the problem of computing maximal polytopes in parameter space, for general root location regions Λ with boundary given either by means of analytical equations or in numerical form. We notice that the solution of the above problem allows also for the solution of the problem of checking if roots of a given family lie or not in a given region Λ. We provide two algorithmic solutions to the maximal polytope problem. The first one leads in general to a family of linear programs, while the second requires a family of computations of segments of the boundary of the convex hull of a planar set of points. In particular, the first algorithmic solution has been investigated more thoroughly and easily computable conditions have been obtained under which the linear program reduces simply to the solution of a system of two linear equations. This new computational simplification, which has been used in implementing a computer code on a personal computer, results in a remarkable computing time reduction. Computational saving is a crucial point especially if the stability robustness analysis algorithm developed is used in certain robustification control problems (see section 5) or as a possible rough tool for robust synthesis.

In a second approach, we assume the system given as a state equation model where the entries of a known stable *nominal* matrix are perturbed by polynomial functions of an uncertain parameter vector p. A method of analysis converting the generalized stability problem in the nonsingularity analysis of a suitable matrix is proposed. This method requires to check positivity of a multinomial form over a hyperrectangular domain in parameter space. This numerical problem can be reduced to finding the real solutions of a system of polynomial equations (see e.g., [26]). Numerical algorithms based on homotopy methods for finding solutions of polynomial systems are available (see [27]); nevertheless, from a practical point of view, these algorithms can be used to solve the original stability problem only when a very limited number of parameters are involved. The proposed method simplifies considerably when considering problems with one or two uncertain parameters. It is shown that if matrix entries depend on one parameter, the generalized stability problem can be given a solution in terms of one eigenvalue problem and that for two uncertain parameters the solution of a finite number of eigenvalue problems is required.

2. NOTATION AND BASIC DEFINITIONS

Let $p = [p_1, p_2, \ldots, p_q]^t$ be the vector of parameters on which the polynomial coefficients depend. Let us consider uncertain polynomials $\Delta(s,p)$ such that

$$\Delta(s,p) = \delta_0(p) + \delta_1(p)s + \cdots + \delta_n(p)s^n, \ p \in \Omega(\rho) \tag{1}$$

where $\Omega(\rho) \subset \mathbf{R}^q$ is a convex polytope and $\delta_i(\cdot) : \Omega(\rho) \to \mathbf{R}$, $i = 0, 1, \ldots, n$ are real continuous functions of the parameter vector p. The set $\Omega(\rho)$, called 'uncertainty set', is given as

$$\Omega(\rho) = \{p \in \mathbf{R}^q : \|T(p - p^o)\|_\infty \leq \rho\} \tag{2}$$

where $p^o \in \Omega(\rho)$ is a given vector called *nominal* parameter vector, corresponding to a *nominal* polynomial $\Delta(s, p^o)$ in the polynomial coefficient space $\mathbf{R}^{n+1}$, ρ is a positive value (called 'radius' of the polytope), $T \in \mathbf{R}^{m,q}$ is a full column rank operator, $\| \cdot \|_\infty$ represents an l_∞ norm. Notice that hyperrectangular uncertainty sets in parameter space can be obtained by assumung T as a (q,q) diagonal matrix $T = diag(w_1^{-1}, \ldots, w_q^{-1})$, where w_i, $i = 1, \ldots, q$ are positive 'weights' determining the ratios of the sides of the hyperrectangular domain. We will often denote the perturbation vector $p - p^o$ by $\tilde{p}$.

The theory in next section 3 is developed for the case in which functions $\delta_i(p), i = 0, 1, \cdots, n$ are *affine* in p, i.e.

$$\delta = Hp + h \tag{3}$$

where $\delta = [\delta_0, \ldots, \delta_n]^t \in \mathbf{R}^{n+1}$, $H \in \mathbf{R}^{n+1,q}$ and $h \in \mathbf{R}^{n+1}$.

For what concerns regions of root location for the uncertain polynomials, we will consider open regions Λ of the complex plane given as the union of a finite number of simply connected regions. In view of the fact that we deal with classes of polynomials with real coefficients, we will assume without loss of generality that Λ is always symmetrical with respect to the real axis. We say that a polynomial is Λ-stable if all its roots lie in Λ. Notice that we do not make any restrictive assumption on the boundary $\partial\Lambda$; for our purposes, it suffices that $\partial\Lambda$ is given either in analytic form (by means of parametric or implicit equations) or in any numerical form. For ease of illustration, we assume only formally that

$$\partial\Lambda = \{s \in \mathbf{C} : s = F(\gamma),\ \gamma \in \mathbf{R}\} \tag{4}$$

where $F(\cdot)$ is a complex valued map, possibly given numerically.

As we will discuss better in next sections, we are able to give a solution to the root location problem in the form of a one parameter optimization problem under the assumptions (2) and (3). For the special case of stability of interval polynomials for continuous time systems, the proposed approach allows to obtain a closed form solution to the problem of computing the maximal stability box in coefficient space, without using the Theorem of Kharitonov (see [18]).

Let us now consider the $n+1$ dimensional polynomial coefficient space. The boundary of the domain of Λ-stable polynomials $\Delta(\Lambda)$ in this space is a subset of the set

$$\Delta(\partial\Lambda) = \left\{\delta \in \mathbf{R}^{n+1} : \delta_0 + \delta_1 s + \ldots + \delta_n s^n = 0, s \in \partial\Lambda \ \ (s = F(\gamma))\right\} . \tag{5}$$

As it can be easily checked, $\Delta(\partial\Lambda)$ is generated by the one degree of freedom movement of a linear manifold according to the sweep of s on $\partial\Lambda$ (or equivalently of the parameter γ on its domain of definition). In particular, we observe that $\Delta(\partial\Lambda)$ is obtained by letting s traverse $\partial\Lambda$ in only one of the upper or lower complex half plane. Thus, the optimization problems obtained for $s \in \partial\Lambda$ will be always intended restricted to only one half plane.

The counterimage of $\Delta(\partial\Lambda)$ in parameter space is given by

$$\Omega(\partial\Lambda) = \{p \in \mathbf{R}^q : \Delta(s,p) = 0,\ s \in \partial\Lambda\ (s = F(\gamma))\} . \tag{6}$$

Again, the boundary of the domain $\Omega(\Lambda)$ of parameters generating Λ-stable polynomials is a subset of $\Omega(\partial\Lambda)$. Linearity of (3) implies that (6) is generated by a hyperplane moving according to the sweep of s on $\partial\Lambda$.

In section 4 we consider families of polynomials whose coefficients are polynomial functions of the parameter vector p. These structured perturbations arise when considering uncertain linear dynamical systems given in state equations

$$\dot{x}(t) = A(p)x(t) \quad (x(t+1) = A(p)x(t)) \tag{7}$$

where

$$A(p) = A_o + \sum_{i=1}^{l} f_i(p - p^o)A_i \tag{8}$$

where $A_o = A(p^o) \in \mathbf{R}^{n,n}$ is the *nominal* matrix, $A_i \in \mathbf{R}^{n,n}$, $f_i(\cdot)$, are scalar polynomial functions such that $f_i(0) = 0$. For this class of perturbations we will consider hyperrectangular uncertainty sets $\Omega^B(\rho)$ in parameter space, i.e., $T = diag(w_1^{-1}, \dots, w_q^{-1})$.

We define the class of matrices $\mathcal{A}(\rho)$ as follows:

$$\mathcal{A}(\rho) = \{A(p) \in \mathbf{R}^{n,n} : p \in \Omega^B(\rho)\} \tag{9}$$

and assume that matrix A_o is Λ-stable, i.e., has eigenvalues in the admissible region Λ.

Now we briefly recall some definitions on matrix Kronecker products which will be used in section 4 (see [28] for details).
Given two matrices $M, \tilde{M} \in \mathbf{R}^{n,n}$, we define the operators $L_1[M, \tilde{M}]$ and $L_2[M, \tilde{M}]$ as

$$L_1[M, \tilde{M}] = E(M \oplus \tilde{M})SE^t \tag{10}$$

$$L_2[M, \tilde{M}] = E(M \otimes \tilde{M})SE^t \tag{11}$$

where $\oplus$ and $\otimes$ denote ordinary Kronecker sum and product respectively. Matrix $E \in \mathbf{R}^{n(n+1)/2, n^2}$ is $E = diag(E_1, \dots, E_n)$ and matrix $S \in \mathbf{R}^{n^2, n^2}$. In particular, $E_i \in \mathbf{R}^{i,n}$ and $E_i = [e_1, \dots, e_i]^t$, while $S = [s_1, \dots, s_{n^2}]$ with

$$s_{n(i-1)+j} = l_{n(i-1)+j} + (1 - \delta_{ij}) l_{n(j-1)+i} \quad , i = 1, \dots, n \quad , j = 1, \dots, n \; . \tag{12}$$

The elements e_i and l_i introduced above represent respectively n and n^2 dimensional column vectors of zeros everywhere except a unit entry in the i-th position; δ_{ij} is the Kronecker delta. For simplicity of notation we will denote $L_1[M, M]$ and $L_2[M, M]$ by $L_1[M]$ and $L_2[M]$ respectively.

3. MAXIMAL DOMAINS AND ROOT LOCATION CHECK IN PARAMETER SPACE

In this section we provide algorithms for determining maximal polytopic domains in parameter space generating only Λ-stable polynomials in the case in which polynomial coefficients are (affine) linear functions of the parameter vector p.

3.1 Problem solution as a family of linear programs

Suppose that a class of admissible perturbation is given, i.e., T, p^o are known in (2), and that a region Λ is assigned. Assuming that p^o generates a Λ-stable *nominal* polynomial, we want to find maximal ρ for which $\Omega(\rho)$ contains only parameters generating Λ-stable polynomials. This is a tangency problem consisting in expanding $\Omega(\rho)$ until at least one point of its boundary reaches one of the surfaces represented by (6). This amounts to solving the minimum norm problem (apart from possible degeneracies which can be considered separately [18])

$$\rho^* = \inf_{p \,:\, p \in \Omega(\partial\Lambda)} \|T(p - p^o)\|_\infty \; . \tag{13}$$

It is easy to check that problem (13) is equivalent to

$$\rho^* = \inf_{p,\gamma,\rho} \rho$$

$$\text{subject to} \quad \begin{cases} \rho \geq 0 \\ -\rho \leq t_i^t(p - p^o) \leq \rho, \quad i = 1, \ldots, m \\ \Delta(s, p) = 0, \; s = F(\gamma) \end{cases} \tag{14}$$

where $t_i^t, i = 1, \ldots, m$ are row vectors of matrix T. For a given γ we define the following function

$$\rho_s(\gamma) = \inf_{p,\rho} \rho$$

$$\text{subject to} \quad \begin{cases} \rho \geq 0 \\ -\rho \leq t_i^t(p - p^o) \leq \rho, \quad i = 1, \ldots, m \\ \Re[\Delta(\gamma, p)] = 0 \\ \Im[\Delta(\gamma, p)] = 0 \end{cases} \tag{15}$$

where $\Re$ and $\Im$ denote real and imaginary parts respectively. If for some γ the set defined by $\Delta(\gamma, p) = 0$ is empty, we set $\rho_s(\gamma) = \infty$. Problem (13) is equivalent to

$$\rho^* = \inf_{\gamma} \rho_s(\gamma) \tag{16}$$

which is a one parameter optimization problem. For each γ, i.e., for each $s = F(\gamma)$, the computation of $\rho_s(\gamma)$ requires in general the solution of a linear programming problem in $q + 1$ parameters and $2m + 3$ constraints.

The above considerations prove constructively the following Theorem.

Theorem 1
Let Λ be a given region of the complex plane. Let p^o be a given nominal parameter vector generating a Λ-stable polynomial and let ρ^* be given by (16). *Then, the polytope $\Omega(\rho^*)$ is maximal in the given class of polytopes generating Λ-stable polynomials.*
□

Notice that the computational burden of solving (16) is acceptable in many practical situations. However, in several applications for robustness analysis of feedback control systems, the solution of families of problems like (16) may be required (see section 5 for details). In these cases, computational efficiency in solving (16) may become a crucial issue. It can be shown, (see [20]) that, provided some easily checkable conditions are met on a given interval of the parameter γ, $\rho_s(\gamma)$ can be computed on that interval by means of a recursive algorithm. In fact, given $\rho_s(\gamma)$, the algorithm allows to compute $\rho_s(\gamma + \Delta\gamma)$ ($\Delta\gamma$ 'sufficiently' small) by a simple updating of $\rho_s(\gamma)$. The updating algorithm consists in solving a *system of two linear equations*, independently of the dimension of the parameter vector p. The general linear program (15) need be solved only for certain 'critical' values of γ, corresponding to situations in which the tangency point solving (15) changes from one exposed edge of the box (or polytope) in parameter space to another one (see [20] for further details).

Remark 1
It is not difficult to show that the problem of checking root location of a given family of polynomials with linearly dependent coefficients in an assigned region Λ of the complex plane, can be always solved by solving a suitable maximal polytope problem like (16) (see [18]).

Remark 2
Connections can be estabilished between problem (14) and the four vertex polynomials in coefficient space of the celebrated Kharitonov's Theorem. In particular, a thorough geometric analysis of (14) shows that the tangency points of the box with the boundary of stability in coefficient space takes place at one of the four Kharitonov vertices. This implies that the maximal stability box in coefficient space can be computed by only checking these four vertices and this in turn requires to compute real roots of at most 4 algebraic equations of order less or equal to $n-1$ (see [18] for more details).

Remark 3
If Λ is unbounded and if $\delta_n(p)$ preserves the same sign for every $p \in \Omega(\rho)$, the one parameter sweep (16) can be restricted to a bounded interval. In fact, in this case it is always possible to find an upper bound on the modulus of the roots of the polynomials of the given family (details can be found in [18,19]).

3.2 An alternative solution algorithm for Λ-stability problems

In this subsection we show how the maximal Λ-stability box problem ($T = diag(w_1^{-1}, \ldots, w_q^{-1})$ in (2)) for families of uncertain polynomials with linearly correlated coefficients may be given a solution alternative to that presented in the preceding section.

Refer to problem (13). In the light of [24,25], this tangency problem can be solved as follows. Consider the admissible solution set of problem (14) for a given $s = z$

$$\Delta(z, p) = 0 \tag{17}$$

with $p \in \partial\Omega^B(\rho)$. To simplify analysis suppose that $\delta_i(p)$ are linear in p, i.e. , $h = 0$ in (3) (similar conclusions may be reached if $h \neq 0$). Equation (17) is equivalent to

$$\frac{\Delta(z, \tilde{p})}{\Delta(z, p^o)} = -1 \ . \tag{18}$$

Consider the linear map $L(z, \cdot) : \Omega^B(\rho) \to \mathbf{C}$ defined by the left hand term of (18). The image of $\partial\Omega^B(\rho)$ under this map is the boundary of the convex hull of the mapped vertices of $\Omega^B(\rho)$; hence, all useful information for our problem is contained in the vertices $V_i(\rho)$ of $\Omega^B(\rho)$. Thus, considering mapping of the vertices, we observe that

$$L(z, V_i(\rho)) = L(z, \rho V_i(1)) = \rho L(z, V_i(1)) \ . \tag{19}$$

The map $L(z, \cdot)$ generates a homothetic polytope $\mathcal{P}(\rho)$ in the complex plane. Hence, it easily follows that solution of (15) can be obtained by computing the intercept (in modulus) k of $\partial\mathcal{P}(\rho)$ with the negative real axis for some fixed ρ, say $\rho = 1$, and taking

$$\rho_s(z) = 1/k \ . \tag{20}$$

Of course, the global problem is solved again by sweeping $\partial\Lambda$ as in (16). Notice that the computational burden of this algorithm essentially depends on the computation of $\partial\mathcal{P}(\rho=1)$ for each $z = F(\gamma)$; several algorithms can be used to the purpose (see for example [30] p. 1330). In particular, due to the specific nature of our problem (finding the intersection point of the boundary of the polytope in complex plane with the negative real axis), we do not need construct the whole $\partial\mathcal{P}$ (see also [18]).

4. ROBUST STABILITY OF UNCERTAIN STATE SPACE MODELS: FAMILIES OF MATRICES WITH POLYNOMIALLY CORRELATED PERTURBATIONS

In this section we derive necessary and sufficient conditions to check if the eigenvalues of $A(p)$ have negative real parts. Moreover, we extend the obtained results for investigating eigenvalue location in different regions Λ of the complex plane.
We recall a Lemma on which rely the results of the present section.

Lemma [31]

Let M be a matrix with eigenvalues λ_i, $i = 1,\dots,n$. The eigenvalues μ_{ij} and η_{ij} of $L_1[M]$ and $L_2[M]$ are given respectively by

$$\mu_{ij} = \lambda_i + \lambda_j \quad ,i = 1,\dots,n \quad ,j = i,\dots,n \tag{21}$$

$$\eta_{ij} = \lambda_i \cdot \lambda_j \quad ,i = 1,\dots,n \quad ,j = i,\dots,n \tag{22}$$

Notice that a matrix $\tilde{L}_1[M] \in \mathbf{R}^{n(n-1)/2,n(n-1)/2}$ depending linearly on M can be always found such that

$$det L_1[M] = det M \cdot det \tilde{L}_1[M] \ . \tag{23}$$

Details on the structure of matrix $\tilde{L}_1[M]$ may be found in [31]. Consider a class of matrices $\mathcal{A}(\rho)$ as defined in (9), such that A_o is stable. We state the following theorem relating stability of a matrix $A(p)$ to the nonsingularity of the Kronecker product of $A(p)$ by itself.

Theorem 2
The class of matrices $\mathcal{A}(\rho)$ contains only stable matrices if and only if

$$det\left[I + \textstyle\sum_{i=1}^{l} f_i(p-p^o)L_1[A_i]\cdot L_1^{-1}[A_o]\right] > 0, \quad \forall p \in \Omega^B(\rho) \ . \tag{24}$$

□

Proof (see [18]).

The above Theorem shows that the robust stability problem can be reduced to the positivity test of a multinomial form over a hyperrectangular domain $\Omega^B(\rho)$ in parameter space. We observe that this problem has been widely studied in the literature. In particular, in [26] it is shown that a positivity test can always be reduced to a suitable problem of checking for the existence or the nonexistence of a real solution of a system of $q+1$ polynomial equations in $q+1$ variables. This is in general a hard problem and it requires reasonable computing times only when a limited number of parameters is involved. In this cases, one may take advantage of recently developed computer packages implementing algorithms based on homotopy methods searching for all the solutions of a system of polynomial equations (see [27]).

We now use the preceding general result to give the stability problem an easy and closed form solution when matrix entries depend polynomially on one or two physical uncertain parameters.

4.1 One parameter perturbations ($q = 1$)

Let us rearrange the summation in (8) as

$$\sum_{i=1}^{l} f_i(\tilde{p})A_i = \sum_{j=1}^{u} \tilde{p}^j B_j \tag{25}$$

where u is the maximum degree of $\tilde{p}$ and B_j are suitable constant matrices. The critical criterion for stability easily derives from (24)

$$det[I + \sum_{j=1}^{u} \tilde{p}^j L_1[B_j] \cdot L_1^{-1}[A_o]] = 0 \tag{26}$$

which, in view of a property of determinants (see [33], p.181), is equivalent to finding maximum and minimum real eigenvalues of a suitable matrix F of order $un(n+1)/2$:

$$det[I + \tilde{p}F] = 0 \tag{27}$$

By denoting by μ_M and μ_m respectively the maxinum and minimum real eigenvalues of F and by Λ_c the left half plane, the domain of continuous time stability $\Omega(\Lambda_c)$ for the uncertain matrix can be expressed as

$$\begin{array}{lll} i) & \Omega(\Lambda_c) = \{\tilde{p} : \tilde{p} \in (-1/\mu_M, \infty)\}, & \text{if } 0 \leq \mu_m \leq \mu_M \\ ii) & \Omega(\Lambda_c) = \{\tilde{p} : \tilde{p} \in (-1/\mu_M, -1/\mu_m)\}, & \text{if } \mu_m \leq 0 \leq \mu_M \\ iii) & \Omega(\Lambda_c) = \{\tilde{p} : \tilde{p} \in (-\infty, -1/\mu_m)\}, & \text{if } \mu_m \leq \mu_M \leq 0 \end{array} \tag{28}$$

A similar result for the special case $u = 1$ (linear perturbation) has been derived in [32], [34].

4.2 Two parameter perturbations ($q = 2$)

In this case summation in (8) can be rearranged as

$$\sum_{i=1}^{l} f_i(\tilde{p})A_i = C_o(\tilde{p}_2) + \sum_{j=1}^{u} \tilde{p}_1^j C_j(\tilde{p}_2) = K_o(\tilde{p}_1) + \sum_{j=1}^{u'} \tilde{p}_2^j K_j(\tilde{p}_1) \tag{29}$$

where u and u' are the maximum degrees of $\tilde{p}_1$ and $\tilde{p}_2$ respectively, C_j and K_j are suitable matrices such that $C_o(0) = K_o(0) = 0$. Hence, the critical criterion for stability deriving from (24) can be expressed in two equivalent forms

$$det[I + \tilde{p}_1 G(0)] \cdot det[I + \tilde{p}_2 H(\tilde{p}_1)] = 0 \tag{30}$$

$$det[I + \tilde{p}_2 H(0)] \cdot det[I + \tilde{p}_1 G(\tilde{p}_2)] = 0 \tag{31}$$

where $G(\tilde{p}_2)$ and $H(\tilde{p}_1)$ can be obtained like matrix F of the one parameter case (see [18] for further details).

To test stability of the class of matrices $\mathcal{A}(\rho)$ over a rectangle in parameter space, we must perform two steps.

1-st step - Check if $\partial\Omega^B(\rho) \subset \Omega(\Lambda_c)$.

This is equivalent to evaluating the extremal real eigenvalues of $G(\rho w_2)$, $G(-\rho w_2)$, $H(\rho w_1)$ and $H(-\rho w_1)$.

2-st step - Check for the non existence of unstable interior points in $\Omega^B(\rho)$.

To check for the absence of unstable points, it suffices to verify that the left hand term of (30) (or (31)), denoted by $det[\tilde{p}_1, \tilde{p}_2]$ for notational convenience, is such that the equation system

$$\left[\begin{array}{l} det[\tilde{p}_1, \tilde{p}_2] = 0 \\ \frac{\partial}{\partial \tilde{p}_1} det[\tilde{p}_1, \tilde{p}_2] = 0 \quad (or \frac{\partial}{\partial \tilde{p}_2} det[\tilde{p}_1, \tilde{p}_2] = 0) \end{array} \right. \tag{32}$$

has no solutions interior to $\Omega^B(\rho)$ [35].

By applying the polynomial resultant theorem [36] and letting

$$det[\tilde{p}_1, \tilde{p}_2] = \sum_{j=0}^{s} a_{s-j}(\tilde{p}_2)\tilde{p}_1^j \tag{33}$$

with $s = un(n+1)/2$, the above condition is satisfied if

$$det R(\tilde{p}_2) \neq 0 \quad , -\rho w_2 \leq \tilde{p}_2 \leq \rho w_2 \tag{34}$$

where matrix R is the Sylvester form of (32) (see [18] for specific details). On the contrary, if there exists some value $\tilde{p}_2$, say $\tilde{p}_2^*$, at which (34) does not hold, the test condition is satisfied provided the relation

$$det[\tilde{p}_1, \tilde{p}_2^*] \neq 0 \quad , -\rho w_1 \leq \tilde{p}_1 \leq \rho w_1 \tag{35}$$

is fulfilled.

We observe that checking stability of $\Omega^B(\rho)$ by means of the proposed method requires the solution of four eigenvalue problems like (27) and to check for the existence or not of real solutions in given intervals of a finite number of polynomial equations.

4.2 Λ-stability robustness analysis

The preceding theory can be extended to deal with regions of the complex plane defined as follows

$$\begin{array}{rcl} \Lambda_s & = & \{s \in \mathbf{C} : s \in Sect[\sigma, \theta]\} \\ \Lambda_f & = & \{s \in \mathbf{C} : |\Im[s]| < \omega_o\} \\ \Lambda_d & = & \{s \in \mathbf{C} : |s - d| < r, d \in \mathbf{R}\} \end{array} \tag{36}$$

where $Sect[\sigma, \theta]$ represents a sector in the complex plane defined by σ (displacement of the vertex with respect to the origin of complex plane) and θ (minimum counterclockwise angle between the vertical upper half-line with origin at the point $(\sigma, 0)$ and the two sector sides).

For example, for what concerns regions Λ_s and Λ_f, consider the transformations

$$D(p) = \begin{bmatrix} \cos\theta & -\sin\theta \\ \sin\theta & \cos\theta \end{bmatrix} \otimes (A(p) - \sigma I) \ . \tag{37}$$

and

$$D(p) = \begin{bmatrix} 0 & -1 \\ 1 & 0 \end{bmatrix} \otimes A(p) - \omega_o I \ . \tag{38}$$

It can be easily proven that (37) and (38) map the n eigenvalues of $A(p)$ in Λ_s or Λ_f respectively to the left half plane.

For what concerns the region of pole location Λ_d, which is of interest in discrete system analysis, it can be verified that the check can be reduced to a positivity test over the box $\Omega^B(\rho)$ of the multinomial form (see [18] for details)

$$det\left[r^2 I - L_2[A(p) - dI]\right] \ . \tag{39}$$

Notice that the domain of stability for discrete time systems ($r = 1$ and $d = 0$ in (36) and (39)) can be easily obtained for one parameter perturbations ($q = 1$). In fact, like for continuous time stability, it is will suffice to compute maximum and minimum real eigenvalues of a suitable matrix, given in this case by

$$\begin{bmatrix} \{L_2[A_o - dI, A_1] + L_2[A_1, A_o - dI]\} \cdot [r^2 I - L_2[A_o - dI]]^{-1} & L_2[A_1] \cdot [r^2 I - L_2[A_o - dI]]^{-1} \\ I & 0 \end{bmatrix} . \tag{40}$$

5. APPLICATION EXAMPLES TO CONTROL PROBLEMS

In this section we report numerical results relative to some applications of the results given in section 3 to robustness analysis of control problems. The presented results have been obtained by means of a general program implemented on a personal computer which has been also specialized to deal with the robustness problems described in the following subsections.

Consider a SISO linear feedback control system with plant tranfer function $G(s; p)$ whose coefficients depend linearly on a set of uncertain physical parameters p and with a fixed compensator $C(s)$ such that

$$G(s; p) = \frac{\sum_{i=0}^{m} n_i(p) s^i}{\sum_{i=0}^{n} d_i(p) s^i} \tag{41}$$

$$C(s) = K_c \frac{1 + \sum_{i=1}^{r} n_i^c s^i}{1 + \sum_{i=1}^{s} d_i^c s^i} \ . \tag{42}$$

It is not difficult to show that the closed loop characteristic polynomial coefficients are affine in p and that this is true also when considering SIMO or MISO systems (see e.g. [12]). Thus, the results obtained in section 3 can be used to compute system stability margins for SISO as well as for SIMO or MISO control systems.

By assuming that the controller $C(s)$ stabilizes the nominal plant $G(s;p^o)$, the results of section 3 allow to compute the stability margin of the closed loop system against physical parameters perturbations according to any polyhedral norm. We recall that stability margins in l_2 norms for the same class of perturbations considered here have been derived in [12].

Example 1
Consider the plant

$$G(s;p) = \frac{1}{s^3 + d_2(p)s^2 + d_1(p)s + d_0(p)} \tag{43}$$

where p is a 3-dimensional physical parameter vector and

$$d_2(p) = p_1 + p_2;\ d_1(p) = 2p_1 - p_3;\ d_0(p) = 1 - p_2 + 2p_3 \tag{44}$$

The nominal parameter vector is $p^o = [3,3,1]^t$ and the controller is

$$C(s) = K_c\frac{1 + .667s}{1 + .0667s} \tag{45}$$

with nominal gain $K_c = 15$. It is required to compute the stability margin according to a weighted l_∞ norm defined by $T = diag(w_1^{-1}, w_2^{-1}, w_3^{-1}) = diag(1,1,10)$. Figure 1 shows the function $\rho_s(\gamma)$ which has absolute minimum $\rho^* = 1.83$ at $\gamma = 3.13$.

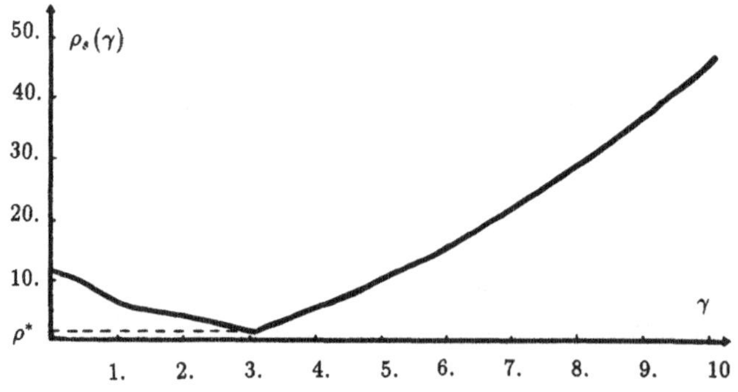

Figure 1. One parameter function $\rho_s(\gamma)$ for the uncertain system of Example 1.

5.2 Pole location region of a feedback control system with a polytope of plants

This problem consists in computing the region $\Psi(\rho)$ in complex plane including all and only the poles of the closed loop system given by (43) and (45), for a given uncertainty polytope $\Omega(\rho)$ in parameter space. $\Psi(\rho)$ is defined as follows

$$\Psi(\rho) = \{s \in \mathbf{C} : \exists p \in \Omega(\rho) | \Delta(s,p) = 0\} \tag{46}$$

The knowledge of this region is of definite interest from a control engineering point of view, because it may give indications on how to adjust the controller parameters in order to confine the uncertain closed loop poles in prescribed regions. The solution of a suitable family of stability margin computations allows one to determine the region $\Psi(\rho)$ for any value of the polytope radius ρ. In fact, consider a family of contours $\partial\Lambda$ covering the whole complex plane. For example, we may consider straight half lines through the origin covering the upper half plane. If we denote by (γ,ϕ) the polar coordinates of a point in the upper half plane, we can consider as family of boundaries the bundle of straight lines through the origin $\{\partial\Lambda(\gamma;\phi) : \gamma \geq 0, 0 \leq \phi \leq \pi\}$. In correspondence to the two dimensional $\partial\Lambda$, a two degrees of freedom function $\rho_s(\gamma,\phi)$ can be defined like in (15). Consider this function for a fixed value ϕ and the line $\rho = \overline{\rho}$ (radius of a given polytope). The possible intersections of these two curves define a set of intervals I_i^ϕ on the γ axis which can be partitioned in two subsets S_1, S_2 such that

$$\begin{aligned} S_1(\phi) &= \{I_i^\phi : \forall\gamma \in I_i^\phi \rightarrow \rho_s(\gamma,\phi) \leq \overline{\rho}\} \\ S_2(\phi) &= \{I_i^\phi : \forall\gamma \in I_i^\phi \rightarrow \rho_s(\gamma,\phi) > \overline{\rho}\} \,. \end{aligned} \tag{47}$$

Notice that intervals belonging to S_1 define points of the complex plane which are roots of at least one polynomial of the given family; the opposite is true for intervals of the set S_2. We observe that the determination of these two sets requires the solution of a one parameter problem.

By allowing ϕ to vary from 0 to π, we are able to construct the region of pole location $\Psi(\overline{\rho})$ as the set

$$\Psi(\overline{\rho}) = \{s \in \mathbf{C} : \gamma \in I_i^\phi \text{ and } I_i^\phi \in S_1(\phi)\} \tag{48}$$

Notice that the determination of regions of pole locations for different values of the radius ρ of the uncertainty polytope does not imply additional computational effort, but only requires to change the threshold value $\overline{\rho}$ in (47).

If $\Psi(\rho)$ belongs to the left half plane, we can define the following quantity

$$\sigma^* = \min_{s\in\Psi(\rho)} |\Re[s]| \,. \tag{49}$$

This quantity, which will be called *degree of stability robustness*, represents meaningful information about a family of uncertain systems, in the sense of measuring how far is the family from instability. Conceptually, it may be considered as a counterpart in the complex plane of the concept of stability margin in parameter space.

Example 1 (continued)
Figure 2 shows two regions of pole location for the closed loop control system given before for two values of the radius $\rho = 1.0$ and $\rho = 2.0$. The obtained degree of stability robustness for the first polytopic family is $\sigma^* = 0.764$.

5.3 Computation of loop gain ranges guaranteeing stability of a polytope of plants

Assume that a nominal plant $G(s;p^o)$ is given with transfer function coefficients subject to polytopic perturbations as described in the preceding subsections. Suppose that there exists a nominal stabilizing controller $C^o(s)$ for the nominal plant. Assume that K_c is the only design parameter of the controller. The problem is to find the set of values of K_c stabilizing the given uncertain family of plants. If we denote by $\overline{\rho}$ the radius of the uncertainty polytope and by $\rho^*(K_c)$ the stability margin of the closed loop system relative to a controller gain K_c, the set of K_c looked for is

$$S_k = \{K_c \in \mathbf{R}^+ : \rho^*(K_c) > \overline{\rho}\} \, .$$

As it can be easily verified, the above set can be computed by solving a family of problems like (16). Notice that the sweep over the parameter K_c can be performed on intervals of K_c which stabilize the nominal plant and which can be computed by an ordinary root locus or Routh-Hurwitz test.

Example 1 (continued)
With reference to the system of Example 1, the stabilizing set S_k obtained for an uncertainty region of radius $\overline{\rho} = 1.0$ is

$$S_k = \{1.2 \leq K_c < 65\}$$

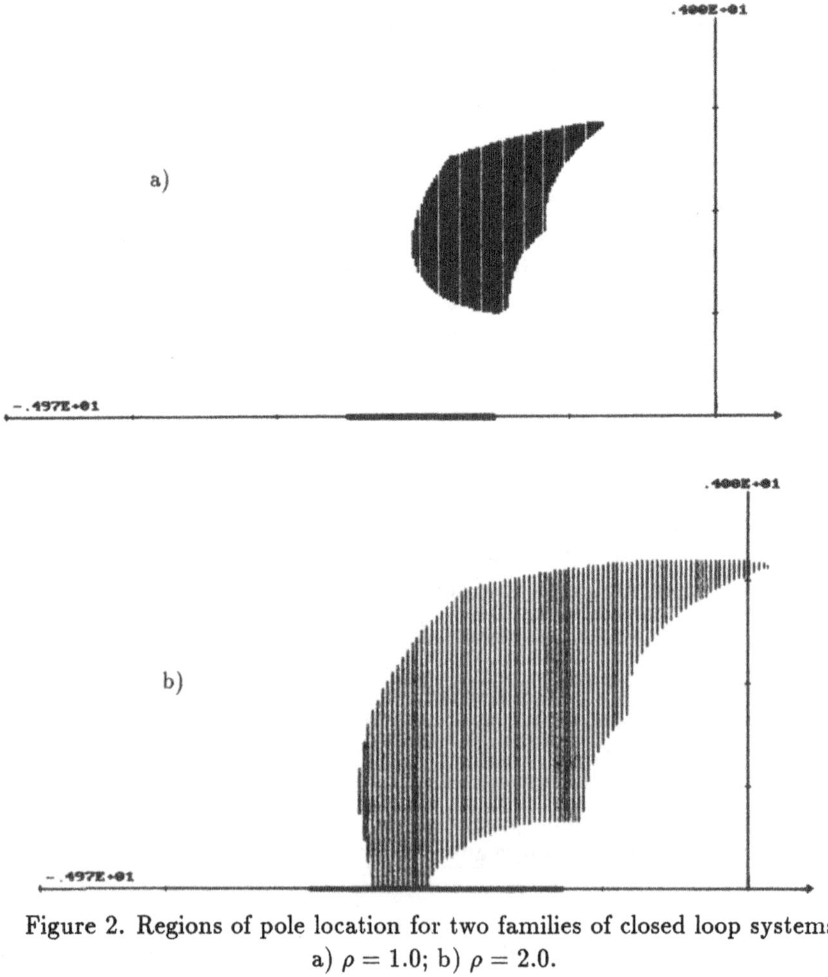

Figure 2. Regions of pole location for two families of closed loop systems: a) $\rho = 1.0$; b) $\rho = 2.0$.

REFERENCES

[1] V. L. Kharitonov, "Asymptotic stability of an equilibrium position of a family of systems of linear differential equations", *Dfferentsial'nye Uravneniya*, vol. 14, pp. 2086-2088, 1978.

[2] A. T. Fam and J. S. Meditch, "A canonical parameter space for linear systems design",*IEEE Trans. on Automat. Contr.*, vol. AC-23, pp. 454-458, 1978

[3] J. Ackermann, " Parameter space design of robust control systems", *IEEE Trans. on Automat. Contr.*, vol. AC-25, pp. 1058-1072, 1980.

[4] B. Ross Barmish, "Invariance of the strict Hurwitz property for polynomials with perturbed coefficients",*IEEE Trans. on Automat. Contr.*, vol. AC-29, pp. 935-936, 1984

[5] Bialas, S. and J. Garloff, " Stability of polynomials under coefficient perturbation", *IEEE Trans. on Automat. Contr.*, vol. AC-30, pp. 310-312, 1985.

[6] C. B. Soh, C. S. Berger and K. P. Dabke, "On the stability properties of polynomials with perturbed coefficients", *IEEE Trans. on Automat. Contr.*, vol. AC-30, pp. 1033-1036, 1985

[7] C. V. Hollot and A. C. Bartlett, "Some discrete-time counterparts to Kharitonov's stability criterion for uncertain systems", *IEEE Trans. on Automat. Contr.*, vol. AC-31, pp. 355-356, 1986

[8] N. K. Bose, E. I. Jury and E. Zeheb, "On robust Hurwitz and Schur polynomials", *Proc. 25-th Conf. on Decision and Control*, Athens(Greece), pp. 739-744, 1986

[9] H. Lin, C. V. Hollot, A. C. Bartlett, "Stability of families of polynomials: geometric considerations in coefficient space",*Int. J. Contr.*, vol. 45, pp. 649-660, 1987

[10] A. C. Bartlett, C. V. Hollot and H. Lin, " Root locations of an entire polytope of polynomials: it suffices to check the edges", *Proc. American Control Conference*, Minneapolis, 1987 and *Mathematics of Controls, Signals and Systems*,1, 1987.

[11] B. R. Barmish and C. L. DeMarco, "Criteria for robust stability with structured uncertainty: a perspective", *Proc. of the American Control Conference*, Minneapolis, 1987.

[12] S. P. Bhattacharyya, *Robust Stabilization Against Structured Perturbations.* Lecture Notes in Control and Information Sciences, 99, Springer Verlag, 1987.

[13] R. M. Biernacki, H. Hwang and S. P. Bhattacharyya, "Robust stability with structured real parameter perturbations" *IEEE Trans. on Automat. Contr.*, vol. AC-32, pp. 495-506, 1987.

[14] H. Chapellat and S. P. Bhattacharyya, "Geometric conditions for the robust stability of interval plants", *TCSP Research Report*, No. 87-020, Texas A&M University, College Station,TX (USA), 1987 and to appear.

[15] B. Ross Barmish, "A generalization of Kharitonov's four polynomial concept for robust stability problems with linearly dependent coefficient perturbations", *Proc. ACC*, Atlanta (USA), 1988.

[16] M. K. Saridereli and F. J. Kern, " The stability of polynomials under correlated coefficient perturbations", *Proc. 26-th Conf. Decision and Control*, Los Angeles (CA), pp. 1618-1621, 1987.

[17] A. Vicino,"Some results on robust stability of discrete time systems", *IEEE Trans. on Automat. Contr.,*, vol. AC-33, pp. 844-847, 1988.

[18] A. Tesi and A. Vicino, "Robustness analysis for uncertain dynamical systems with structured perturbations", *Proc. 27-th Conf. Decision and Control*, Austin (USA), 1988.

[19] A. Vicino, "Results on robustness of pole location in perturbed systems", *Proc. 1988 IFAC Symposium on Identification and System Parameter Estimation*, Beijing (China), pp. 1147-1152, 1988 and to appear in *Automatica*, January 1989.

[20] A. Tesi and A. Vicino, "An efficient algorithm for robust stability analysis of linear control systems with linearly correlated parametric uncertainties", *Res. Rep. , Dipartimento di Sistemi e Informatica, Universitá di Firenze*, Firenze (Italy), 1988.

[21] R. K. Yedavalli, "Improved measures of stability robustness for linear state spce models", *IEEE Trans. on Automat. Contr.*, vol. AC-30, pp. 577-579, 1985.

[22] M. B. Argoun, "On sufficient conditions for the stability of interval matrices", *Int. J. Contr.*, vol. 44, pp. 1245-1250, 1986.

[23] K. Zhou and P. Khargonekar, "Stability robustness bounds for linear state-space models with structured uncertainty", *IEEE Trans. on Automat. Contr.*, vol. AC-32, pp. 621-623, 1987.

[24] A. Sideris and R. R. E. de Gaston, "Multivariable stability margin calculation with uncertain correlated parameters", *Proc. 25-th Conf. Decision and Control*, Athens (Greece), pp. 766-771, 1986.

[25] R. R. E. de Gaston and M. G. Safonov, "Exact calculation of the multiloop stability margin", *IEEE Trans. on Automat. Contr.*, vol. AC-33, pp. 156-171, 1988.

[26] T. A. Bickart and E. I. Jury, "Real polynomials: nonnegativity and positivity", *IEEE Trans. Circuits Syst.*, vol. CAS-25, pp. 676-683, 1978.

[27] L. T. Watson, S. C. Billups and A. P. Morgan, " Hompack: A suite of codes for global convergent homotopy algorithms", *ACM Trans. Mathematical Softw.*, vol. 13, pp. 281-310.

[28] A. Graham, *Kronecker Products and Matrix Calculus With Applications*,Ellis Horwood Ltd., Chichester, 1981.

[29] M. J. Dieudonné, " La théorie analytique des polynomes d'une variable (à coefficients quelconques)", *Memorial des Sciences Mathem.*, Fasc. 93, Paris, 1938.

[30] G. T. Toussaint, "Pattern recognition and geometrical complexity", *Proc. 5-th Int. Conference on Pattern Recognition*, pp. 1324-1347, 1980.

[31] A. T. Fuller, "Conditions for a matrix to have only characteristic roots with negative real parts", *J. Math. Anal. Applic.*, vol. 23, pp. 71-98, 1968.

[32] S. Bialas, "A necessary and sufficient condition for the stability of convex combinations of stable polynomials or matrices", *Bulletin Polish Ac. of Sci.*, vol. 33, pp. 473-480, 1985.

[33] R. Bellman, *Introduction to Matrix Analysis*, McGraw-Hill, New York, 1974.

[34] M. Fu and B. R. Barmish, "Stability of convex and linear combinations of polynomials and matrices arising in robustness problems", *Proc. Conf. on Information Sci. and Systems*, Johns Hopkins University, Baltimore, 1987.

[35] E. Walach and E. Zeheb, "Sign-Test of multivariable real polynomials", *IEEE Trans. on Circuits and Systems*, vol. CAS-27, pp. 619-625, 1980.

[36] B. D. O. Anderson and R. W. Scott, "Output feedback stabilization - Solution by algebraic methods", *Proceedings IEEE*, vol. 65, pp. 849-861, 1977.

[37] D. D. Šiljak, *Large-Scale Dynamic Systems: Stability and Structure*, North Holland, New York, 1978.

[38] Liao Xiao Xin, "Stability of interval matrices", *Int. J. Control*, vol. 45, pp. 203-210, 1987.

MARKOV'S THEOREM OF DETERMINANTS AND THE STABILITY OF FAMILIES OF POLYNOMIALS

C.V. Hollot

Department of Electrical and Computer Engineering
University of Massachusetts
Amherst, MA 01003

I. INTRODUCTION

Amid growing interest in Kharitonov's stability result [4]; e.g., see [7], a theorem due to Markov seems to have been overlooked (at least in this author's opinion.) Markov's "Theorem on Determinants" (see page 241 of [1]) leads to a simple condition for a family of polynomials to be Hurwitz. It requires only two members of the family to be Hurwitz; recall that Kharitonov's Theorem requires four.

There are two possible explanations for this oversight. First, Markov's Theorem was originally motivated by so-called "moment problems" (see Chapter 16 in [1] and [5] for further details) and not by stability problems. Indeed, its not clear just when Markov's result was interpreted from a stability viewpoint, though it appears that this connection was appreciated in the Russian literature as early as 1936; e.g., see [8]. Secondly, Markov's Theorem doesn't work in polynomial coefficient space. Rather, polynomials must be expressed in terms of their associated Markov parameters. As an illustration of such representations, consider the polynomial

$$f(\lambda) = \lambda^4 + 5\lambda^3 + 8\lambda^2 + 8\lambda + 3 = (\lambda^4 + 8\lambda^2 + 3) + \lambda(5\lambda^2 + 8)$$

and form the expansion

$$(5\lambda + 8)/(\lambda^2 + 8\lambda + 3) = 5\lambda^{-1} - 32\lambda^{-2} + 241\lambda^{-3} - 1832\lambda^{-4} + \dots .$$

The four leading coefficients in this series (5, 32, 241, 1832) are the Markov parameters for this fourth degree polynomial. In general, for an nth-degree real polynomial, the n leading coefficients in such an expansion constitute the Markov parameters. Now, its in this "space of Markov parameters" that Markov's theorem is in force. That is, all the polynomials associated with a "box of Markov parameters" are Hurwitz if and only if two vertices (of Markov parameters) are Hurwitz. Thus, to exploit Markov's result, one must work in the space of Markov parameters rather than polynomial coefficient space.

Despite this inconvenience, its felt that Markov's result is important. Variations in physical parameters, (which gives rise to polynomial families) don't respect whether an analyst models a polynomial family in its coefficient space or in its space of Markov parameters. Indeed, for some examples, a box in Markov space may better model the effects of parameter variations than a box in polynomial coefficient space.

In this paper, we (re)expose Markov's stability result and examine its implications in light of Kharitonov's stability theorem. In particular we'll determine the "largest stability box" in the space of Markov parameters and compare it with its "Kharitonov counterpart" in polynomial coefficient space. Perhaps the main contribution of this work is to create an awareness to Markov's Theorem and to motivate applications of this result in the robustness area.

II. MARKOV PARAMETERS OF A POLYNOMIAL

Consider an nth-degree, real polynomial

$$f(\lambda) = a_0\lambda^n + a_1\lambda^{n-1} + \dots + a_n. \tag{2.1}$$

Traditionally, we view the polynomial $f(\lambda)$ as a vector (a_0, a_1,

..., a_n) in its (n+1)-dimensional space of coefficients. Alternatively, we can express $f(\lambda)$ in terms of its so-called Markov parameters. To do this, we first write

$$f(\lambda) = h(\lambda^2) + \lambda g(\lambda^2). \tag{2.2}$$

Assuming that $h(\lambda)$ and $g(\lambda)$ are coprime, we then expand the irreducible rational fraction $g(\lambda)/h(\lambda)$ in a series of decreasing powers of λ

$$\frac{g(\lambda)}{h(\lambda)} = s_{-1} + \frac{s_0}{\lambda} - \frac{s_1}{\lambda^2} + \frac{s_2}{\lambda^3} - \cdots . \tag{2.3}$$

Remark 2.1: If $f(\lambda)$ is Hurwitz; i.e., if $f(\lambda)$ has only roots with negative real parts, then $h(\lambda)$ and $g(\lambda)$ are automatically coprime. This follows since (h,g) must form a positive pair; e.g., see Theorem 13, page 228 of [1], and therefore must have only interlacing roots.

Definition 2.1: Let m=[n/2]. If n=2m, then $(s_0, s_1, \ldots, s_{2m-1})$ are said to be the Markov parameters of $f(\lambda)$. If n=2m+1, then $(s_{-1}, s_0, s_1, \ldots, s_{2m-1})$ constitute the Markov parameters.

It is useful to characterize the relationship between the space of polynomial coefficients $(a_0, a_1, \ldots, a_n)$ and the space of Markov parameters $(s_{-1}, s_0, s_1, \ldots, s_{2m-1})$. In the following we'll assume that n is even and hence $s_{-1}=0$.

Let $A \subset R^{n+1}$ denote the set of all polynomial coefficients for which $h(\lambda)$ and $g(\lambda)$ are coprime. That is, $(a_0, a_1, \ldots, a_n) \varepsilon A$ implies that $h(\lambda)$ and $g(\lambda)$ are coprime and

$$a_0\lambda^n + a_1\lambda^{n-1} + \ldots + a_n = h(\lambda^2) + \lambda g(\lambda^2). \tag{2.4}$$

Define the mapping $\phi: A \subset R^{n+1} \rightarrow R(\phi) \subset R^n$ by

$$\phi[(a_0, a_1, \ldots, a_n)] = (s_0, s_1, \ldots, s_{2m-1}) \tag{2.5}$$

where $R(\phi)$ denotes the range of ϕ and where the s_i, $i=0,1,\ldots,2m-1$ are the leading, 2m coefficients in the expansion (2.3) and h and g are given in (2.4).

Remarks 2.2: (i) Mapping ϕ gives the transformation from the space of polynomial coefficients (for those polynomials with g and h coprime) to the space of Markov parameters.

(ii) Each vector $(s_0,s_1,\ldots,s_{2m-1})\varepsilon R(\phi)$ generates a (finite) Hankel matrix

$$S_m \triangleq \begin{bmatrix} s_0 & s_1 & \cdots & s_{m-1} \\ s_1 & s_2 & & \\ \vdots & & & \\ s_{m-1} & s_m & \cdots & s_{2m-2} \end{bmatrix} \tag{2.6}$$

of rank m; see Theorem 8 on page 207 of [1]. Using this fact it follows from Theorem 7 on page 205 of [1] that the subsequent coefficients s_{2m}, $s_{2m+1},\ldots$ in series (2.3) are uniquely determined by the 2m numbers $s_0,s_1,\ldots,s_{2m-1}$. Thus, an nth-degree real polynomial $f(\lambda)$, with h and g coprime, is uniquely determined (to within a constant factor) by its Markov parameters. In other words, if A is equipped with a suitable equivalance relation, then ϕ is one-to-one.

(iii) Let $B \subset R^n$ be all those vectors $(s_0,s_1,\ldots,s_{2m-1})$ for which the corresponding S_m in (2.6) has rank m. We claim that ϕ is onto B; i.e., $R(\phi)=B$. To see this, let some arbitrary $(s_0,s_1,\ldots,s_{2m-1})\varepsilon B$ be given. Since S_m in (2.6) has rank m, then these numbers uniquely determine coefficients $\alpha_1,\alpha_2,\ldots,\alpha_m$ through

$$s_q = \sum_{g=1}^{m} \alpha_g s_{q-g}, \quad q = m, m+1,\ldots,2m-1. \tag{2.7}$$

Now, let s_{2m}, $s_{2m+1},\ldots$ be generated from this recursion; i.e., take

$$s_q = \sum_{g=1}^{m} \alpha_g s_{q-g}, \quad q = 2m, 2m+1, \ldots . \tag{2.8}$$

Theorem 8 on page 207 of [1] states that the sum of the series

$$R(\lambda) = \frac{s_0}{\lambda} - \frac{s_1}{\lambda^2} + \frac{s_2}{\lambda^3} - \ldots$$

is a <u>rational</u> <u>function</u> of λ. Thus, we can write $R(\lambda) = g(\lambda)/h(\lambda)$ and form

$$f(\lambda) = h(\lambda^2) + \lambda g(\lambda^2) = a_0\lambda^n + a_1\lambda^{n-1} + \ldots + a_n. \tag{2.9}$$

Hence, $\phi[(a_0,a_1,\ldots,a_n)]=(s_0,s_1,\ldots,s_{2m-1})$ and ϕ is onto B. Moreover, if the polynomials h and g in (2.9) are

$$h(\lambda) = d_0\lambda^m + d_1\lambda^{m-1} + \ldots + d_m \tag{2.10}$$

and

$$g(\lambda) = c_1\lambda^{m-1} + c_2\lambda^{m-2} + \ldots + c_m \tag{2.11}$$

then the c_i and d_i are related to the Markov parameters via the following relations:

$$\begin{bmatrix} d_m/d_0 \\ d_{m-1}/d_0 \\ \vdots \\ d_1/d_0 \end{bmatrix} = \begin{bmatrix} s_0 & -s_1 & \ldots & (-1)^{m-1}s_{m-1} \\ -s_1 & s_2 & & \\ \vdots & & & \\ (-1)^{m-1}s_{m-1} & (-1)^m s_m & \ldots & s_{2m-2} \end{bmatrix}^{-1} \begin{bmatrix} (-1)^m s_m \\ (-1)^{m+1}s_{m+1} \\ \vdots \\ (-1)^{2m}s_{2m-1} \end{bmatrix}$$

$$\begin{aligned} c_1 &= d_0 s_0; \\ c_2 &= -d_0 s_1 + d_1 s_0; \\ &\vdots \\ c_m &= (-1)^{m-1} d_0 s_{m-1} + (-1)^{m-2} d_1 s_{m-2} + \ldots + d_{m-1}s_0. \end{aligned} \tag{2.12}$$

•

We collect these facts in the next lemma.

Lemma 2.1: Consider sets A and B as described in Remarks 2.2. The mapping ϕ defined in (2.3) - (2.5), which transforms the space of polynomial coefficients to the space of Markov parameters, is one-to-one and onto B. The inverse of ϕ is determined from (2.9) - (2.12).

∇∇∇

III. CONVEXITY OF THE HURWITZ REGION IN THE SPACE OF MARKOV PARAMETERS

It is known; e.g., see [2], that the Hurwitz region in the space of polynomial coefficients is not convex. In contrast, the Hurwitz region in the space of Markov parameters is.

Definition 3.1: The Markov parameters $(s_0, s_1, \ldots, s_{2m-1})$ (n=2m) or $(s_{-1}, s_0, \ldots, s_{2m})$ (n=2m+1) are said to be Hurwitz if the real polynomial $f(\lambda)=a_0\lambda^n+a_1\lambda^{n-1}+\ldots+a_n$ is Hurwitz where $\phi(a_0,a_1,\ldots,a_n)]=(s_0,s_1,\ldots, s_{2m-1})$.

The key result in showing the convexity of the Hurwitz region in Markov space is contained in the next lemma.

Lemma 3.1 (see Theorem 17, page 235 of [1] for proof): The Markov parameters $(s_0, s_1, \ldots, s_{2m-1})$ (n=2m) or $(s_{-1}, s_0, \ldots, s_{2m-1})$ (n=2m+1) is Hurwitz if and only if the two finite Hankel matrices

$$S_m \triangleq \begin{bmatrix} s_0 & s_1 & \cdots & s_{m-1} \\ s_1 & s_2 & & \\ \vdots & & & \\ s_{m-1} & s_m & \cdots & s_{2m-2} \end{bmatrix} ; \quad S_m^{(1)} \triangleq \begin{bmatrix} s_1 & s_2 & \cdots & s_m \\ s_2 & s_3 & & \\ \vdots & & & \\ s_m & s_{m+1} & \cdots & s_{2m-1} \end{bmatrix} \tag{3.1}$$

are positive-definite (and $s_{-1}>0$ when n=2m+1).

∇∇∇

We now have the following.

Theorem 3.1: The space of all Hurwitz Markov parameters is a convex cone.

Proof: Since the space of positive-definite matrices is a convex cone and since the entries of S_m and $S_m^{(1)}$ in (3.1) depend linearly on the Markov parameters then Theorem 3.1 follows immediately from Lemma 3.1. ∇∇∇

A consequence of this theorem is that a polytope (of Markov parameters) is Hurwitz if and only if the polytope's vertices are stable. To be precise, let Ω be the convex hull of a finite set of points (vertices) ω_i, $i=1,2,\ldots,l$ in Markov space.

Corollary 3.1: The polytope Ω is Hurwitz if and only if each vertex ω_i, $i=1,2,\ldots,l$ (of Markov parameters) is Hurwitz.

IV. LARGEST STABILITY BOX IN THE SPACE OF MARKOV PARAMETERS: AN APPLICATION OF MARKOV'S THEOREM OF DETERMINANTS

In [3], Barmish shows how the largest stability box in the space of polynomial coefficients can be determined. Envoking the remarkable stability result of Kharitonov [4], he demonstrates that the dimensions of such a stability box can be deduced from only four, uncoupled, one-parameter problems. Recall that Kharitonov's theorem states that a box of polynomials (in polynomial coefficient space) is Hurwitz if and only if four vertex polynomials are Hurwitz.

As a counterpart to [3], we'll now show that the largest stability box (in the space of Markov parameters) can be deduced from two, uncoupled, one-parameter problems. This result follows from a straightforward application of yet another remarkable stability theorem - Markov's Theorem; e.g., see the "Theorem of Determinants" and Theorem 21 on pages 241 and 242 of [1]. Markov's Theorem states that a box in the space of Markov parameters is Hurwitz if and only if two vertices of Markov parameters are Hurwitz.

The problem of determining the largest stability box in the space of Markov parameters begins by assuming some Hurwitz Markov parameters $(s_0,s_1,\ldots,s_{2m-1})$; for simplicity we will restrict our attention to the case when n is even. Given some $\varepsilon>0$ we define a box in the space of Markov parameters by

$$M_\varepsilon \overset{\Delta}{=} \{\sigma: |s_i - \sigma_i| < \varepsilon, \ i = 0,2,\ldots,2m-1\} \tag{4.1}$$

Our goal is to find the largest number ε, defined ε_{max}, for which $M_{\varepsilon_{max}}$ contains only Hurwitz Markov parameters.

Remark 4.1: (i) For $\varepsilon=0$, M_ε reduces to the "nominal" Markov parameters $(s_0,s_1,\ldots,s_{2m-1})$ which by assumption are Hurwitz.

(ii) The box M_ε given in (4.1) is less general than those considered in [3]. Presently, M_ε allows for only equally weighted perturbations in all the Markov parameters while in [3] unequal weightings in the polynomial coefficients are admissible. We confine ourselves to the special case of equal weightings for the sake of notational conciseness and do so without loss of generality since the following theorem is also valid for these more general boxes.

Theorem 4.1: *Let $\underline{\varepsilon}$ and $\bar{\varepsilon}$ be the largest numbers ε for which the two respective sets of Markov parameters*

$$\underline{s} \overset{\Delta}{=} (s_0-\varepsilon,\ s_1+\varepsilon,\ s_2-\varepsilon,\ \ldots,\ s_{2m-1}+\varepsilon); \tag{4.2}$$

$$\bar{s} \overset{\Delta}{=} (s_0+\varepsilon,\ s_1-\varepsilon,\ s_1+\varepsilon,\ \ldots,\ s_{2m-1}-\varepsilon) \tag{4.3}$$

are Hurwitz. Then,

$$\varepsilon_{max} = \min\{\underline{\varepsilon},\ \bar{\varepsilon}\}. \tag{4.4}$$

Proof: The proof follows immediately from a version of Markov's Theorem (see Theorem 21, page 242 of [1]) which can be paraphrased in the present context as follows. Let any $\varepsilon>0$ be given. Then, the box M_ε contains only Hurwitz Markov parameters if and only if the two sets of Markov parameters, $(s_0-\varepsilon, s_1+\varepsilon, s_2-\varepsilon, \ldots, s_{2m-1}+\varepsilon)$ and $(s_0+\varepsilon, s_1-\varepsilon, s_2+\varepsilon, \ldots, s_{2m-1}-\varepsilon)$ are Hurwitz. Its now clear that ε_{max} is given by (4.4). ∇∇∇

Remarks 4.2: (i) To determine the $\underline{\varepsilon}$ and $\bar{\varepsilon}$ required in Theorem 4.1, one need only execute some one-parameter problems. Using Lemma 3.1 we see that $\underline{\varepsilon}$ is the largest ε for which

$$\begin{bmatrix} s_0-\varepsilon & s_1+\varepsilon & \cdots & s_{m-1}+\varepsilon \\ s_1+\varepsilon & s_2-\varepsilon & & \\ \vdots & & & \\ s_{m-1}+\varepsilon & s_m-\varepsilon & \cdots & s_{2m-1}-\varepsilon \end{bmatrix} ; \begin{bmatrix} s_1+\varepsilon & s_2-\varepsilon & \cdots & s_m-\varepsilon \\ s_2-\varepsilon & s_3+\varepsilon & & \\ \vdots & & & \\ s_m-\varepsilon & s_{m+1}+\varepsilon & \cdots & s_m+\varepsilon \end{bmatrix} \tag{4.5}$$

are both positive-definite. Similarly, $\bar{\varepsilon}$ is the largest ε such that

$$\begin{bmatrix} s_0+\varepsilon & s_1-\varepsilon & \cdots & s_{m-1}-\varepsilon \\ s_1-\varepsilon & s_2+\varepsilon & & \\ \vdots & & & \\ s_{m-1}-\varepsilon & s_m+\varepsilon & \cdots & s_{2m-1}+\varepsilon \end{bmatrix} ; \begin{bmatrix} s_1-\varepsilon & s_2+\varepsilon & \cdots & s_m+\varepsilon \\ s_2+\varepsilon & s_3-\varepsilon & & \\ \vdots & & & \\ s_m+\varepsilon & s_{m+1}-\varepsilon & \cdots & s_m-\varepsilon \end{bmatrix} \tag{4.6}$$

are both positive-definite.

(ii) Compared to computing the largest stability box in polynomial coefficient space, the computational burden in determining the largest box in the space of Markov parameters is roughly one-half. In coefficient space one must determine whether all the leading principal minors of four, n-dimensional Hurwitz testing matrices are positive. In contrast, Theorem 4.1 requires one to check the positivity of all the leading principal minors of four, $\frac{n}{2}$ - dimensional Hankel matrices.

(iii) Perhaps more important than these computational savings is the <u>difference</u> between the largest stability boxes in polynomial coefficient space and the space of Markov parameters. That is, suppose that P_{max} and $M_{\varepsilon_{max}}$ denote the largest stability boxes in polynomial coefficient and Markov parameter space respectively. Furthermore, assume that these boxes are generated from the same "nominal" polynomial. Then, the image $\phi(P_{max})$ (ϕ is described in equations (2.3)-(2.5)) neither contains nor is contained in $M_{\varepsilon_{max}}$. This fact will be illustrated in the following example.

V. EXAMPLE

In this section we will use Theorem 4.1 to determine the largest stability box in the space of Markov parameters. To make comparison with [3] we choose

$$f(\lambda) = \lambda^4 + 5\lambda^3 + 8\lambda^2 + 8\lambda + 3 \qquad (5.1)$$

as the nominal Hurwitz polynomial. In [3], the largest stability box in polynomial coefficient space (relative to this $f(\lambda)$) was determined to be

$$P_{max} \triangleq \{(\alpha_1,\alpha_2,\alpha_3,\alpha_4) : |\alpha_i - a_i| < 1.81\}. \qquad (5.2)$$

Using (2.2) and (2.3) the Markov parameters for $f(\lambda)$ are

$$(s_0,s_1,\ldots,s_{2m-1}) = (5,\ 32,\ 241,\ 1832). \qquad (5.3)$$

To find the largest stability box in Markov space we use Remark 4.2(i) and take $\underline{\varepsilon}$ to be the largest number ε such that

$$\begin{bmatrix} 5-\varepsilon & 32+\varepsilon \\ 32+\varepsilon & 241-\varepsilon \end{bmatrix} ; \quad \begin{bmatrix} 32+\varepsilon & 241-\varepsilon \\ 241-\varepsilon & 1832+\varepsilon \end{bmatrix} \tag{5.4}$$

are both positive-definite and $\bar{\varepsilon}$ to be the largest ε for which

$$\begin{bmatrix} 5+\varepsilon & 32-\varepsilon \\ 32-\varepsilon & 241+\varepsilon \end{bmatrix} ; \quad \begin{bmatrix} 32-\varepsilon & 241+\varepsilon \\ 241+\varepsilon & 1832-\varepsilon \end{bmatrix} \tag{5.5}$$

are both positive-definite. Computation gives

$$\underline{\varepsilon} \tilde{=} .584 ; \quad \bar{\varepsilon} \tilde{=} .2314. \tag{5.6}$$

From (4.4), $\varepsilon_{max} \tilde{=} .2314$ so that from (4.1)

$$M_{\varepsilon_{max}} = \{(\sigma_0, \sigma_1, \sigma_2, \sigma_3) : |\sigma_i - s_i| < .2314\}. \tag{5.7}$$

To compare P_{max} and $M_{\varepsilon_{max}}$, we first compute $\phi^{-1}(M_{\varepsilon_{max}})$; that is, using (2.9)-(2.12) we determine those polynomial coefficients corresponding to all Markov parameters in $M_{\varepsilon_{max}}$. We then project the sets $\phi^{-1}(M_{\varepsilon_{max}})$ and P_{max} onto the (a_3, a_4) plane; see Figure 1. From this figure we see that P_{max} neither contains nor is contained in $\phi^{-1}(M_{\varepsilon_{max}})$. This is a useful observation; it indicates that for certain problems its possible to get "tighter" stability estimates using this Markov space approach.

VI. THE CHEBYSHEV-MARKOV THEOREM OF ROOTS

The Chebyshev-Markov Theorem (of roots) gives further insight into the relationship between a polynomial's Markov parameters and the zeroes of key polynomials. Specifically, this result shows how the

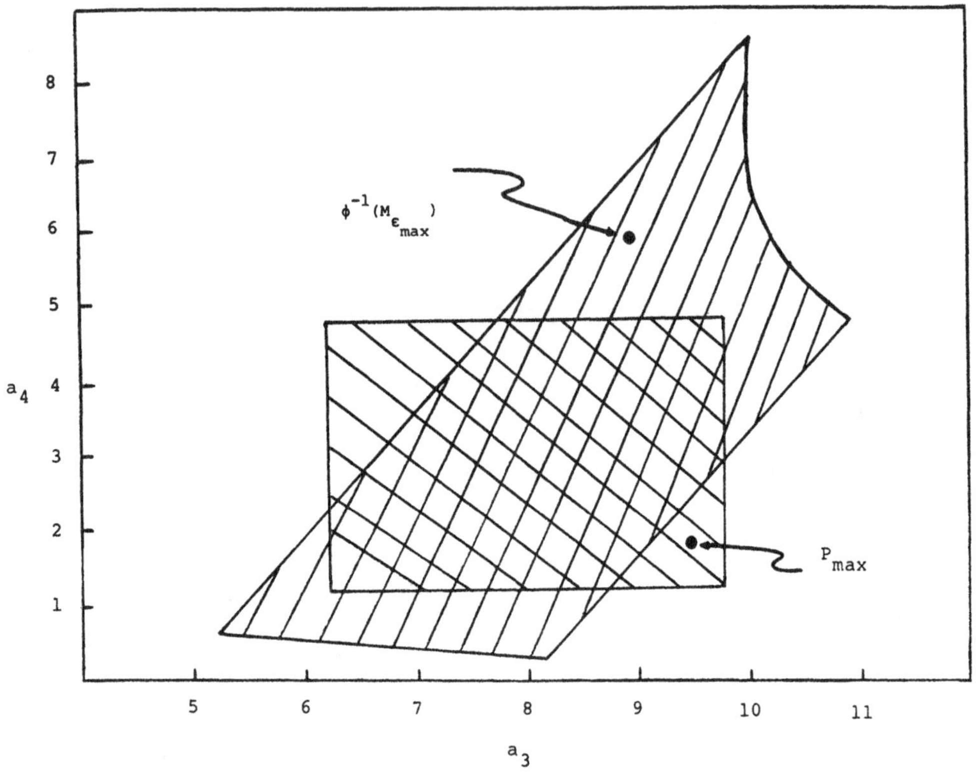

Figure 1. In Section V we found the largest stable box of Markov parameters $M_{\varepsilon_{max}}$. The corresponding largest stable box of polynomial coefficients P_{max} was determined in [3]. In this figure we compare these boxes in coefficient space. Projecting these solids onto the a3 - a4 coefficient plane we see that the Kharitonov box P_{max} neither contains nor is contained in the pre-image of the Markov box $M_{\varepsilon_{max}}$.

zeroes of the "even portion" of a Hurwitz polynomial changes as a function of variations in the corresponding Markov parameters. In the following we'll state this result, illustrate it and draw comparisons with similar behavior found in Kharitonov's stable boxes.

To begin, assume n=2m and let

$$f(\lambda) = a_0\lambda^n + a_1\lambda^{n-1} + \ldots + a_n$$
$$= h(\lambda^2) + \lambda g(\lambda^2)$$

and

$$\phi[(a_0,a_1, \ldots, a_n)] = (s_0,s_1, \ldots, s_{2m-1}).$$

With $f(\lambda)$ Hurwitz, it follows from the Hermite-Biehler Theorem (see [1]) that the zeroes of h(u) are real, negative and distinct. We order these zeroes as

$$u_m < u_{m-1} < \ldots < u_1 < 0$$

and state the Chebyshev-Markov Theorem - it's proof can be found on page 247 of [1].

Theorem 6.1 (Chebyshev-Markov Theorem of Roots): *If* $f(\lambda)$ *is Hurwitz, then for* i=1,2, ..., m

$$(-1)^k \frac{du_i}{ds_k} > 0, \quad k = 1,2, \ldots, 2m-1. \tag{6.1}$$

∇∇∇

Remarks 6.1: (i) This theorem says that the roots of h(u) increase with increasing s_0, s_2, ..., s_{2m-2} and with decreasing s_1, s_3, ..., s_{2m-1}.

(ii) The preceding remark has particular significance for a box of Hurwitz Markov parameters. For example, consider the box M_ε in (4.1) for some $\varepsilon>0$ for which $\underline{s}$ and $\overline{s}$ are both Hurwitz. This implies, using Theorem 4.1, that all of M_ε is Hurwitz. Now, let

$$\phi^{-1}[\underline{s}] \overset{\Delta}{=} h_{\underline{s}}(\lambda^2) + \lambda g_{\underline{s}}(\lambda^2); \qquad \phi^{-1}[\bar{s}] \overset{\Delta}{=} h_{\bar{s}}(\lambda^2) + \lambda g_{\bar{s}}(\lambda^2).$$

Since $\underline{s}$ and $\bar{s}$ are both Hurwitz, then the zeroes of $h_{\underline{s}}$ and $h_{\bar{s}}$ are real, negative and distinct. Order the zeroes of $h_{\underline{s}}$ and $h_{\bar{s}}$ as

$$\underline{u}_m < \underline{u}_{m-1} < \dots < \underline{u}_1 < 0; \quad \bar{u}_m < \bar{u}_{m-1} < \dots < \bar{u}_1 < 0$$

respectively. Now, any Markov parameter $s \varepsilon M_\varepsilon$, has components s_0, s_2, ..., s_{2m-2} larger than the corresponding components of $\underline{s}$. Similarly, this Markov parameter s has components s_1, s_3, ..., s_{2m-1} smaller than the corresponding components of $\underline{s}$. It thus follows from the preceding remark that if

$$\phi^{-1}[s] = h_s(\lambda^2) + \lambda g_s(\lambda^2)$$

with the zeroes of h_s ordered as

$$u_m < u_{m-1} < \dots < u_1 < 0,$$

then

$$\underline{u}_i < u_i < \bar{u}_i, \quad i = 1,2, \dots, m. \tag{6.2}$$

This relationship is depicted in Figure 2a.

(iii) Remark (ii) is especially interesting in light of Kharitonov's result. To illustrate, consider a Hurwitz box of polynomials in coefficient space. The four Kharitonov polynomials can be written as

$$K_1(\lambda) = h_+(\lambda^2) + \lambda g_+(\lambda^2),$$
$$K_2(\lambda) = h_+(\lambda^2) + \lambda g_-(\lambda^2),$$
$$K_3(\lambda) = h_-(\lambda^2) + \lambda g_-(\lambda^2)$$

and

$$K_4(\lambda) = h_-(\lambda^2) + \lambda g_+(\lambda^2)$$

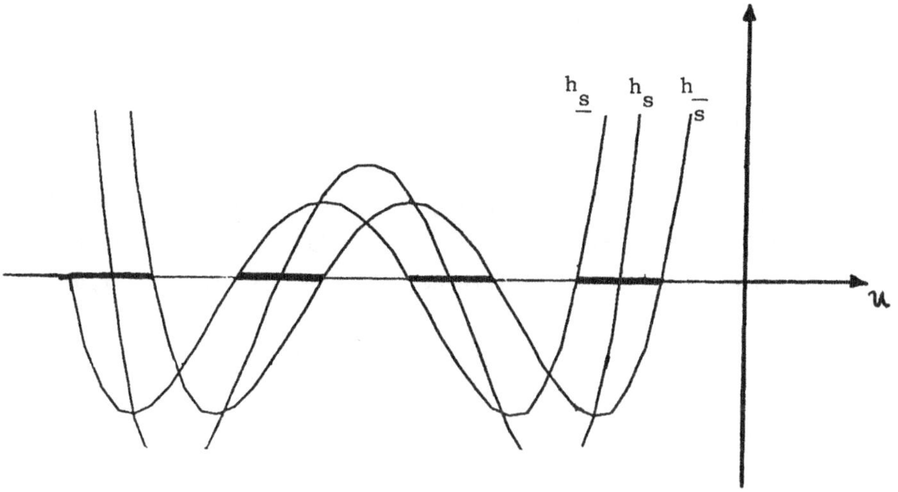

Figure 2a. The Chebyshev-Markov Theorem of Roots shows how the zeroes of h_s (the even portion of any Markov-box polynomial) lie in intervals defined by the zeroes of $h_{\underline{s}}$ and $h_{\bar{s}}$ (even portions of $\underline{s}$ and $\bar{s}$, the special vertices of a Markov box). Compare this figure to Kharitonov's result illustrated in Figure 2b.

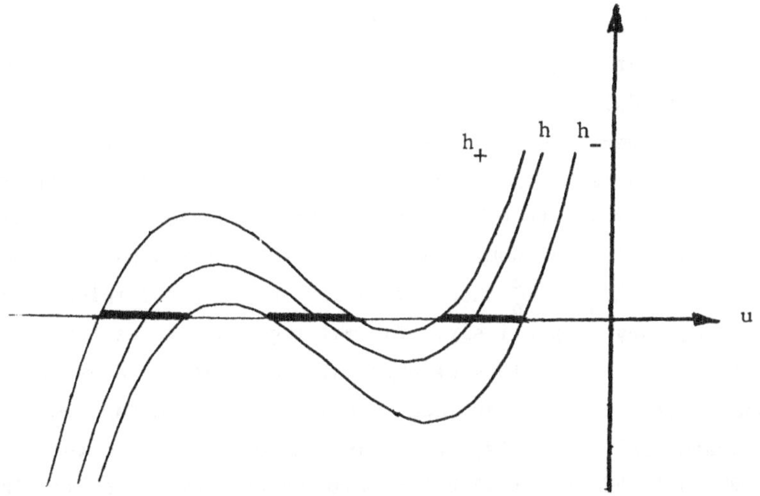

Figure 2b. The even portion h(u) of any polynomial in a box of Hurwitz polynomials in coefficient space is bounded by $h_-(u)$ and $h_+(u)$. Thus, the zeroes of h(u) are defined by the zeroes of $h_-(u)$ and $h_+(u)$. These last two polynomials are the even portions of the Kharitonov polynomials. Compare this fact to the Chebyshev-Markov Theorem illustrated in Figure 2a.

where $h_-(u)$, $h_+(u)$, $g_-(u)$ and $g_+(u)$ have the following property. Any polynomial $f(\lambda)=h(\lambda^2)+\lambda g(\lambda^2)$ in this box satisfies

$$h_-(u) \leq h(u) \leq h_+(u); \qquad g_-(u) \leq g(u) \leq g_+(u).$$

Consequently, the roots of h(u) and g(u) lie in intervals defined by $h_-(u)$, $h_+(u)$, $g_-(u)$ and $g_+(u)$. This is illustrated in Figure 2b - notice the similarities and differences to the Markov couterpart in Figure 2a.

(iv) Finally, we remark that a version of the Chebyshev-Markov Theorem does not hold for for the odd polynomials $g_s(u)$. This fact was pointed out by Anderson [10].

FINAL REMARKS

In this paper we have placed Markov's Theorem (of Determinants) in context with Kharitonov's stability result. It will be interesting to see its impact in the robustness area; will we find it useful to pose polynomial problems in the space of Markov parameters? When this paper was presented at the Torino Workshop, Professors C.A. Desoer (University of California, Berkeley) and M. Mansour (ETH, Zurich) made some pointed comments to this last question. First, Professor Desoer noted that physical significance must be attached to the Markov parameters if they are to prove useful. For example, in coefficient space a second-order polynomial $\lambda^2 + a_1\lambda + a_2$ admits a physical parameterization $\lambda^2 + 2\zeta\omega_n\lambda + \omega_n^2$ where $\zeta\omega_n$ and ω_n represent damping and the natural frequency respectively. The damping and natural frequency can be directly related to values of physical components such as resistors and capacitors or inertias and springs. Can the same be done for Markov parameters? Secondly, Professor Mansour pointed to a "box" result which is "four times" better than Kharitonov's result! Instead of considering polynomials in coefficient or Markov space, he suggests expressing an nth-degree polynomial in terms of its so-called n-dimensional "Hurwitz parameters." The Hurwitz parameters are the values of the n leading principal minors of the corresponding Hurwitz matrix. Clearly, a box of Hurwitz parameters is stable; i.e., positive, if and only if the vertex closest to the origin is stable! This is an important point since it illustrates the potential weakness of Markov (and Hurwitz parameters) relative to the power of Kharitonov's result. That is, systems and control problems appear to be most easily stated and analyzed in terms of polynomial coefficients - the space where Kharitonov's result is in force. In contrast, the computational burden or conservatism encountered in translating given system parameters to Markov or Hurwitz parameters may outweigh the "twice" or "four times" niceness recorded here.

REFERENCES

[1] F.R. Gantmacher, The Theory of Matrices, Vol. 2, Chelsea, New York, 1960.

[2] S. Bialas and J. Garloff, "Convex Combinations of Stable Polynomials," Journal of the Franklin Institute, Vol. 319, pp. 373-377, 1985.

[3] B.R. Barmish, "Invariance of the Strict Hurwitz Property for Polynomials With Perturbed Coefficients," IEEE Transactions on Automatic Control, Vol. 29, pp.935-936, 1984.

[4] V.L. Kharitonov, "Asymptotic Stability of an Equilibrium Position of a Family of Systems of Linear Differential Equations," Differential'nye Uravneniya, Vol. 14, pp. 2086-2088, 1978.

[5] M.G. Krein and A.A. Nudel'man, The Markov Moment Problem and Extremal Problems, Translations of Mathematical Monographs, Vol. 50, American Mathematical Society, Providence, Rhode Island, 1977.

[6] A.A. Markov, Collected Works, Nauka, Moscow, pp. 78-105, 1948.

[7] B.R. Barmish and C.L. Demarco, "Criteria for Robust Stability of Systems With Structured Uncertainty: A Perspective," Proceedings of the 1987 American Control Conference, Minneapolis, pp. 476-481, 1987.

[8] M.G. Krein and M.A. Naimark, The Method of Symmetric and Hermetian Forms in the Theory of Separation of Roots of Algebraic Equations, Kharkov, GNTI, 1936 (in Russian).

[9] M. Vidyasagar and N. Viswanadham, "Algebraic Design Techniques for Reliable Stabilization," IEEE Transactions on Automatic Control, Vol. 27, pp. 1085-1095, 1982.

[10] B.D.O. Anderson, Private Communication, June, 1988.

AN APPLICATION OF STATE SPACE METHODS TO OBTAIN EXPLICIT FORMULAE FOR ROBUSTNESS MEASURES OF POLYNOMIALS

D. Hinrichsen
Institute for Dynamical Systems
University of Bremen
2800 Bremen 33, FRG

A.J. Pritchard
Control Theory Centre
University of Warwick
Coventry CV4 7AL, UK

Abstract

In this paper we study the stability radii of polynomials under structured perturbations of the coefficient vector. Given an open subset $\mathbf{C}_g$ of the complex plane the stability radius measures the size of the smallest complex or real perturbation that moves at least one root of the polynomial out of $\mathbf{C}_g$. New formulae for both the complex and the real case are derived and specialized, for various perturbation structures and perturbation norms. Moreover it is shown how to compute the stability radii of Hurwitz polynomials under structured perturbations. The results are illustrated and compared with existing robustness criteria by a number of examples.

1. INTRODUCTION

Many desirable properties of linear feedback systems can be expressed by the requirement that the closed loop characteristic polynomial has all its roots in a prescribed open subset $\mathbf{C}_g$ of the complex plane. Since the coefficient vector of this polynomial depends upon the physical parameters of a plant, it will be subject to perturbations and uncertainties. A basic task of robustness analysis is to determine which variations of the coefficient vector a given nominal polynomial can tolerate without loosing the property that all its roots are in $\mathbf{C}_g$.

This problem has received a good deal of attention in the recent literature, where the main emphasis has been on the two special cases of *Hurwitz* and *Schur* polynomials (i.e. $\mathbf{C}_g = \mathbf{C}_-$, the open left half plane or $\mathbf{C}_g = \mathbf{C}_1$, the open unit disc).

One way of deriving sufficient conditions for certain *sets of polnomials* is via a careful analysis of existing stability criteria for single polynomials. The most prominent of this type of result is Kharitonov's Theorem [1] which is based on the so-called Hermite-Biehler stability criterion, see [2, p.228]. Extensions and system theoretic applications of this theorem have recently been given e.g. in [3] - [8]. Other stability results for sets of polynomials have been derived from the Nyquist stability criterion (see [9],[10]) or from more recent sufficient stability criteria due to Lipatov and Sokolov [11] and Nie and Xie [12] (see [8], [13]).

A different approach to robust stability analysis of polynomials is based on optimization ideas. A class of special subsets in the coefficient space (e.g. ellipsoids or polytopes) is parametrized by a positive real number, and the supremum of all parameter values for which the corresponding subset consists only of Hurwitz (or Schur) polynomials, is determined. In the context of Kharitonov's Theorem optimization problems are considered in [14],[15]. An independent approach was pursued by Soh et al.[16] who characterized the distance of a Schur (or Hurwitz) polynomial from the set of non-Schur (resp. non-Hurwitz) polynomials in the coefficient space. Extensions of their formulae to other stability domains and to structured perturbations can be found in [17] and [18]. Mathematically these investigations are based on a paper of Fam and Meditch [19] describing the topological boundary of the set of real Schur polynomials in the coefficient space.

In view of the significant recent progress in the stability analysis of uncertain polynomials, several authors have tried to generalize these results to uncertain *matrices* and *systems*. It was soon recognized that a direct extension of Kharitonov's result to interval matrices [20] was not feasible [21].The results of Soh et al.[16] were extended to single input or single output systems in [18].

In the present paper we proceed in the reverse direction and derive new robustness results for polynomials from a general theory of the *stability radius* of linear state space systems. This theory of stability radii has been developed over the last three years, see [22]-[29]. The results of this paper are based on [23] and [29]. We hope that the new formulae that we present and the ease by which they are obtained will demonstrate the applicability of the general theory. It yields a unifying framework for the robustness analysis of polynomials. For instance, the radius of the largest stability hypersphere studied in [16] is a special case of the unstructured real stability radius whereas the radius investigated in [18] is a special case of the structured real stability radius.

One of the main advantages of our approach is that the reliable and efficient algorithm developed in [26],[28] for computing the complex stability radius of stable systems can now be applied to determine the stability radii of Hurwitz polynomials. The question of how to solve numerically the global minimization problems involved in the formulae characterizing the largest stability hyperspheres [16],[18] has not yet received due attention in the literature.

The outline of the paper is as follows. In Section 2 we introduce the general concept of the structured real or complex stability radius for polynomials and discuss briefly various special cases. In Section 3 we study the *complex* stability radius for various perturbation norms and illustrate the results by several examples. The examples include well- and ill-conditioned Hurwitz polynomials and the computations are carried out via the algorithm Stabrad described in [28]. In Section 4 new formulae for the unstructured and various types of structured *real* stability radii are derived. As an easy consequence we get a necessary and sufficient criterion under which a segment in the coefficient space consists only of Hurwitz polynomials. The distance of a real Hurwitz polynomial from instability is determined for different perturbation norms, and it is shown that under certain conditions the *real unstructured* stability radius of a polynomial is equal to a *structured complex* stability radius of an associated polynomial. Some remarks concerning the computation of the real stability radius and a series of examples conclude the paper.

2. PROBLEM FORMULATION

Throughout the paper we suppose that $\mathbf{K}$ is the field of real or the field of complex numbers ($\mathbf{K} = \mathbf{R}$ or $\mathbf{C}$) and that

$$\mathbf{C} = \mathbf{C}_g \cup \mathbf{C}_b \tag{2.1}$$

is a partition of the complex plane into a "good" part which is open and a "bad" part which is a closed subset of $\mathbf{C}$. By $\partial\mathbf{C}_b = \bar{\mathbf{C}}_g \cap \mathbf{C}_b$ we denote the boundary of $\mathbf{C}_b$ (and $\mathbf{C}_g$) in $\mathbf{C}$.

We identify every monic polynomial of degree $n \geq 1$

$$p(s,a) = s^n + a_{n-1} s^{n-1} + \ldots + a_1 s + a_0 \tag{2.2}$$

with its coefficient vector $a = [a_0,\ldots,a_{n-1}] \in \mathbf{K}^{1\times n}$, viewed as a row vector. Now assume that $p(s,a)$ is a nominal polynomial with all its roots in $\mathbf{C}_g$ and that the coefficients a_{j-1} are perturbed to

$$a_{j-1}(d) = a_{j-1} - \sum_{i=1}^{\ell} d_i c_{ij}\,, \qquad j \in \underline{n} = \{1,\ldots,n\} \tag{2.3}$$

where $C = (c_{ij}) \in \mathbf{K}^{\ell\times n}$ is a given matrix. The coordinates of the unknown *disturbance vector* $d = [d_1,\ldots,d_\ell] \in \mathbf{K}^{1\times\ell}$ (row vector) represent the deviations of the system parameters from their nominal values. (2.3) allows for arbitrary affine dependencies of the coefficients on any number of system parameters. Moreover, even if the coefficients are non-linear functions of the physical parameters of the system, it is often possible to introduce artificial parameters d_i so that the parameter uncertainty can adequately be represented in the form (2.3).

Definition 2.1
Given a partition (2.1) of the complex plane, a norm $\|\cdot\|$ on $\mathbf{K}^{1\times\ell}$ and perturbations of the form (2.3), the stability radius of a polynomial $p(s,a)$ of the form (2.2) is defined by

$$r_{\mathbf{K}}(a,C;\mathbf{C}_b) = \inf\{\|d\|;\ d\in\mathbf{K}^{1\times\ell},\ \exists\lambda\in\mathbf{C}_b:\ p(\lambda,a(d)) = 0\}. \tag{2.4}$$

By definition $r_{\mathbf{K}}(a,C;\mathbf{C}_b) = \infty$ iff there does not exist $d \in \mathbf{K}^{1\times\ell}$ such that $p(\lambda,a(d)) = 0$ for some $\lambda \in \mathbf{C}_b$. An easy compactness argument proves the following lemma.

Lemma 2.2
If $r_{\mathbf{K}}(a,C;\mathbf{C}_b) < \infty$ then there exists a minimal norm destabilizing perturbation $d \in \mathbf{K}^{1\times\ell}$ such that

$$\|d\| = r_{\mathbf{K}}(a,C;\mathbf{C}_b) \quad \text{and} \quad p(\lambda,a(d)) = 0 \quad \text{for some} \quad \lambda \in \mathbf{C}_b. \tag{2.5}$$

Conversely, if $d \in \mathbf{K}^{1\times\ell}$, $\|d\| < r_{\mathbf{K}}$ then the perturbed polynomial $p(s,a(d))$ has all its roots in $\mathbf{C}_g$. Hence, knowledge of $r_{\mathbf{K}}(a,C;\mathbf{C}_b)$ for some given $p(s,a)$, C and $\mathbf{C}_b$ implies both a stability result for a *set* of polynomials and an instability result.

Geometrically, the parameter set $\{d\in \mathbf{K}^{1\times\ell};\ \|d\| < r_{\mathbf{K}}\}$ is the largest open ball B, centre 0 in the normed space $(\mathbf{K}^{1\times\ell},\|\cdot\|)$ which guarantees that all the roots of the perturbed polynomials $p(s,a(d))$, $d \in B$ remain in $\mathbf{C}_g$. Depending on the norm $\|\cdot\|$, the corresponding set of "stable" polynomials

$$\{a(d);\ \|d\| < r_{\mathbf{K}}\} \tag{2.6}$$

has different geometric forms. If $\|\cdot\| = \|\cdot\|_\infty$ is the maximum norm and $\mathbf{K} = \mathbf{R}$, the set (2.6) has the form of a symmetric polytope centered at a. The choice of this norm allows to study Kharitonov's problem in our framework. In fact, an interval $[\underline{a},\bar{a}] = \{p(s,a);\ \underline{a}_i \le a_i \le \bar{a}_i,\ i = 0,\dots,n-1\}$ of real polynomials consists only of Hurwitz polynomials iff $r_{\mathbf{R}}(a,C;\mathbf{C}_-) > 1$ where $a = (\underline{a}+\bar{a})/2$ and $C = \mathrm{diag}[(\bar{a}_0 - \underline{a}_0)/2,\dots,(\bar{a}_{n-1} - \underline{a}_{n-1})/2]$. If $\|\cdot\| = \|\cdot\|_2$ is the usual Hilbert norm on $\mathbf{K}^{1\times\ell}$, the set (2.6) has the shape of an ellipsoid in the affine subspace $a + \mathbf{K}^{1\times\ell}C$ of $\mathbf{K}^{1\times n}$.

By choice of the partition (2.1), of the norm $\|\cdot\|$ on $\mathbf{K}^{1\times\ell}$ and the structure matrix $C \in \mathbf{K}^{\ell\times n}$, the stability radius becomes a very versatile tool of robustness analysis. The most important choices of $\mathbf{C}_g$ are clearly $\mathbf{C}_g = \mathbf{C}_-$ and $\mathbf{C}_g = \mathbf{C}_1$, the cases of Hurwitz and Schur polynomials. We denote the corresponding radii by $r_{\mathbf{K}}^-(a,C)$ and $r_{\mathbf{K}}^1(a,C)$, respectively.

The matrix $C \in \mathbf{K}^{\ell\times n}$ determines the *structure* of the perturbations. The case which has been studied most in the literature, is the unstructured case where $C = I_n$. The *unstructured* stability radii

$$d_{\mathbf{K}}^-(a) = r_{\mathbf{K}}^-(a,I_n) \quad \text{and} \quad d_{\mathbf{K}}^1(a) = r_{\mathbf{K}}^1(a,I_n) \tag{2.7}$$

represent the distance of a Hurwitz resp. Schur polynomial $p(s,a)$ from the set of non-Hurwitz (resp. non-Schur) polynomials in the coefficient space $\mathbf{K}^{1\times n}$. Another special case of interest is obtained when one coefficient a_{j-1} is perturbed while all the other coefficients remain unchanged. This case is represented by the structure matrix

$$C = e^j = [0,\dots,0,1,0,\dots,0]$$

where e^j is the j-th row of the identity matrix I_n. The corresponding stability radius $r_{\mathbf{K}}^-(a,e^j)$ (resp. $r_{\mathbf{K}}^1(a,e^j)$) is the absolute value of the smallest perturbation d_{j-1} of the coefficient a_{j-1} for which the perturbed polynomial

$$s^n + a_{n-1}s^{n-1} + \dots + (a_{j-1}-d_{j-1})s^{j-1} + \dots + a_1 s + a_0$$

has a root on the imaginary axis (resp. the unit circle).

3. THE COMPLEX STABILITY RADIUS

Throughout this section we suppose that $\mathbf{K} = \mathbf{C}$, $C \in \mathbf{C}^{\ell\times n}$ is a given matrix and $\|\cdot\|$ any norm on $\mathbf{C}^{1\times\ell}$. If $\|\cdot\|_*$ denotes the norm on $\mathbf{C}^\ell = \mathbf{C}^{\ell\times 1}$ which is dual to $\|\cdot\|$, then $\|\cdot\|$ is conversely the dual norm of $\|\cdot\|_*$ (see [31], §5.6]), i.e. $\|d\|$ is the operator norm of the linear form $y \to dy$ on $(\mathbb{C}^\ell, \|\cdot\|_*)$:

$$\|d\| = \max\{|dy|;\ y \in \mathbb{C}^\ell,\ \|y\|_* = 1\}.$$

We will often specialize to the $1,2,\infty$ norms on $\mathbb{C}^{1\times\ell}$:

$$\|d\| = \|d\|_1 = \sum_{i=1}^{\ell} |d_i| , \qquad \|y\|_* = \|y\|_\infty = \max_{i\in\underline{\ell}} |y_i|$$

$$\|d\| = \|d\|_2 = \left[\sum_{i=1}^{\ell} |d_i|^2\right]^{\frac{1}{2}} , \qquad \|y\|_* = \|y\|_2 = \left[\sum_{i=1}^{\ell} |y_i|^2\right]^{\frac{1}{2}}$$

$$\|d\| = \|d\|_\infty = \max_{i\in\underline{\ell}} |d_i| , \qquad \|y\|_* = \|y\|_1 = \sum_{i=1}^{\ell} |y_i| .$$

The following proposition holds for arbitrary norms on $\mathbb{C}^{1\times\ell}$.

Proposition 3.1
Suppose that $p(s,a)$ is a complex polynomial with all its roots in $\mathbb{C}_g$ and let

$$G(s) = \frac{1}{p(s,a)} [c_1(s),\dots,c_\ell(s)]^T , \quad c_i(s) = \sum_{j=1}^{n} c_{ij}s^{j-1}, \quad i\in\underline{\ell} . \tag{3.1}$$

Then

$$r_{\mathbb{C}}(a,C;\mathbb{C}_b) = \left[\max_{s\in\partial\mathbb{C}_b} \|G(s)\|_*\right]^{-1} = \left[\max_{s\in\mathbb{C}_b} \|G(s)\|_*\right]^{-1}. \tag{3.2}$$

Proof: For every $d \in \mathbb{C}^{1\times\ell}$, the roots of $p(\cdot,a(d))$ coincide with the eigenvalues of the matrix $A+BdC$ where

$$A = \begin{bmatrix} 0 & 1 & 0 & \cdots & 0 \\ 0 & 0 & 1 & \cdots & 0 \\ \vdots & \vdots & \vdots & \cdots & \vdots \\ 0 & 0 & 0 & \cdots & 1 \\ -a_0 & -a_1 & -a_2 & \cdots & -a_{n-1} \end{bmatrix}_{n\times n} , \quad B = \begin{bmatrix} 0 \\ \vdots \\ \vdots \\ 0 \\ 1 \end{bmatrix}_{n\times 1} , \quad C = (c_{ij})_{\ell\times n}. \tag{3.3}$$

Hence

$$r_{\mathbb{C}}(a,C;\mathbb{C}_b) = r_{\mathbb{C}}(A,B,C;\mathbb{C}_b) \tag{3.4}$$

where

$$r_{\mathbb{C}}(A,B,C;\mathbb{C}_b) = \inf\{\|d\|_{\mathfrak{L}(\mathbb{C}^\ell,\mathbb{C})} ;\ d\in\mathbb{C}^{1\times\ell},\ \sigma(A+BdC) \cap \mathbb{C}_b \neq \emptyset\} \tag{3.5}$$

is the complex stability radius of the matrix A with respect to the perturbation structure (B,C), see [23]. Note that $\|d\|_{\mathfrak{L}(\mathbb{C}^\ell,\mathbb{C})}$ in (3.5) is the operator norm of d as a linear map from $(\mathbb{C}^\ell, \|\cdot\|_*)$ into $(\mathbb{C}, |\cdot|)$ and hence coincides with $\|d\|$. Since

$$(sI_n-A)^{-1}B = \frac{1}{p(s,a)} [1,s,\dots,s^{n-1}]^T$$

we have

$$G(s) = C(sI_n-A)^{-1}B.$$

So (3.2) is a special case of the general formula for the complex structured stability radius, see [23],[29]:

$$r_{\mathbb{C}}(A,B,C;\mathbb{C}_b) = \left[\max_{s\in\partial\mathbb{C}_b} \|G(s)\|_*\right]^{-1} = \left[\max_{s\in\mathbb{C}_b} \|G(s)\|_*\right]^{-1} . \quad \square$$

If we assume $r_{\mathbb{C}}(a,C;\mathbb{C}_b) < \infty$ it is possible to construct a minimal norm destabilizing perturbation $d \in \mathbb{C}^{1\times\ell}$. Suppose that $s_0 \in \partial\mathbb{C}_b$ maximizes $\|G(s)\|_*$:

$$\|G(s_0)\|_* = \max_{s\in\partial\mathbb{C}_b} \|G(s)\|_* = r_{\mathbb{C}}^{-1} > 0 . \tag{3.6}$$

As a consequence of the Hahn-Banach Theorem there exists $d\in\mathbb{C}^{1\times\ell}$ aligned with $G(s_0)$ [31, §5.7] such that

$$dG(s_0) = 1 \quad \text{and} \quad \|d\| = \|G(s_0)\|_*^{-1} \tag{3.7}$$

Any such d is a minimum norm destabilizing perturbation. In fact, if (A,B,C) is defined by (3.3) then $dG(s_0) = 1$ implies

$$(s_0I_n-A)^{-1}BdC(s_0I_n-A)^{-1}B = (s_0I_n-A)^{-1}B$$

and hence, for $z = (s_0I_n-A)^{-1}B \neq 0$,

$$BdCz = (s_0I_n-A)z, \text{ i.e. } [s_0I_n-(A+BdC)]z = 0.$$

Thus

$$dG(s_0) = 1 \Rightarrow s_0 \in \sigma(A+BdC). \tag{3.8}$$

For the three norms $\|\cdot\|_q$, $q = 1,2,\infty$ the minimum norm disturbance vectors d (3.7) are easily determined once $G(s_0)$ is known.

Proposition 3.2

Suppose $q = 1,2,\infty$ and $1/q + 1/q^* = 1$. If $r_{\mathbb{C}}(a,C;\mathbb{C}_b) = \|G(s_0)\|_{q^*}^{-1} < \infty$, $G(s_0) = [\gamma_1,\dots,\gamma_\ell]^T$ and $|\gamma_k| = \max_{j\in\underline{\ell}} |\gamma_j|$ then a minimum destabilizing perturbation d_q with regard to the norm $\|\cdot\|_q$ is given, respectively, by

$$d_1 = \left[0,\dots,0,\frac{\bar\gamma_k}{|\gamma_k|},\ 0,\dots,0\right] \|G(s_0)\|_\infty^{-1} \tag{3.9a}$$

$$d_2 = [\bar\gamma_1,\dots,\bar\gamma_\ell]\ \|G(s_0)\|_2^{-2} \tag{3.9b}$$

$$d_\infty = \left[\frac{\bar\gamma_1}{|\gamma_1|},\dots,\frac{\bar\gamma_\ell}{|\gamma_\ell|}\right] \|G(s_0)\|_1^{-1}, \quad \frac{\bar\gamma_i}{|\gamma_i|} := 0 \text{ if } \gamma_i = 0 \tag{3.9c}$$

Proof: It is straightforward to show that the above d's satisfy (3.7). □

It is interesting that in the unstructured case ($C = I_n$) with norm $||\cdot||_1$ a perturbation of a *single* coefficient a_k can be found which is destabilizing and minimal. This will be confirmed in Corollaries 3.4 and 3.5 where we consider distances from instability (i.e. $C = I_n$).

Choosing $\mathbf{C}_g = \mathbf{C}_-$ or $\mathbf{C}_g = \mathbf{C}_1$ (3.2) we obtain formulae for the structured complex stability radii of a Hurwitz or Schur polynomial.

Corollary 3.3
If $p(s,a)$, $a \in \mathbf{C}^{1\times n}$ is a Hurwitz (Schur) polynomial and $G(s)$ defined by (3.1) then

$$r_{\mathbf{C}}^{-}(a,C) = \left[\max_{\omega\in\mathbf{R}} \|G(i\omega)\|_*\right]^{-1} \tag{3.10}$$

$$r_{\mathbf{C}}^{1}(a,C) = \left[\max_{\theta\in[0,2\pi]} \|G(e^{i\theta})\|_*\right]^{-1} . \tag{3.11}$$

In the unstructured case (ℓ=n, $C=I_n$),

$$G(s) = \frac{1}{p(s,a)} [1,s,s^2,\dots,s^{n-1}]^T. \tag{3.12}$$

The following specializations of Corollary 3.3 yield explicit formulae for the $\|\cdot\|_q$-distance of Hurwitz or Schur polynomials from the set of non-Hurwitz resp. non-Schur polynomials, $q = 1,2,\infty$.

Corollary 3.4
Suppose that $p(\cdot,a)$, $a \in \mathbf{C}^{1\times n}$ is Hurwitz. Then

1-norm: $$d_{\mathbf{C}}^{-}(a) = \left[\max_{\omega\in\mathbf{R}} \|G(i\omega)\|_\infty\right]^{-1} = \min_{\omega\in\mathbf{R}} \min_{0\le j\le n-1} \frac{|p(i\omega,a)|}{|\omega^j|} \tag{3.13a}$$

2-norm: $$d_{\mathbf{C}}^{-}(a) = \left[\max_{\omega\in\mathbf{R}} \|G(i\omega)\|_2\right]^{-1} = \min_{\omega\in\mathbf{R}} \frac{|p(i\omega,a)|}{(1+\omega^2+\dots+\omega^{2n-2})^{1/2}} \tag{3.13b}$$

∞-norm: $$d_{\mathbf{C}}^{-}(a) = \left[\max_{\omega\in\mathbf{R}} \|G(i\omega)\|_1\right]^{-1} = \min_{\omega\in\mathbf{R}} \frac{|p(i\omega,a)|}{(1+|\omega|+\dots+|\omega|^{n-1})} . \tag{3.13c}$$

Corollary 3.5
If $p(\cdot,a)$, $a \in \mathbf{C}^{1\times n}$ is Schur, then

1-norm: $$d_{\mathbf{C}}^{1}(a) = \left[\max_{\theta\in[0,2\pi]} \|G(e^{i\theta})\|_\infty\right]^{-1} = \min_{\theta\in[0,2\pi]} |p(e^{i\theta},a)| \tag{3.14a}$$

2-norm: $$d_{\mathbf{C}}^{1}(a) = \left[\max_{\theta\in[0,2\pi]} \|G(e^{i\theta})\|_2\right]^{-1} = \min_{\theta\in[0,2\pi]} \frac{|p(e^{i\theta},a)|}{\sqrt{n}} \tag{3.14b}$$

∞-norm: $$d_{\mathbf{C}}^{1}(a) = \left[\max_{\theta\in[0,2\pi]} \|G(e^{i\theta})\|_1\right]^{-1} = \min_{\theta\in[0,2\pi]} \frac{|p(e^{i\theta},a)|}{n} . \tag{3.14c}$$

The distances $d_{\mathbf{C}}^{-}(a)$, $d_{\mathbf{C}}^{1}(a)$ yield adequate robustness measures if all the coefficients of $p(s,a)$ are subject to independent perturbations of equal weight. On the other hand it is interesting to consider the case where the coefficients of $p(s,a)$ all depend on one and the same unknown parameter $d \in \mathbf{C}$ (i.e. $\ell = 1$, $C = [c_1,\dots,c_n] \in \mathbf{C}^{1\times n}$). This case has received special attention in perturbation theory and numerical analysis.

Corollary 3.6

Suppose that all the roots of the polynomial $p(s,a)$ are in $\mathbb{C}_g$ and $c = [c_1,\dots,c_n] \in \mathbb{C}^{1\times n}$. Then

$$r_{\mathbb{C}}(a,c;\mathbb{C}_b) = \min_{s\in\partial\mathbb{C}_b} \frac{|p(s,a)|}{|c(s)|} \tag{3.15}$$

where

$$c(s) = c_n s^{n-1} + \dots + c_2 s + c_1 . \tag{3.16}$$

Of special interest is the case where only one coefficient is perturbed, i.e. $c = e^j$. If $p(\cdot,a)$, $a \in \mathbb{C}^{1\times n}$ is Hurwitz then

$$r_{\mathbb{C}}^{-}(a,e^j) = \min_{\omega\in\mathbb{R}} \frac{|p(i\omega,a)|}{|\omega|^{j-1}}, \quad j \in \underline{n} . \tag{3.17}$$

If $p(\cdot,a)$ is Schur then, by (3.15) and (3.14a),

$$r_{\mathbb{C}}^{1}(a,e^j) = \min_{\theta\in[0,2\pi]} |p(e^{i\theta},a)| = d_{\mathbb{C}}^{1}(a) \tag{3.18}$$

where $d_{\mathbb{C}}^{1}(a)$ is taken with respect to the norm $\|\cdot\|_1$. Note that in the Schur case the stability radii $d_{\mathbb{C}}^{1}(a,e^j)$ do not depend upon $j \in \underline{n}$.

We conclude this section with two examples. Since the evaluation of the formulae in Proposition 3.1 and Corollaries 3.3 - 3.6 involve the solution of global non-convex optimization problems their application to concrete examples is a nontrivial task. To solve these computational problems in the case $\|\cdot\| = \|\cdot\|_2$ we recommend that one uses the matrices A,B,C defined in (3.3) and applies the algorithm Stabrad 2 described in [28]. The algorithm computes

$$r_{\mathbb{C}}^{-}(A,B,C) = r_{\mathbb{C}}^{-}(a,C)$$

for arbitrary structure matrices $C \in \mathbb{C}^{\ell\times n}$. Moreover it determines a maximizing ω_0 and hence via (3.9b) a minimum norm destabilizing disturbance vector $d \in \mathbb{C}^{1\times\ell}$ (in the Hilbert case).

In the first example we illustrate the relationship between the complex stability radii $r_{\mathbb{C}}^{-}(a,e^j)$ and the root sensitivities with respect to variations in single coefficients. Let $p(s) = \sum_{i=0}^{n} a_i s^i$, $q(s) = \sum_{i=1}^{n} c_i s^{i-1}$, $a_n = 1$ and consider the perturbed polynomial

$$p(s,a(\varepsilon)) = p(s) + \varepsilon q(s), \quad \varepsilon \in \mathbb{C}.$$

If s_k is a simple root of $p(s)$ and $s_k(\varepsilon)$ is the corresponding simple root of $p(\cdot,a(\varepsilon))$ (for small $|\varepsilon|$) then up to first order

$$s_k(\varepsilon) \approx s_k + \zeta_k\varepsilon \tag{3.19}$$

where ζ_k is the *sensitivity* of s_k with respect to variations of ε about 0:

$$\zeta_k = \frac{ds_k(\varepsilon)}{d\varepsilon}\Big|_{\varepsilon=0} = -\frac{q(s_k)}{p'(s_k)} \tag{3.20}$$

(see[30]). While (3.19) yields good estimates of the roots of $p(s,a(\varepsilon))$

for *small* $|\varepsilon|$ it is not clear what happens for large values of $|\varepsilon|$. On the other hand the stability radius $r_C(a,C;C_b)$ provides information about *large* parameter variations.

The following example illustrates that an *ill-conditioned* Hurwitz polynomial, having large root sensitivities with respect to changes in single coefficients may nevertheless possess a relatively high robustness of stability.

Example 3.7
A standard ill-conditioned polynomial in Numerical Analysis (see e.g. [30],p.82) is the seemingly innocent Hurwitz polynomial

$$\begin{aligned} p(s) &= p(s,a) = (s+1)(s+2)\dots(s+7) \\ &= s^7 + 28s^6 + 322s^5 + 1960s^4 + 6769s^3 + 13132s^2 + 13068s + 5040. \end{aligned}$$

Suppose that only the coefficient $a_6 = 28$ is perturbed, i.e. $q(s) = s^6$ and $p(s,a(\varepsilon)) = p(s) + \varepsilon s^6$. The corresponding sensitivities of the roots $s_k = -k$, $k = 1,\dots,7$ are

$$\zeta_k = -\frac{q(s_k)}{p'(s_k)} = -\frac{k^6}{\prod\limits_{i=1,\, i\neq k}^{7}(-k+i)} = (-1)^k \frac{k^6}{(k-1)!(7-k)!} \tag{3.21}$$

e.g.

$$\zeta_1 = -\frac{1}{6!} = -\frac{1}{720},\quad \zeta_7 = -\frac{7^6}{6!} \approx -163.4.$$

In order to examine the effect of "large" parameter variations, we let ∂C_b be the circle centred at -4 with radius R and calculate $r_C(a,e^7;C_b)$ and $r_C(a,I_n;C_b)$ for the norms $\|\cdot\|_q$, $q = 1,2,\infty$. Using (3.2) and (3.15) with $s = -4 + Re^{i\theta}$, $\theta \in [0,2\pi]$ we obtain the results shown in Tabelle 3.1. Because of the high sensitivity of the roots $s_7 = -7$ it is not surprising that the stability radii are small. For $R = 4.5$ linear extrapolation via (3.19) would mean that the root $s_7(\varepsilon)$ hits the circle at -8.5 for $\varepsilon = 1.5/163.4 \approx .0092$. Thus the actual stability radius is nearly five times larger than predicted by formula (3.19). The discrepancy between local sensitivity and global robustness becomes even more evident when we consider the Hurwitz partition where $C_g = C_-$. In fact, following the linear extrapolation formula (3.19) the root $s_7(\varepsilon)$ should hit the imaginary axis for $\varepsilon = -7/163.4 \approx -0.0428$. But applying the algorithm Stabrad 2 as described in [28], we obtain $r_C^-(a,e^7) = 18.3194$. Thus robustness of stability of $p(s,a)$ with respect to perturbation of the coefficient a_6 is about 400 times larger than the sensitivities indicate. A perturbation of $a_6 = 28$ must attain a size of about 65 % of the coefficient value before it destabilizes the polynomial.

Table 3.1 Stability radii of p(s) with respect to different regions C_b

R	$r_C(a,e^7;C_b)$	$r_C(a,I_n;C_b)$		
		$q = 1$	$q = 2$	$q = \infty$
3.5	.00593	.00593	.00587	.0051
4.0	.0192	.0192	.0191	.0168
4.5	.0420	.0420	.0417	.0371

Table 3.2 Distances of p(s) from instability and associated minimum norm destabilizing perturbations

norm	$d_{\mathbf{C}}^{-}(a)$	ω_0	perturbation vector d
1-norm	18.3194	10.40	[0,0,0,0,0,0,11.0−14.65i]
2-norm	18.234	10.34	[0,0,0,0,−.10+.133i,1.43+1.03i,10.71−14.66i]
∞-norm	16.4946	9.69	[0,0,0,0,−8.49+14.14i,14.63+7.61i,7.73−14.57i].

Nevertheless a_6 is the most critical coefficient of p(s,a). This can also be seen by the fact that the stability radius is hardly reduced if all the coefficients are perturbed independently, cf. Table 3.2.
The right hand column of Table 3.2 contains minimal destabilizing perturbations. The first few terms in d_2 and d_∞ are not strictly zero but small in comparison with the others.

□

In the next example we consider a Hurwitz polynomial which has been studied by other authors. Note that Kharitonov's theorem as well as the propositions of Fam and Meditch are essentially results on *real* polynomials so that the robustness papers based on these results ([3]-[7],[14]-[18]) are only applicable to polynomials with real coefficients and real valued perturbations.

Example 3.8
In [7] it was shown that the polynomials

$$p(s,a(d)) = s^3 + 2s^2 + 4s + 2 - d(s^2 + 2s + 1)$$

are Hurwitz for all $d \in [-1,1]$ but that the Kharitonov test fails to give this result, since e.g. the boundary polynomial $s^3 + s^2 + 2s + 3$ is not Hurwitz. Computing the structured complex stability radius for $p(s,a) = s^3 + 2s^2 + 4s + 2$ with structure matrix $c = [1,2,1]$ one obtains by Corollary 3.6

$$r_{\mathbf{C}}^{-}(a,c) = \left[\max_{\omega\in\mathbf{R}} \left| \frac{(i\omega)^2+2i\omega+1}{(i\omega)^3+2(i\omega)^2+4i\omega+2} \right| \right]^{-1} = 1.08$$

and hence the stronger result: p(s,a(d)) is Hurwitz for all complex perturbations d such that $|d| < 1.08$. Moreover we know that there is a disturbance $d \in \mathbf{C}$, $|d| = 1.08$ such that p(s,a(d)) has an imaginary root. In fact, Stabrad 2 yields a maximizing frequency $\omega_0 = 1.6649$ and hence by (3.9a) the disturbance

$$d = 1.08^2 \frac{1-\omega_0^2-2\omega_0 i}{2-2\omega_0^2-(4\omega_0-\omega_0^3)i} = 0.9199 + 0.5748i$$

destabilizes p(s,a).

□

4. THE REAL STABILITY RADIUS

In this section we suppose that $\mathbf{K} = \mathbf{R}$, $C \in \mathbf{R}^{\ell\times n}$ is a given matrix, $\|\cdot\|$ a norm on $\mathbf{R}^{1\times\ell}$ and $\mathbf{C} = \mathbf{C}_g \cup \mathbf{C}_b$ is a partition of the complex plane as in the previous sections. Moreover, we only consider *real* polynomials (of degree $n \geq 1$)

$$p(s,a) = s^n+a_{n-1}s^{n-1}+\ldots+a_1s+a_0, \quad a \in \mathbf{R}^{1\times n}. \tag{4.1}$$

For these polynomials both the real and the complex stability radii $r_{\mathbf{K}}(a,C;\mathbf{C}_b)$, $\mathbf{K} = \mathbf{R}, \mathbf{C}$ are well defined by (2.4), but in most applications only real valued perturbations are of interest. In these cases the complex stability radius, although a tight upper bound for non-destabilizing complex perturbations, is a conservative measure of robustness:

$$r_{\mathbf{C}}(a,C;\mathbf{C}_b) \;\leq\; r_{\mathbf{R}}(a,C;\mathbf{C}_b). \tag{4.2}$$

To characterize the *real* stability radius we denote by $d(y,\mathbf{R}v)$ the distance of a point $y \in \mathbf{R}^{\ell}$ from the linear space $\mathbf{R}v$ spanned by $v \in \mathbf{R}^{\ell}$ in the normed space $(\mathbf{R}^{\ell}, \|\cdot\|_*)$:

$$d(y,\mathbf{R}v) \;=\; \min_{\alpha\in\mathbf{R}} \|y - \alpha v\|_* \tag{4.3}$$

where $\|\cdot\|_*$ is the dual norm of $\|\cdot\|$ on $\mathbf{R}^{\ell}$.

Remark 4.1
In the Hilbert space case ($\|\cdot\| = \|\cdot\|_* = \|\cdot\|_2$) it is easy to see that

$$d^2(y,\mathbf{R}v) \;=\; \begin{cases} \|y\|^2 - \langle y,v\rangle^2/\|v\|^2, & v \neq 0 \\ \|y\|^2 \qquad\qquad\qquad\;\;, & v = 0 \end{cases} \tag{4.4}$$

see Fig. 4.1. Analogous general formulae for the norms $\|\cdot\|_1$ and $\|\cdot\|_\infty$ are not available. □

Now choose A,B,C as in (3.3). Defining the real stability radius $r_{\mathbf{R}}(A,B,C;\mathbf{C}_b)$ analogously to the complex one, see (3.5), it follows as in the proof of Proposition 3.1 that

$$r_{\mathbf{R}}(a,C;\mathbf{C}_b) \;=\; r_{\mathbf{R}}(A,B,C;\mathbf{C}_b). \tag{4.5}$$

In [29] we show that

$$r_{\mathbf{R}}(A,B,C;\mathbf{C}_b) \;=\; \left[\max_{s\in\partial\mathbf{C}_b} d(G_R(s),\mathbf{R}G_I(s))\right]^{-1} \tag{4.6}$$

where

$$G(s) \;=\; C(sI-A)^{-1}B \;=\; G_R(s) + iG_I(s), \quad G_R(s),\; G_I(s) \in \mathbf{R}^{\ell} \tag{4.7}$$

is the associated transfer function and, by definition, $0^{-1} = \infty$.

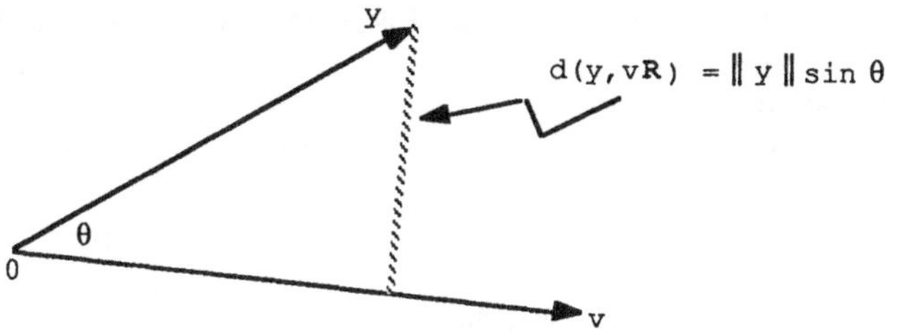

Fig. 4.1 $d(y,v\mathbf{R})$ in the Hilbert space case if $v \neq 0$

Proceeding as in the proof of Proposition 3.1 we get

Proposition 4.2
Suppose $(a,C) \in \mathbf{R}^{1\times n} \times \mathbf{R}^{\ell\times n}$ and that all the roots of the polynomials $p(s,a)$ lie in $\mathbf{C}_g$. Then

$$r_{\mathbf{R}}(a,C;\mathbf{C}_b) = \left[\max_{s\in\partial\mathbf{C}_b} d(G_R(s),\mathbf{R}G_I(s))\right]^{-1} \tag{4.8}$$

where $d(\cdot,\cdot)$ is defined by (4.3) and $G_R(s)$, $G_I(s) \in \mathbf{R}^{\ell}$ are the real and imaginary parts of

$$G(s) = \frac{1}{p(s,a)}\begin{bmatrix} c_1(s) \\ \vdots \\ c_\ell(s)\end{bmatrix}, \quad c_i(s) = \sum_{j=1}^{n} c_{ij}s^{j-1}, \; i \in \underline{\ell}\,. \tag{4.9}$$

In the Hilbert space case ($\|\cdot\| = \|\cdot\|_2$), formula (4.8) can be written in the following more explicit form (see Remark 4.1):

$$r_{\mathbf{R}}(a,C;\mathbf{C}_b) = \min\left\{\left[\max_{s\in\partial\mathbf{C}_b,\,G_I(s)=0}\|G(s)\|\right]^{-1}, \right. \tag{4.10}$$
$$\left.\left[\sup_{s\in\partial\mathbf{C}_b,\,G_I(s)\neq 0}\left[\|G_R(s)\|^2 - \frac{\langle G_R(s),G_I(s)\rangle^2}{\|G_I(s)\|^2}\right]\right]^{-1/2}\right\}.$$

Here as elsewhere in this paper we set $[\max \emptyset]^{-1} = 0$, by a slight abuse of notation, when there is no $s \in \partial\mathbf{C}_b$ such that $G_I(s) = 0$.

To obtain - in the general case - a minimum norm destabilizing disturbance $d \in \mathbf{R}^{1\times\ell}$ if $r_{\mathbf{R}} < \infty$ one first has to determine a distance maximizing $s_0 \in \partial\mathbf{C}_b$:

$$d(G_R(s_0),\mathbf{R}G_I(s_0)) = r_{\mathbf{R}}^{-1}(a,C;\mathbf{C}_b). \tag{4.11}$$

If $G_I(s_0)$, $G_R(s_0)$ are linearly dependent then necessarily $G_I(s_0) = 0$ (since otherwise $d(G_R(s_0),\mathbf{R}G_I(s_0)) = 0$) and in this case it suffices to choose any $d \in \mathbf{R}^{1\times\ell}$ aligned with $G(s_0) = G_R(s_0)$ such that

$$dG(s_0) = 1 \quad\text{and}\quad \|d\| = \|G(s_0)\|_*^{-1} \tag{4.12}$$

(see Proposition 3.2).

If $G_R(s_0)$ and $G_I(s_0)$ are linearly independent, it follows from a well-known duality theorem in optimization theory (see [31], §5.8) that there exists $d \in \mathbf{R}^{1\times\ell}$ satisfying

$$dG_R(s_0) = 1,\; dG_I(s_0) = 0 \;\text{ and }\; \|d\| = [d(G_R(s_0),\mathbf{R}G_I(s_0))]^{-1}. \tag{4.13}$$

The first two conditions in (4.13) are equivalent to $dG(s_0) = 1$ and so by (3.8) d is a minimum norm destabilizing disturbance vector.

To determine a vector $d \in \mathbf{R}^{1\times\ell}$ satisfying (4.13) suppose that $\hat{\alpha}$ has been found such that

$$\|G_R(s_0) - \hat{\alpha}G_I(s_0)\|_* = d(G_R(s_0),\mathbf{R}G_I(s_0))$$

$d \in \mathbf{R}^{1\times \ell}$ satisfies (4.13) if and only if

$$dG_I(s_0) = 0 \quad \text{and} \quad d[G_R(s_0) - \hat{\alpha}G_I(s_0)] = \|d\| \, \|G_R(s_0) - \hat{\alpha}G_I(s_0)\|_* = 1 \tag{4.14}$$

i.e. d vanishes on $G_I(s_0)$ and is aligned with $G_R(s_0) - \hat{\alpha}G_I(s_0)$. Such a row vector d always exists and in the next remark we show how to find it in case $\|\cdot\| = \|\cdot\|_q$, $q = 1,2,\infty$.

Remark 4.3

Suppose $q = 1,2,\infty$, $\frac{1}{q} + \frac{1}{q^*} = 1$ and $r_{\mathbf{R}}(a,C;\mathbf{C}_b) = \|G_R(s_0) - \hat{\alpha}G_I(s_0)\|_*^{-1}$ where $G_R(s_0) - \hat{\alpha}G_I(s_0) = [\alpha_1,\dots,\alpha_\ell]^T$, $G(s_0) = [\beta_1,\dots,\beta_\ell]^T \neq 0$.
If $q = 2$ a straightforward calculation shows that

$$d = \frac{\|G_I(s_0)\|^2 G_R^T(s_0) - \langle G_I(s_0), G_R(s_0)\rangle G_I^T(s_0)}{\|G_I(s_0)\|^2 \|G_R(s_0)\|^2 - \langle G_I(s_0), G_R(s_0)\rangle^2} \tag{4.15}$$

satisfies (4.13). If $q = 1$ the situation is slightly more complicated. Let $K = \left\{ k \in \underline{\ell} : |\alpha_k| = \max_{j\in\underline{\ell}} |\alpha_j| \right\}$. $d \in \mathbf{R}^{1\times\ell}$ satisfies the second condition in (4.14) if and only if

$$d_j = 0,\ j \in \underline{\ell}\backslash K,\ \operatorname{sgn} d_k = \operatorname{sgn}\alpha_k,\ k \in K \text{ and } \sum_{k\in K} |d_k| = \left[\max_{j\in\underline{\ell}} |\alpha_j|\right]^{-1} \tag{4.16}$$

where $\operatorname{sgn}\alpha_k = 1,0,-1$ if $\alpha_k > 0$, $= 0$, < 0, respectively. The remaining freedom in the choice of $d \in \mathbf{R}^{1\times\ell}$ is used to satisfy

$$\sum_{k=1}^{\ell} d_k\beta_k = 0. \tag{4.17}$$

Similarly if $q = \infty$, let $J = \{j \in \underline{\ell};\ a_j \neq 0\}$. $d \in \mathbf{R}^{1\times\ell}$ satisfies the second condition in (4.14) if and only if

$$d_j = \left[\sum_{i=1}^{\ell} |\alpha_i|\right]^{-1} \operatorname{sgn}\alpha_j \quad \text{for} \quad j \in J. \tag{4.18}$$

The d_i, $i \in \underline{\ell}\setminus J$ are chosen so that (4.17) is satisfied. □

Replacing $\mathbf{C}_g$ by $\mathbf{C}_-$ or $\mathbf{C}_1$, the above results yield formulae for the real stability radii of Hurwitz and Schur polynomials. These specializations are straight forward and are omitted.

We now derive more explicit formulae for special perturbation structures $C \in \mathbf{R}^{\ell\times n}$ and begin with the scalar case ($\ell = 1$, $C = c = [c_1,\dots,c_n]$) where

$$G(s) = G_R(s) + iG_I(s) = \frac{c(s)}{p(s,a)}\ ,,\ c(s) = \sum_{j=1}^{n} c_j s^{j-i}. \tag{4.19}$$

In this case only *one* norm on the perturbation space $\mathbf{R}^\ell = \mathbf{R}$ is of interest ($\|\cdot\| = \|\cdot\|_q = |\cdot|$, $q = 1, 2,\infty$). Moreover the second term on the RHS of (4.10) is ∞ so that (4.10) implies the following real counterpart of Corollary 3.6.

Corollary 4.4
Suppose that all the roots of the polynomial $p(s,a)$, $a \in \mathbf{R}^{1\times n}$ are in $\mathbf{C}_g$ and $c = [c_1,\dots,c_n] \in \mathbf{R}^{1\times n}$. Then

$$r_{\mathbf{R}}(a,c;\mathbf{C}_b) = \min \{|G(s)|^{-1};\ s \in \partial\mathbf{C}_b,\ G_I(s) = 0\} \tag{4.20}$$

where G is defined by (4.19) (and, by definition, $\min \emptyset := \infty$).

□

Note that, generically, (4.20) is a minimization problem over a finite set, the set of zeros of the harmonic function G_I on $\partial\mathbf{C}_b$.

The following specialization of Corollary 4.4 deals with the problem of determining the size of the smallest real perturbation of a *single* coefficient which destabilizes a given Hurwitz polynomial.

Corollary 4.5
Suppose that $p(s,a)$, $a \in \mathbf{R}^{1\times n}$ is a Hurwitz polynomial and $p(i\omega,a) = p_1(\omega^2) + i\omega\, p_2(\omega^2)$, where $p_j(\omega^2)$, $j = 1,2$ are real polynomials of degree $\le n/2$ in ω^2. Then for $j \in \underline{n}$

$$r_{\mathbf{R}}^{-}(a,e^j) = \min \left\{ \left|\frac{p_2(\omega^2)}{\omega^{j-2}}\right|;\ \omega^2 > 0,\ p_1(\omega^2) = 0 \right\}, \quad j \text{ even} \tag{4.21}$$

$$r_{\mathbf{R}}^{-}(a,e^j) = \min \left\{ \left|\frac{p_1(\omega^2)}{\omega^{j-1}}\right|;\ \omega^2 \ge 0,\ \omega p_2(\omega^2) = 0 \right\}, \quad j \text{ odd} \tag{4.22}$$

where $0^0 = 1$.

Proof: Since in this case $G(s) = \dfrac{s^{j-1}}{p(s,a)}$, we have

$$G(i\omega) = \frac{i^{j-1}\omega^{j-1}}{|p(i\omega,a)|^2}\,(p_1(\omega^2) - i\omega p_2(\omega^2)).$$

Hence if j is even

$$G_R(i\omega) = \frac{(-1)^{j/2+1}\omega^j p_2(\omega^2)}{|p(i\omega,a)|^2}, \qquad G_I(i\omega) = \frac{(-1)^{j/2+1}\omega^{j-1} p_1(\omega^2)}{|p(i\omega,a)|^2}.$$

Since $|G_R(i\omega)| = \dfrac{\omega^j |p_2(\omega^2)|}{\omega^2 p_2(\omega^2)^2} = \dfrac{\omega^{j-2}}{|p_2(\omega^2)|}$ if $p_1(\omega^2) = 0$, and $|G_R(i\omega)| = 0$ if $\omega = 0$, (4.21) follows from (4.20). Similar calculations yield (4.22) when j is odd.

□

Many intricacies of stability theory are due to the fact that stability is a nonconvex property. In particular, the convex combinations

$$p(s,\gamma a + (1-\gamma)b), \quad 0 \le \gamma \le 1 \tag{4.23}$$

are not necessarily Hurwitz if $p(s,a)$, $p(s,b)$ are Hurwitz. A natural question is: Under which conditions on the coefficient vectors a and b can it be asserted that the segment (4.23) only consists of Hurwitz polynomials. The next corollary answers this question.

Corollary 4.6

Given $a,b \in \mathbf{R}^{1\times n}$, all the polynomials in (4.23) have all their roots in $\mathbf{C}_g$ if and only if

(i) $p\left(s,\frac{a+b}{2}\right)$ has all its roots in $\mathbf{C}_g$;

(ii) $$\min\{|G_R(s)|^{-1};\ s \in \partial\mathbf{C}_b,\ G_I(s) = 0\} > \frac{1}{2} \tag{4.24}$$

where $G_R(s), G_I(s) \in \mathbf{R}$ are defined by

$$G_R(s) + iG_I(s) = \frac{c(s)}{p\left(s,\frac{1}{2}(a+b)\right)},\quad c(s) = \sum_{j=0}^{n-1} (a_j-b_j)s^j. \tag{4.25}$$

Proof: The polynomials in (4.23) have all their roots in $\mathbf{C}_g$ iff this holds for all polynomials of the form

$$p\left(s,\frac{a+b}{2} - \varepsilon(a-b)\right),\qquad \varepsilon \in \left[-\frac{1}{2},\frac{1}{2}\right].$$

But this is equivalent to

$$r_{\mathbf{R}}\left(\frac{a+b}{2}, a-b;\ \mathbf{C}_b\right) > \frac{1}{2}\ .$$

Hence Corollary 4.6 follows from Corollary 4.4. □

As a last application of Proposition 4.1 we now determine the distances of a real Hurwitz polynomial from the set of real non Hurwitz ones. We do this for each of the three norms $\|\cdot\|_q$, $q = 1,2,\infty$.

Proposition 4.7

If $p(\cdot,a)$, $a \in \mathbf{R}^{1\times n}$ is Hurwitz, $p(s,a) = p_1(-s^2) + sp_2(-s^2)$ where $p_j(-s^2)$, $j = 1,2$ are real polynomials in $-s^2$, then with respect to the Euclidean norm $\|\cdot\|_2$

$$d_{\mathbf{R}}^{-}(a) = \min\left\{a_0, \left[\max_{\omega^2\in\mathbf{R}_+} \frac{1+\omega^4+\ldots+\omega^{2n-4}}{p_1^2(\omega^2)+p_2^2(\omega^2)}\right]^{-\frac{1}{2}}\right\},\quad n \text{ even} \tag{4.26}$$

$$d_{\mathbf{R}}^{-}(a) = \tag{4.27}$$

$$\min\left\{a_0, \left[\max_{\omega^2\in\mathbf{R}_+} \frac{(1+\omega^4+\ldots+\omega^{2n-6})(1+\omega^4+\ldots+\omega^{2n-2})}{p_1^2(\omega^2)(1+\omega^4+\cdots+\omega^{2n-6})+p_2^2(\omega^2)(1+\omega^4+\cdots+\omega^{2n-2})}\right]^{-\frac{1}{2}}\right\},\quad n \text{ odd}.$$

Proof: The proof is for $n > 1$ odd which is slightly more difficult. Recall

$G(s) = \frac{1}{p(s,a)}[1,s,\ldots s^{n-1}]^T$ and $p(i\omega,a) = p_1(\omega^2) + i\omega p_2(\omega^2)$, so that

$$|p(i\omega,a)|^2G_R(i\omega) = [p_1(\omega^2), \omega^2p_2(\omega^2), -\omega^2p_1(\omega^2), -\omega^4p_2(\omega^2), \cdots, (-1)^{\frac{n-1}{2}}\omega^{n-1}p_1(\omega^2)]^T$$

$$|p(i\omega,a)|^2G_I(i\omega) = [-\omega p_2(\omega^2), \omega p_1(\omega^2), \omega^3p_2(\omega^2), -\omega^3p_1(\omega^2), \cdots, (-1)^{\frac{n+1}{2}}\omega^np_2(\omega^2)]^T.$$

Thus

$$|p(i\omega,a)|^4\|G_R(i\omega)\|^2 = (p_1^2(\omega^2) + \omega^4 p_2^2(\omega^2))\,(1+\omega^4+\ldots+\omega^{2n-6}) + \omega^{2n-2}\, p_1^2(\omega^2)$$

$$|p(i\omega,a)|^4\|G_I(i\omega)\|^2 = \omega^2(p_1^2(\omega^2) + p_2^2(\omega^2))\,(1+\omega^4+\ldots+\omega^{2n-6}) + \omega^{2n}\, p_2^2(\omega^2)$$

$$|p(i\omega,a)|^8 \langle G_R(i\omega),\ G_I(i\omega)\rangle^2 = \omega^2 p_1^2(\omega^2)\, p_2^2(\omega^2)\, [(\omega^2-1)(1+\omega^4+\cdots+\omega^{2n-2}) - \omega^{2n-2}]^2.$$

A simple calculation yields

$$|p(i\omega,a)|^4[\|G_R(i\omega)\|^2\|G_I(i\omega)\|^2 - \langle G_R(i\omega),G_I(i\omega)\rangle^2] = \omega^2(1+\omega^4+\ldots+\omega^{2n-6})(1+\omega^4+\ldots+\omega^{2n-2}).$$

Hence

$$\left[\|G_R(i\omega)\|^2 - \frac{\langle G_R(i\omega),G_I(i\omega)\rangle^2}{\|G_I(i\omega)\|^2}\right]^{-\frac{1}{2}}$$

$$= \left[\frac{(1+\omega^4+\ldots+\omega^{2n-6})(1+\omega^4+\ldots+\omega^{2n-2})}{p_1^2(\omega^2)(1+\omega^4+\ldots+\omega^{2n-6}) + p_2^2(\omega^2)(1+\omega^4+\ldots+\omega^{2n-2})}\right]^{-\frac{1}{2}}.$$

Now $G_I(i\omega) = 0$ if and only if $\omega = 0$. Since $\|G_R(0)\| = 1/a_0$, (4.27) follows from (4.10).

□

As a consequence of this proposition we obtain the following interesting result which shows that the real unstructured stability radius of a real Hurwitz polynomial $p(s,a)$ can be expressed via the complex structured stability radius $r_{\mathbf{C}}^{-}(\tilde{a},C)$ of an associated complex polynomial.

Corollary 4.8
If $p(s,a)$, $a \in \mathbf{R}^{1\times n}$ is a Hurwitz polynomial, n even and

$$\tilde{a} = [a_0+ia_1, 0, a_2+ia_3, 0, \ldots, 0, a_{n-2} + ia_{n-1}] \tag{4.28a}$$

$$C = \begin{bmatrix} 1 & 0 & 0 & 0 & 0 & \cdots & 0 \\ 0 & 0 & 1 & 0 & 0 & \cdots & 0 \\ 0 & 0 & 0 & 0 & 1 & \cdots & 0 \\ \cdot & \cdot & \cdot & \cdot & \cdot & \cdots & \cdot \\ 0 & 0 & 0 & 0 & 0 & \cdots 1 & 0 \end{bmatrix}_{\frac{n}{2}\times n} . \tag{4.28b}$$

Then with respect to the Euclidean norm $\|\cdot\|_2$

$$d_{\mathbf{R}}^{-}(a) = \min\{a_0, r_{\mathbf{C}}^{-}(\tilde{a},C)\}. \tag{4.29}$$

Proof: By (4.26)

$$d_{\mathbf{R}}^{-}(a) = \min\left\{a_0, \left[\max_{\omega\in\mathbf{R}} \|\tilde{G}(i\omega)\|\right]^{-1}\right\}$$

where

$$\tilde{G}(i\omega) = \frac{1}{p_1(\omega^2)+ip_2(\omega^2)} \begin{bmatrix} 1 \\ (i\omega)^2 \\ \vdots \\ [(i\omega)^2]^{\frac{n-2}{2}} \end{bmatrix}_{\frac{n}{2}\times 1} \tag{4.30}$$

Using the notation of Proposition 4.7 we have

$$p_1(\omega^2) = a_0 - a_2\omega^2 + a_4\omega^4 - a_6\omega^6 + - \dots + (-1)^{\frac{n}{2}}\omega^n$$

$$p_2(\omega^2) = a_1 - a_3\omega^2 + a_5\omega^4 - a_7\omega^6 + - \dots + (-1)^{\frac{n-2}{2}} a_{n-1}\omega^{n-2}$$

and so

$$p_1(\omega^2) + ip_2(\omega^2) = (a_0+ia_1) + (a_2+ia_3)(i\omega)^2 + \dots + (a_{n-2}+ia_{n-1})(i\omega)^{n-2} + (i\omega)^n.$$

Hence $p(i\omega,\tilde{a}) = p_1(\omega^2) + ip_2(\omega^2)$ and so (4.29) follows by application of Corollary 3.3 to $\tilde{G}(i\omega)$. □

Unfortunately, we have not been able to obtain an analogous result for the case where n is odd.

Proposition 4.9
Under the same assumptions as in Proposition 4.7, but now with respect to the maximum norm, we have

$$d_{\mathbf{R}}^{-}(a) = \min\left\{a_0, \min_{\omega\in\mathbf{R}}\left[\frac{1}{1+\omega^2+\dots+\omega^{n-2}}\max\{|p_1(\omega^2)|,|p_2(\omega^2)|\}\right]\right\}, \quad n \text{ even}. \tag{4.31}$$

$$d_{\mathbf{R}}^{-}(a) = \min\left\{a_0, \min_{\omega\in\mathbf{R}}\max\left\{\frac{|p_1(\omega^2)|}{1+\omega^2+\dots+\omega^{n-1}}, \frac{|p_2(\omega^2)|}{1+\omega^2+\dots+\omega^{n-3}}\right\}\right\}, \quad n \text{ odd}. \tag{4.32}$$

Proof: The proof is for the case n odd. Using the formulae in the proof of Proposition 4.7 it is easy to see that

$$|p(i\omega,a)|^2\, \|G_R(i\omega) - \alpha G_I(i\omega)\|_1 = |p_1(\omega^2) + \alpha\omega p_2(\omega^2)|(1+\omega^2+\dots+\omega^{n-1}) \tag{4.33}$$
$$+ |\omega^2 p_2(\omega^2) - \alpha\omega p_1(\omega^2)|(1+\omega^2+\dots+\omega^{n-3}).$$

If $\omega \in \mathbf{R}$ is fixed, a minimum over $\alpha \in \mathbf{R}$ occurs when either $p_1(\omega^2) + \alpha\omega p_2(\omega^2) = 0$ or $\omega^2 p_2(\omega^2) - \alpha\omega p_1(\omega^2) = 0$. Solving for α and evaluating the RHS of (4.33) for this value of α yields

$$d(G_R(i\omega), \mathbf{R}G_I(i\omega)) = \min\left\{\frac{1+\omega^2+\dots+\omega^{n-1}}{|p_1(\omega^2)|}, \frac{1+\omega^2+\dots+\omega^{n-3}}{|p_2(\omega^2)|}\right\}$$

where the distance is taken with respect to the norm $\|\cdot\|_* = \|\cdot\|_1$.

Hence (4.32) follows from (4.8). □

$d_{\mathbf{R}}^{-}$ is the largest $\rho > 0$ such that all the polynomials in the cube

$$\{p(s,b);\quad a_i - \rho < b_i < a_i + \rho \quad \text{for} \quad i \in \underline{n}\}$$

are Hurwitz. The problem to determine the maximal ρ has been investigated in [14],[15] using Kharitonov's Theorem (see also [32] for an analysis of the quartic case (n=4)). Equations (4.31) and (4.32) yield - to our knowledge for the first time - explicit general formulae for $d_{\mathbf{R}}^{-}(a) = \rho_{max}$. It is noteworty that the above derivation of these formulae has not made any use of Kharitonov's theorem.

Finally we have

Proposition 4.10
Under the same assumptions as in Proposition 4.7, but now with respect to the norm $\|\cdot\|_1$, we have

$$d_{\mathbf{R}}^-(a) = \min\left\{a_0, \min_{\omega\in\mathbf{R}} f(\omega)\right\} \tag{4.34}$$

where

$$f(\omega) = \begin{cases} \max\{|p_2(\omega^2) - p_1(\omega^2)|, |p_2(\omega^2) + p_1(\omega^2)|\} & \text{if } |\omega| \le 1,\ n \text{ arbitrary} \\[2ex] \max\left\{\dfrac{|p_2(\omega^2)-p_1(\omega^2)|}{|\omega|^{n-2}}, \dfrac{|p_2(\omega^2)+p_1(\omega^2)|}{|\omega|^{n-2}}\right\} & \text{if } |\omega| > 1,\ n \text{ even} \\[2ex] \max\left\{\dfrac{|p_1(\omega^2) - \omega^2 p_2(\omega^2)|}{|\omega|^{n-1}}, \dfrac{|p_1(\omega^2) + \omega^2 p_2(\omega^2)|}{|\omega|^{n-1}}\right\} & \text{if } |\omega| > 1,\ n \text{ odd} \end{cases} \tag{4.35}$$

Proof: The proof is for the case n even. Using the formulae in the proof of Proposition 4.7 it is easy to see that

$$|p(i\omega,a)|^2 \, \|G_R(i\omega) - \alpha G_I(i\omega)\|_\infty$$

$$= \begin{cases} \max\{|p_1(\omega^2) + \alpha\omega p_2(\omega^2)|, |\omega^2 p_2(\omega^2) - \alpha\omega p_1(\omega^2)|\} & \text{if } |\omega| \le 1 \\[2ex] |\omega|^{n-2}\max\{|p_1(\omega^2) + \alpha\omega p_2(\omega^2)|, |\omega^2 p_2(\omega^2) - \alpha\omega p_1(\omega^2)|\} & \text{if } |\omega| > 1. \end{cases}$$

Here the upper formula holds for arbitrary $n \ge 1$. If $\omega \ne 0$ is fixed, α minimizes the maxima on the RHS if

$$|p_1(\omega^2) + \alpha\omega p_2(\omega^2)| = |\omega^2 p_2(\omega^2) - \alpha\omega p_1(\omega^2)|.$$

Since $(p_1(\omega), p_2(\omega)) \ne (0,0)$ this equation has at most two and at least one solution for α. Substituting for α yields

$$|p(i\omega,a)|^2 d(G_R(i\omega), \mathbf{R}G_I(i\omega)) = \frac{|p(i\omega,a)|^2}{|p_2(\omega^2) - p_1(\omega^2)|} \quad \text{or} \quad \frac{|p(i\omega,a)|^2}{|p_2(\omega^2) + p_1(\omega^2)|}$$

where the distance is taken with respect to $\|\cdot\|_* = \|\cdot\|_\infty$. Hence the result follows from (4.8). □

Before we conclude this paper with some illustrative examples, we briefly comment on the computation of the real stability radii via the formulae presented in this section.

To compute $d(y,\mathbf{R}v)$, $v \ne 0$, via (4.3) for the ∞-norm it is sufficient (as an easy argument shows) to search for α in the finite set

$$\{\alpha \in \mathbf{R}: |y_i - \alpha v_i| = |y_j - \alpha v_j| \text{ for some } i,j \in \underline{\ell},\ i \ne j\}.$$

For the 1-norm the search may be restricted to the set

$$\{\alpha \in \mathbf{R}: |y_i - \alpha v_i| = 0 \text{ for some } i \in \underline{\ell}\}.$$

In general, most of our computations have been carried out by crude search methods for a maximizing $s \in \partial \mathbb{C}_b$. However in some cases the algorithm Stabrad 2 can again be applied. For example to compute the unstructured stability radius $d_{\mathbf{R}}^{-}(a)$ with respect to the 2-norm via (4.26) or (4.27) one must determine the global maximum of a strictly proper rational function $f(\omega^2)$ over $\mathbf{R}_+$. The numerator and denominator are both positive on $\mathbf{R}_+$ so this can be carried out by the following three steps:

1. Compute a Cholesky factorization of $f(\omega^2)$, i.e.a strictly proper real rational function $g(s)$ which has all its poles and zeros in $\mathbf{C}_-$ such that

$$f(\omega^2) \quad = \quad g(-i\omega)g(i\omega) \quad = \quad |g(i\omega)|^2.$$

2. Determine a realization $(\tilde{A},\tilde{b},\tilde{c})$ of $g(s)$.
3. Compute $r_{\mathbf{C}}^{-}(\tilde{A};\tilde{b},\tilde{c})$ by means of the algorithm Stabrad 2, see [28].

As a result one obtains

$$d_{\mathbf{R}}^{-}(a) = \min\ \{a_0, r_{\mathbf{C}}^{-}(\tilde{A};\tilde{b},\tilde{c})\}. \tag{4.36}$$

In the scalar case (Corollary 4.4) if $G(s) = c(s)/p(s,a)$ and $p(s,a)$ is Hurwitz, write

$$c(s) = c_1(-s^2) + sc_2(-s^2), \quad p(s,a) = p_1(-s^2) + sp_2(-s^2)$$

where $c_1(-s^2)$, $c_2(-s^2)$, $p_1(-s^2)$, $p_2(-s^2)$ are real polynomials in $-s^2$. $c_1(-s^2)$, $p_1(-s^2)$ contain all the even power terms of $c(s)$ resp. $p(s,a)$ and $sc_2(-s^2)$, $sp_2(-s^2)$ contain all the odd-power terms in $c(s)$, resp. $p(s,a)$. Since

$$G(i\omega) \quad = \quad \frac{c_1(\omega^2) + i\omega\ c_2(\omega^2)}{p_1(\omega^2) + i\omega\ p_2(\omega^2)} \tag{4.37}$$

we have

$$G_R(i\omega) \quad = \quad \frac{c_1(\omega^2)p_1(\omega^2) + \omega^2 c_2(\omega^2)p_2(\omega^2)}{p_1^2(\omega^2) + \omega^2\ p_2^2(\omega^2)} \tag{4.38a}$$

$$G_I(i\omega) \quad = \quad \frac{\omega[c_2(\omega^2)p_1(\omega^2) - c_1(\omega^2)p_2(\omega^2)]}{p_1^2(\omega^2) + \omega^2\ p_2^2(\omega^2)}\ . \tag{4.38b}$$

By (4.20)

$$r_{\mathbf{R}}^{-}(a,c) = \min\{|G(i\omega)|^{-1};\quad \omega \in \mathbf{R},\quad G_I(i\omega) = 0\}. \tag{4.39}$$

Now $G_I(i\omega) = 0$ is equivalent to

$$\omega = 0 \quad \text{or} \quad [c_2(\omega^2)p_1(\omega^2) - c_1(\omega^2)p_2(\omega^2)] = 0 \tag{4.40}$$

where the expression in brackets is a real polynomial of degree < n in ω^2. This polynomial cannot be identically zero in ω^2 since otherwise

$$G(i\omega) = \frac{c_1(\omega^2)p_1(\omega^2) + i\omega\ c_1(\omega^2)p_2(\omega^2)}{p_1(\omega^2)[p_1(\omega^2) + i\omega\ p_2(\omega^2)]} = \frac{c_1(\omega^2)}{p_1(\omega^2)}, \quad \omega \in \mathbf{R}$$

hence by the identity theorem $G(s) = c_1(-s^2)/p_1(-s^2)$. But this contradicts the assumption that all the poles of G(s) lie in $\mathbf{C}_-$. Therefore the set Ω^2 of all $\omega^2 \geq 0$ satisfying (4.40) has at most n elements. Thus it simply remains to determine the minimum of a set of at most n real numbers:

$$r_{\mathbf{R}}^-(a,c) = \min_{\omega^2 \in \Omega^2} |G(i\omega)|^{-1}. \tag{4.41}$$

Example 4.11
Consider the Hurwitz polynomial

$$p(s,a) = s^4 + 5s^3 + 8s^2 + 8s + 3, \quad a = [3,8,8,5].$$

Applying Kharitonov's theorem Barmish [14] determined the largest $\varepsilon > 0$ for which the open cube in $\mathbf{R}^4$ with centre a and radius ε

$$\{p(s,b) : |b_i - a_i| < \varepsilon, \quad i = 0,1,2,3\} \tag{4.42}$$

only consists of Hurwitz polynomials. He obtained $\varepsilon_{max} = 1.81$. Since ε_{max} is the real stability distance $d_{\mathbf{R}}^-(a)$ with respect to the ∞-norm, we may use (4.31) to compute it. We have

$$d_{\mathbf{R}}^-(a) = \min \left\{ 3, \min_{\omega \in \mathbf{R}} \frac{1}{1+\omega^2} \max\{|\omega^4 - 8\omega^2 + 3|, |5\omega^2 - 3|\} \right\}.$$

Computing the RHS yields $d_{\mathbf{R}}^-(a) = 1.807$, so confirming the Barmish result. If instead we use the Euclidean norm, from (3.13a) and (4.26) we have

$$d_{\mathbf{C}}^-(a) = \min_{\omega \in \mathbf{R}} \left[\frac{(\omega^4 - 8\omega^2 + 3)^2 + (8\omega - 5\omega^3)^2}{1 + \omega^2 + \omega^4 + \omega^6} \right]^{1/2}$$

$$d_{\mathbf{R}}^-(a) = \min \left\{ 3, \min_{\omega^2 \in \mathbf{R}_+} \left[\frac{(\omega^4 - 8\omega^2 + 3)^2 + (8 - 5\omega^2)^2}{1 + \omega^4} \right]^{1/2} \right\}.$$

Applying Stabrad 2 as described above and in Section 2 one computes $d_{\mathbf{C}}^-(a) = 2.3776$, $d_{\mathbf{R}}^-(a) = 3$. The cube (4.42) with $\varepsilon = \varepsilon_{max}$ is not contained in the $\|\cdot\|_2$-ball with radius $d_{\mathbf{R}}^-(a) = 3$ and centre a, and vice versa.

With respect to the 1-norm we may use (4.34) but since $d = [-3,0,0,0]$ is destabilizing it is clear that we again have $d_{\mathbf{R}}^-(a) = 3$.

The stability radii of p(s,a) for perturbations of the single coefficients a_0, a_1, a_2, a_3 are, respectively

$r_{\mathbf{C}}^-(a,e^1) = 3$ $\quad r_{\mathbf{C}}^-(a,e^2) = 5$ $\quad r_{\mathbf{C}}^-(a,e^3) = 4.52$ $\quad r_{\mathbf{C}}^-(a,e^4) = 3.26$

$r_{\mathbf{R}}^-(a,e^1) = 3$ $\quad r_{\mathbf{R}}^-(a,e^2) = 6.03$ $\quad r_{\mathbf{R}}^-(a,e^3) = 4.53$ $\quad r_{\mathbf{R}}^-(a,e^4) = 3.95$.

Clearly, for any unit row vector $c \in \mathbf{K}^{1\times n}$, $\|c\| = 1$, $d_{\mathbf{K}}^-(a) \leq r_{\mathbf{K}}^-(a,c)$.
In the present case

$$d_{\mathbf{C}}^-(a) < \min_{j=1,\ldots,4} r_{\mathbf{C}}^-(a,e^j) \quad \text{but} \quad d_{\mathbf{R}}^-(a) = \min_{j=1,\ldots,4} r_{\mathbf{R}}^-(a,e^j).$$

□

Table 4.1 Real stability radii of $p(s,a) = (s+1)\ \ldots\ (s+7)$

norm	$d_{\mathbf{R}}^{-}(a)$	ω_0	d
1-norm	21.686	17.31	[0,0,0,0,0,0,1] 21.686
2-norm	21.597	17.29	[0,0,-.0002,.0019,.0722,-.5591,-21.591]
∞-norm	21.016	16.64	[-1,1,1,-1,-1,1,1] 21.016

In the next two examples we determine the real stability radii corresponding to some of the complex stability radii computed in Section 3.

Example 4.12
Consider the Hurwitz polynomial $p(s,a) = (s+1)(s+2)\ldots(s+7)$ analyzed in Example 3.7. By Corollary 4.5

$$r_{\mathbf{R}}^{-}(a,e^7) = \min \left\{ \left|\frac{p_1(\omega^2)}{\omega^6}\right| ;\quad \omega^2 \geq 0, \quad \omega\ p_2(\omega^2) = 0 \right\}$$

where (cf. Example 3.7)

$$\begin{aligned} p_1(\omega^2) &= -28\ \omega^6 + 1960\ \omega^4 - 13132\ \omega^2 + 5040 \\ p_1(\omega^2) &= -\omega^6 + 322\ \omega^4 - 6769\ \omega^2 + 13068. \end{aligned}$$

We compute $\Omega^2 = \{\omega^2 \in \mathbf{R}_+;\ \omega p_2(\omega^2) = 0\} = \{0, 1.47^2, 4.51^2, 17.31^2\}$ and hence

$$r_{\mathbf{R}}^{-}(a,e^7) = 21.60 \geq 18.3194 = r_{\mathbf{C}}^{-}(a,e^7).$$

By (4.27) we obtain for the distance of $p(s,a)$ from the set of real non-Hurwitz polynomials with respect to the 2-norm

$$d_{\mathbf{R}}^{-}(a) = \min \left\{ 5040, \left[\max_{\omega^2 \in \mathbf{R}_+} \frac{(1+\omega^4+\omega^8)(1+\omega^4+\omega^8+\omega^{12})}{p_1^2(\omega^2)(1+\omega^4+\omega^8) + p_2^2(\omega^2)(1+\omega^4+\omega^8+\omega^{12})} \right]^{-1/2} \right\}.$$

Similar formulae can be obtained from (4.32) and (4.34) for the unstructured stability radii with respect to the 1- and ∞-norms. Computation yields the results in Table 4.1 where the right hand column contains minimal destabilizing perturbations.

□

Example 4.13
Consider the perturbed polynomial

$$p(s,a(d)) = s^3 + 2s^2 + 4s + 2 - d(s^2 + 2s + 1)$$

studied in Example 3.8. By Corollary 4.4 the associated structured real stability radius is given by

$$r_{\mathbf{R}}^{-}(a,c) = \min \{ |G(i\omega)|^{-1};\ \omega \in \mathbf{R},\ G_I(i\omega) = 0 \}$$

where $a = [2,4,2]$, $c = [1,2,1]$ and (see (4.37),(4.38))

$$G(i\omega) = \frac{-\omega^2+1 + 2i\omega}{-2\omega^2+2 + i\omega(-\omega^2+4)}, \quad G_I(i\omega) = \frac{\omega^3(1-\omega^2)}{\omega^6-4\omega^4 + 8\omega^2+4}.$$

We compute $\Omega^2 = \{\omega^2 \in \mathbf{R}_+;\ G_I(i\omega) = 0\} = \{0,1\}$ and so

$$r_{\mathbf{R}}^-(a,c) = 1.5 > 1.08 = r_{\mathbf{C}}^-(a,c).$$

□

We end with an example illustrating Corollary 4.6

Example 4.14
By the Routh criterion a cubic polynomial

$$p(s,a) = s^3 + a_2 s^2 + a_1 s + a_0$$

is Hurwitz if and only if

$$a_0 > 0,\ a_1 > 0,\ a_2 > 0,\ a_1 a_2 > a_0.$$

Consider first the two Hurwitz polynomials

$$p(s,a) = s^3 + s^2 + 2s + 1, \quad p(s,b) = s^3 + 5s^2 + 10s + 13.$$

We have

$$p\left(s, \frac{1}{2}(a+b)\right) = s^3 + 3s^2 + 6s + 7, \quad c(s) = -(4s^2+8s+12))$$

hence

$$c_1(\omega^2) = 4\omega^2 - 12, \qquad c_2(\omega^2) = -8$$
$$p_1(\omega^2) = -3\omega^2 + 7, \qquad p_2(\omega^2) = -\omega^2 + 6.$$

Condition (4.40) has the form

$$\omega = 0 \quad \text{or} \quad -8(7-3\omega^2) - (4\omega^2-12)(6-\omega^2) = 0$$

so that $\Omega^2 = \{0\}$ and, by (4.39),

$$r_{\mathbf{R}}\left(\frac{a+b}{2}; a-b\right) = |G(0)|^{-1} = \frac{7}{12} > \frac{1}{2}.$$

Thus the segment of all convex combinations $\gamma p(s,a) + (1-\gamma)p(s,b)$, $0 \le \gamma \le 1$ consists of Hurwitz polynomials.

Now choose $p(s,a)$ as before but $p(s,b) = s^3 + 5s^2 + 10s + 29$.

Proceeding as above one obtains $\Omega^2 = \{0,3,4\}$ and

$$r_{\mathbf{R}}\left(\frac{a+b}{2}, b-a\right) = \min\left\{\left|\frac{-4\omega^2 + 8i\omega + 28}{-\omega^3 i - 3\omega^2 + 6\omega i + 15}\right|^{-1};\ \omega^2 \in \Omega^2\right\} = \frac{1}{4}.$$

Therefore, in this case the segment between $p(s,a)$ and $p(s,b)$ does not consist of Hurwitz polynomials only. In fact the closest non-Hurwitz polynomial to $p\left(s, \frac{a+b}{2}\right)$ on the line $p(s,a) + \mathbf{R}[p(s,b) - p(s,a)]$ is

$$p\left(s, \frac{a+b}{2} - \frac{1}{4}[p(s,b)-p(s,a)]\right) = p\left(s, \frac{3}{4}a + \frac{1}{4}b\right) = s^3 - 2s^2 + 4s + 8.$$

It has the roots -2 and ±2i.

□

Acknowledgement
We would like to thank Miss Jitske Pijnacker for performing the computations in the examples. This work was supported by the EEC "Stimulation action" under grant ST2J-0066-2.

References

[1] V.L. Kharitonov, Asymptotic stability of an equilibrium position of a family of systems of linear differential equations, *Differential Equations*, Plenum Publishing Corp. 14, 1483-1485 (1979).

[2] F.R. Gantmacher, The Theory of Matrices, vol. 2, Chelsea Publ. Co. (1959).

[3] N.K. Bose, A system-theoretic approach to stability of sets of polynomials, *Contemporary Math.*, vol. 47, 25-34 (1985).

[4] C. Hollot and A. Bartlett, Some discrete-time counterparts to Kharitonov's stability criterion for uncertain systems, *IEEE Trans. Aut. Control*, AC-31, 355-357 (1986).

[5] N.K. Bose and E. Zeheb, Kharitonov's theorem and stability test of multidimensional digital filters, *in*: Proc. IEE Circuits and System, London (1986).

[6] J. Cieslik, On possibilities of the extension of Kharitonov's stability test for interval polynomials to the discrete time case, *IEEE Trans. Aut. Control*, AC-32, 237-238 (1987).

[7] K.W. Wei and R.K. Yedavalli, Invariance of strict Hurwitz property for uncertain polynomials with dependent coefficients, *IEEE Trans. Aut. Control*, AC-32, 907-909 (1987).

[8] B.D.O. Anderson, E.I. Jury and M. Mansour, On robust Hurwitz polynomials, *IEEE Trans. Aut. Control*, AC-32, 909-913 (1987).

[9] K.S. Yeung, Linear system stability under parameter uncertainties, *Int. J. Control*, vol. 38, 459-468, (1983).

[10] M.B. Argoun, Stability of a Hurwitz polynomial under coefficient perturbations: necessary and sufficient conditions, *Int. J. Control*, vol. 45, 739-744 (1987).

[11] A.V. Lipatov and N.I. Sokolov, Some sufficient conditions for stability and instability of continuous linear stationary systems, *Aut. and Remote Control* 39, 1285-1291 (1979).

[12] Y.Y. Nie and X.K. Xie, New criteria of polynomial stability, to appear in: *Int. J. Control*.

[13] N.K. Bose, E.I. Jury and E. Zeheb, On robust Hurwitz and Schur polynomials, Proc. 25th Conference on Decision and Control, Athens, 739-744 (1986).

[14] B.R. Barmish, Invariance of the strict Hurwitz property for polynomials with perturbed coefficients, *IEEE Trans. Aut. Control*, AC-29, 935-937 (1984).

[15] S. Bialas and J. Garloff, Stability of the strict Hurwitz property for polynomials with perturbed coefficients, *IEEE Trans. Aut. Control*, AC-30, 935-936 (1985).

[16] C.B. Soh, C.S. Berger and K.P. Dabke, On the stability properties of polynomials with perturbed coefficients, *IEEE Trans. Aut. Control* AC-30, 1033-1036 (1985).

[17] C.B. Soh, C.S. Berger and K.P. Dabke, Addendum to "On the stability properties of polynomials with perturbed coefficients", *Trans. Aut. Control*, AC-32 (1987).

[18] R.M. Biernacki, H. Hwang and S.P. Bhattacharyya, Robust stability with structured real parameter perturbations, *IEEE Trans. Aut. Control*, AC-32, 495-506 (1987).

[19] A.T. Fam and I.S. Meditch, A canonical parameter space for linear systems design, *IEEE Trans. Aut. Control*, AC-23, 454-458 (1978).

[20] S. Bialas, A necessary and sufficient condition for the stability of interval matrices, *Int. J. Control*, vol. 37, 717-722 (1983).

[21] B.R. Barmish and C.V. Hollot, Counter-example to a recent result on the stability of interval matrices by S. Bialas, *Int. J. Control*, vol. 39, 1103-1104 (1984).

[22] D. Hinrichsen and A.J. Pritchard, Stability radii of linear systems, *Systems and Control Letters*, vol. 7, 1-10 (1986a).

[23] D. Hinrichsen and A.J. Pritchard, Stability radius for structured perturbations and the algebraic Riccati equation, *Systems and Control Letters*, vol. 8, 105-113 (1986b).

[24] A.J. Pritchard and S. Townley, A stability radius for infinite dimensional systems, *in*: Proc. Conf. of Distributed Parameter Systems, Vorau, 1986, Lecture Notes in Control and Information Sciences, vol. 102 (1987).

[25] D. Hinrichsen, A. Ilchmann and A.J. Pritchard, Robustness of stability of time-varying linear systems, Institut für Dynamische Systeme, Report No. 161, Universität Bremen (1987), to appear in: *J. Diff. Equ.*

[26] D. Hinrichsen and M. Motscha, Optimization problems in the robustness analysis of linear state space systems, Inst. für Dynamische Systeme, Report No. 169, U. Bremen 1987, to appear in: Proc. Seminar Approximation and Optimization, Habana 1987, Lecture Notes in Mathematics, Springer Verlag.

[27] A. Pritchard and S. Townley, Robustness of linear systems, Control Theory Centre, Report 141, U. Warwick, 1987, to appear in: *J. Diff. Equ.*

[28] D. Hinrichsen, B. Kelb and A. Linnemann, An algorithm for the computation of the structured stability radius with applications, Inst. für Dynamische Systeme, Report No. 182, U. Bremen, 1987, submitted.

[29] D. Hinrichsen and A.J. Pritchard, New robustness results for linear systems under real perturbations, *in:* Proc. 27th IEEE, Conference on Decision and Control, Austin, 1375-1379 (1988)

[30] K.E. Atkinson, An Introduction to Numerical Analysis, J. Wiley (1978).

[31] D.G. Luenberger, Optimization by Vector Space Methods, J. Wiley, New York (1969).

[32] J.P. Guiver and N.K. Bose, Strictly Hurwitz property invariance of quartics under coefficient perturbation, *IEEE Trans. Aut. Control*, AC-28, 106-107, (1983).

ROBUST STABILITY AND STABILIZATION OF INTERVAL PLANTS

Hervé Chapellat and S. P. Bhattacharyya

Department of Electrical Engineering, Texas A&M University

College Station, TX 77843, USA

1. ABSTRACT

In this paper we describe some new results on robust stability and stabilization of control systems under unknown but bounded parameter perturbations, using a polynomial framework. We first described, without proof, a recent generalization of Kharitonov's Theorem that solves the problem of checking the robust stability of a control system containing an interval plant. Next we present some efficient formulas for the ℓ^2 stability margin in parameter space. Finally a robust state feedback stabilization problem and a robust output feedback stabilization problem are solved. The results are illustrated by examples.

2. INTRODUCTION

The robust stability of control systems subject to bounded parameter perturbations is an area of practical importance. Here we present some new results on this problem. Proofs of some of the results are not included and the reader is referred to the appropriate sources. The paper is organized as follows. In the first part, some analysis results are given. We begin by describing a generalization of Kharitonov's Theorem [1]. This generalization, called the Box Theorem, gives necessary and sufficient conditions for the Hurwitz stability of a control system containing a family of plants. The family of plants in question is generated by the variation, within given intervals, of the coefficients of certain prescribed polynomials. For example, these could consist of some or all of the coefficients of the transfer functions describing the plant (interval plant). Such a formulation captures mathematically many practical cases and can overcome the basic limitation of Kharitonov's original theorem arising from the assumption of independence of the polynomial coefficient perturbations.

The Box Theorem prescribes that a certain number of line segments in the parameter space of the plant must be checked for stability. This result is Kharitonov-like in the sense that this number is independent of the order of the system and the number of parameters. The latter also makes this result computationally attractive. Next for this same case of interval plants we present, also without proof, some computationally efficient formulas to calculate exactly the radius of the largest stability hypershpere in parameter space (ℓ^2 -stability margin). The above results are new and we expect them to be useful in the analysis and design of robust control systems. In the second part of the paper we present solutions to two synthesis problems. The first problem can be interpreted as a robust state feedback stabilization problem; our result shows how the robust gain can be calculated. The second problem deals with the robust output feedback stabilization of a class of interval plants; our results show how to calculate a robust feedback controller. These results are also new and we believe that they will play an important role in the development of a complete theory of synthesis of robust controllers.

3. THE BOX PROBLEM IN PARAMETER SPACE

Let the transfer function of a single input multi output plant of order q be described by,

$$G(s) = \frac{1}{d^p(s)} \begin{pmatrix} n_1^p(s) \\ \cdot \\ \cdot \\ \cdot \\ n_m^p(s) \end{pmatrix}.$$

We suppose, for the sake of being specific, that the parameter vector subject to perturbation is the set of transfer function coefficients

$$\underline{P} := [n_{1,0}^p, \ldots, n_{1,q}^p, \ldots, n_{m,0}^p, \ldots, n_{m,q}^p, d_0^p, \ldots, d_m^p],$$

so that

$$n_{i,j}^p \in [\alpha_{i,j}, \beta_{i,j}] \text{ for } i = 1, \ldots, m; \quad j = 0, \ldots, q \tag{3.1}$$

and

$$d_j^p \in [\gamma_j, \kappa_j] \text{ for } j = 0, \ldots, q. \tag{3.2}$$

Thus each coefficient of the $m+1$ polynomials $n_1^p(s), \ldots, n_m^p(s), d^p(s)$, varies in a prescribed arbitrary interval, and the corresponding set of transfer functions $\{G(s)\}$ constitutes the given "interval plant". Of course this includes the case where some coefficients are fixed. Suppose now that a feedback controller with transfer function

$$C(s) = \frac{1}{d^c(s)}(n_1^c(s), \ldots, n_m^c(s)),$$

is proposed. Our problem is to determine wether or not this controller stabilizes the given family of interval plants $\{G(s)\}$. It is obvious that Kharitonov's theorem on interval polynomials does not apply here. As an example consider the following:

$$G(s) = \frac{n^p(s)}{d^p(s)} = \frac{s}{1 - s + \alpha s^2 + s^3}, \text{ where } \alpha \in [3.4, 5],$$

and has a nominal value

$$\alpha^0 = 4.$$

We know that the controller $C(s) = \frac{3}{s+1}$ stabilizes the nominal plant, yielding the nominal closed-loop characteristic polynomial,

$$\delta_4(s) = 1 + 3s + 3s^2 + 5s^3 + s^4.$$

The question of interest is to determine whether $C(s)$ also stabilizes the family of perturbed plants. For a perturbed plant the characteristic polynomial is

$$\delta_\alpha(s) = 1 + 3s + (\alpha - 1)s^2 + (\alpha + 1)s^3 + s^4.$$

In the space (δ_2, δ_3), the coefficients of s^2 and s^3 describe a line segment. To apply Kharitonov's theorem here we have to enclose this segment in a box $\mathcal{B}$ defined by the two 'real' points R_1 and R_2 and two 'artificial' points A_1 and A_2.
However,

$$\delta_{A_1}(s) = 1 + 3s + 2.4s^2 + 6s^3 + s^4,$$

is unstable because its third Hurwitz determinant H_3 is

$$H_3 = \begin{vmatrix} 6 & 3 & 0 \\ 1 & 2.4 & 1 \\ 0 & 6 & 3 \end{vmatrix} = -1.8 < 0.$$

Therefore, Kharitonov's theorem here does not allow us to conclude the stability of the entire family of closed-loop systems. And yet if one checks the values of the Hurwitz determinants along the segment $[R_1, R_2]$ one finds:

$$H = \begin{vmatrix} 1+\alpha & 3 & 0 & 0 \\ 1 & \alpha - 1 & 1 & 0 \\ 0 & 1+\alpha & 3 & 0 \\ 0 & 1 & \alpha - 1 & 1 \end{vmatrix}$$

and

$$\begin{cases} H_1 = 1 + \alpha \\ H_2 = \alpha^2 - 4 \\ H_3 = 2\alpha^2 - 2\alpha - 13 \\ H_4 = H_3 \end{cases} \quad \text{all positive for } \alpha \in [3.4, 5].$$

We therefore see that Kharitonov's original theorem provides only sufficient conditions for our control problem which may sometimes be too restrictive.

An alternative that we do have, using the presently available results, is to apply the Edge theorem of [2]. Since the parameters of the plant lie within a box and the coefficients of the characteristic polynomial depend linearly on the plant parameters, they are certainly also inscribed within a polytope. Consequently the Edge theorem does provide a set of necessary and sufficient conditions in this case. However, let us see what computations are involved in applying the Edge theorem. The plant parameter vector is of dimension $(m+1)(q+1)$, and a box in $R^{(m+1)(q+1)}$, has exactly

$$e = (m+1)(q+1)2^{(m+1)(q+1)-1} \text{ edges.}$$

For a 3rd order plant with 2 outputs, $m = 2, q = 3$, and we get

$$e = 3 \times 4 \times 2^{11} = 24576,$$

and therefore we need to carry out 24576 root loci which is a rather Moreover, this solution using the Edge theorem does not generalize Kharitonov's result. The characteristic polynomial of the closed loop system is given by

$$\delta(s) = d^c(s)d^p(s) + n_m^c(s)n_m^p(s) + \ldots + n_1^c(s)n_1^p(s).$$

Our task is to study the stability of such polynomials $\delta(s)$, where the polynomials $n_i^c(s), d^c(s)$ are fixed and the polynomials $n_i^p(s), d^p(s)$ are interval polynomials. The solution of this problem is given in the following section without proof.

4. A GENERALIZATION OF KHARITONOV'S THEOREM: THE BOX THEOREM

Let m be an arbitrary integer and let

$$\underline{P} = \big(P_1(s), P_2(s), \ldots, P_m(s)\big), \tag{4.1}$$

be an m-tuple of real polynomials where each coefficient $p_{i,j}$ of $P_i(s)$ belongs to a given interval,

$$p_{i,j} \in [\alpha_{i,j}, \beta_{i,j}] \quad i = 1, \ldots, m \quad j = 0, \ldots, d^o(P_i), \tag{4.2}$$

where $d^o(P_i)$ stands for the degree of the polynomial $P_i(s)$.

Let $\mathcal{F}$ denote the family of all possible m-tuples corresponding to (4.2). Each individual polynomial $P_i(s)$ in (4.1) can itself be considered as an interval polynomial and therefore we can define

$$\begin{aligned}
K_i^1(s) &= \alpha_{i,0} + \alpha_{i,1}s + \beta_{i,2}s^2 + \beta_{i,3}s^3 + \ldots \\
K_i^2(s) &= \alpha_{i,0} + \beta_{i,1}s + \beta_{i,2}s^2 + \alpha_{i,3}s^3 + \ldots \\
K_i^3(s) &= \beta_{i,0} + \alpha_{i,1}s + \alpha_{i,2}s^2 + \beta_{i,3}s^3 + \ldots \\
K_i^4(s) &= \beta_{i,0} + \beta_{i,1}s + \alpha_{i,2}s^2 + \alpha_{i,3}s^3 + \ldots,
\end{aligned}$$

the four Kharitonov polynomials associated with the family of interval polynomials corresponding to $P_i(s)$.

Now, define a family of $m4^m$ segments as follows: For any fixed integer l between 1 and m, set

$$P_i(s) = K_i^k(s), \text{ for } i \neq l \text{ and for some } k = 1, 2, 3, 4,$$

and for l, suppose that $P_l(s)$ varies in one of the four segments

$$[K_l^1(s), K_l^2(s)] \text{ or } [K_l^1(s), K_l^3(s)] \text{ or } [K_l^2(s), K_l^4(s)] \text{ or } [K_l^3(s), K_l^4(s)],$$

which we call the Kharitonov segments. By segment $[K_l^1(s), K_l^2(s)]$, we mean of course all convex combinations of the form,

$$(1 - \lambda)K_l^1(s) + \lambda K_l^2(s), \ \lambda \in [0, 1].$$

There are clearly $m4^m$ such segments and we will denote by $\mathcal{S}_m$ the family of all these segments. Any one of these segments is the set of all convex combinations of two m-tuples of polynomials, as for example

$$\underline{P}_\lambda = \left(K_1^{j_1}(s), K_2^{j_2}(s), \ldots, K_{l-1}^{j_{l-1}}(s), (1-\lambda)K_l^1(s)+\lambda K_l^2(s), K_{l+1}^{j_{l+1}}(s), \ldots, K_m^{j_m}(s)\right), \tag{4.3}$$

which can be rewritten as,

$$\underline{P}_\lambda = (1-\lambda)\left(K_1^{j_1}(s), K_2^{j_2}(s), \ldots, K_{l-1}^{j_{l-1}}(s), K_l^1(s), K_{l+1}^{j_{l+1}}(s), \ldots, K_m^{j_m}(s)\right)+$$
$$\lambda\left(K_1^{j_1}(s), K_2^{j_2}(s), \ldots, K_{l-1}^{j_{l-1}}(s), K_l^2(s), K_{l+1}^{j_{l+1}}(s), \ldots, K_m^{j_m}(s)\right).$$

Let us also define $\mathcal{K}_m$ as the finite set of all possible m-tuples where each polynomial is equal to one of the four corresponding Kharitonov polynomials. $\mathcal{K}_m$ contains (in general) 4^m m-tuples, as for example when $\lambda = 0$ or $\lambda = 1$ in (4.3)

Now let $\underline{Q} = (Q_1(s), \ldots, Q_m(s))$ be any given m-tuple of polynomials. We will say that $\underline{Q}$ stabilizes another given m-tuple $\underline{R} = (R_1(s), \ldots, R_m(s))$, if the polynomial

$$Q_1(s)R_1(s) + Q_2(s)R_2(s) + \ldots + Q_m(s)R_m(s),$$

is stable. Similarly we will say that $\underline{Q}$ stabilizes the segment in (4.3) if $\underline{Q}$ stabilizes $\underline{P}_\lambda$, for all λ in $[0,1]$. We can now enunciate the following theorem.

Theorem 4.1: (The Box Theorem.)

For any given m-tuple $\underline{Q} = (Q_1(s), \ldots, Q_m(s))$,

I) $\underline{Q}$ stabilizes the entire family $\mathcal{F}$ of m-tuples if and only if $\underline{Q}$ stabilizes every segment in $\mathcal{S}_m$.

II) Moreover, if for each polynomial $Q_i(s)$, $Q_i(s)$ is either even or odd, then it is enough that $\underline{Q}$ stabilizes the finite set of m-tuples $\mathcal{K}_m$.

III) Finally, stabilizing the finite set $\mathcal{K}_m$ is not sufficient to stabilize $\mathcal{F}$ when the polynomials $Q_i(s)$ do not satisfy the restrictions of II).

The proof of this result is omitted and may be found in [3] and [4].

Remarks: 1) One can immediately see that in the particular case $m = 1$, and $Q_1(s) = 1$, the Box Theorem reduces to Kharitonov's theorem because $Q_1(s) = 1$ is obviously even and part II) of the theorem applies.

2) In the simple case $m = 2, q = 3$ that we considered before, $\mathcal{S}_3$ contains

$$3 \times 4^3 = 192 \text{ segments},$$

and therefore we need only carry out 192 root loci to answer our problem, which is significantly less than the 24576 that were necessary when using the Edge theorem. This improvment is of course mainly due to the fact that the number of elements in $\mathcal{S}_{m+1}$ depends only on m and not on the number of varying parameters, whereas the corresponding number for the Edge theorem depends exponentially on this number.

3) It is also clear that in a practical situation not all the coefficients of the polynomials are necessarily going to vary. Therefore the number of root loci to

be checked may happen to be much smaller than the maximum theoretical number of $m4^m$.
4) This result clearly solves completely the problem of checking wheter or not a prescribed box in parameter space is stabilized by a given controller as shown by the following example.

Example:

$$G(s) = \frac{n^p(s)}{d^p(s)} = \frac{s^3 + \alpha s^2 - 2s + \beta}{s^4 + 2s^3 - s^2 + \gamma s + 1},$$

where

$$\alpha \in [-1, -2], \quad \beta \in [0.5, 1], \quad \gamma \in [0, 1].$$

There are two Kharitonov polynomials associated with $n^p(s)$, namely

$$K^{n,1}(s) = K^{n,2}(s) = 0.5 - 2s - s^2 + s^3, \text{ and }, K^{n,3}(s) = K^{n,4}(s) = 1 - 2s - 2s^2 + s^3,$$

and also two Kharitonov polynomials associated with $d^p(s)$,

$$K^{d,1}(s) = K^{d,3}(s) = 1 - s^2 + 2s^3 + s^4, \text{ and }, K^{d,2}(s) = K^{d,4}(s) = 1 + s - s^2 + 2s^3 + s^4,$$

In order to check that a given controller $C(s)$ stabilizes the entire family of plants, we only need to check that the controller stabilizes the following four segments:

$$\underline{P}_{\lambda,1} = \left(0.5(1+\lambda) - 2s - (1+2\lambda)s^2 + s^3, 1 - s^2 + 2s^3 + s^4\right),$$

$$\underline{P}_{\lambda,2} = \left(0.5(1+\lambda) - 2s + (1+2\lambda)s^2 + s^3, 1 + s - s^2 + 2s^3 + s^4\right),$$

$$\underline{P}_{\lambda,3} = \left(0.5 - 2s - s^2 + s^3, 1 + \lambda s - s^2 + 2s^3 + s^4\right),$$

$$\underline{P}_{\lambda,4} = \left(1 - 2s - 2s^2 + s^3, 1 + \lambda s - s^2 + 2s^3 + s^4\right).$$

5. EXACT CALCULATION OF THE ℓ^2 STABILITY MARGIN

In this section we continue to deal with interval plants but turn to a different type of robustness question. Given a system which is stable at the nominal operating point, we are interested in determining the distance from instability, or equivalently, a stability margin for such control systems. The stability margin can be used to rank the robustness provided by alternative controllers and is therefore of obvious importance in design.

The formulas that are given here without proof are derived by applying the orthogonal projection theorem in the appropriate Euclidean vector space of polynomial m-tuples. This results provide quasi closed form expressions for the stability margin, constitute an improvement over existing computational procedures and also provide deeper insight.

Letting $\underline{X}$ and $\underline{P}$ denote the controller and plant parameter vectors respectively, we consider as before the case in which the characteristic polynomial coefficients $\delta_i(\underline{X}, \underline{P})$ are linear functions of the plant parameter vector $\underline{P}$. Although this is, mathematically, a special case, it will always hold in single input (multi-output) or single output (multi-input) systems if the parameter vector $\underline{P}$ is taken to be the list of plant transfer function coefficients. Since the theory is similar for the two cases we restrict our considerations to the single input case.

Let

$$G(s) = \begin{pmatrix} \frac{\hat{n}_1^p(s)}{\hat{d}_1^p(s)} \\ \cdot \\ \cdot \\ \cdot \\ \frac{\hat{n}_m^p(s)}{\hat{d}_m^p(s)} \end{pmatrix} = \frac{1}{d^p(s)} \begin{pmatrix} n_1^p(s) \\ \cdot \\ \cdot \\ \cdot \\ n_m^p(s) \end{pmatrix},$$

where $d^p(s)$ is the least common denominator of all elements of $G(s)$ and $(n_1^p(s), n_2^p(s), \cdots, n_m^p(s), d^p(s))$ are assumed to be relatively prime. The order of the plant is q and

$$d^p(s) = d_q^p s^q + \cdots + d_0^p ,$$

$$n_i^p(s) = n_{i,q}^p s^q + \cdots + n_{i,0}^p , \quad i = 1, \cdots, m.$$

The plant parameter vector is taken to be:

$$\underline{P} := (n_{1,0}^p, \cdots, n_{1,q}^p, n_{2,0}^p, \cdots, n_{2,q}^p, \cdots, n_{m,0}^p, \cdots, n_{m,q}^p, d_0^p, \cdots, d_q^p),$$

and is a vector of $R^{(m+1)(q+1)}$, or equivalently:

$$\underline{P} := (n_1^p(s), n_2^p(s), \cdots, n_m^p(s), d^p(s)).$$

The length of the perturbation of the plant parameter vector, is measured by its Euclidean norm, that is:

$$\|\Delta \underline{P}\|^2 = \sum_{i=1}^{m} \sum_{j=0}^{q} \Delta n_{i,j}^{p\ 2} \quad + \quad \sum_{j=0}^{q} \Delta d_j^{p2}. \tag{5.1}$$

The controller transfer function is of order r and is described by:

$$C(s) = \frac{1}{d^c(s)} (n_1^c(s), \cdots, n_m^c(s)),$$

where $(n_1^c(s), n_2^c(s), \cdots, n_m^c(s), d^c(s))$ are assumed to be relatively prime, and

$$d^c(s) = d_r^c s^r + \cdots + d_0^c ,$$

$$n_i^c(s) = n_{i,r}^c s^r + \cdots + n_{i,0}^c , \quad i = 0, \cdots, m.$$

Similarly we can define the controller parameter vector as

$$\underline{X} := (n_{1,0}^c, \cdots, n_{1,r}^c, n_{2,0}^c, \cdots, n_{2,r}^c, \cdots, n_{m,0}^c, \cdots, n_{m,r}^c, d_0^c, \cdots, d_r^c),$$

and it is a vector of $R^{(m+1)(r+1)}$, or equivalently:

$$\underline{X} := (n_1^c(s), n_2^c(s), \cdots, n_m^c(s), d^c(s)).$$

The characteristic polynomial of the closed loop system is then given by the polynomial $\delta(s)$ of degree $n = q + r$:

$$\delta(s) = d^c(s)d^p(s) + n_m^c(s)n_m^p(s) + \cdots + n_1^c(s)n_1^p(s). \tag{5.2}$$

Let $C(s)$ be a fixed controller which stabilizes the nominal plant $G(s, \underline{P})$, and consider perturbations on the plant parameter vector $\Delta\underline{P}$. It is of interest in control system design to find the largest stability ball in this space, as it serves as a stability margin for the system. A solution to this problem has already been proposed in [5]. That solution is computationally unattractive because it involves the solution of a linear equation at each frequency. The new formulas given here are efficient and in closed form.

Introduce $\mathcal{P}_n$, the vector space of all real polynomials of degree less than or equal to n with its natural inner product defined as follows:

$$\text{If } \; P(s) = p_0 + p_1 s + \cdots + p_n s^n, \quad \text{and} \quad R(s) = r_0 + r_1 s + \cdots + r_n s^n,$$

then:

$$< P(s), R(s) > := p_0 r_0 + p_1 r_1 + \cdots + p_n r_n = \sum_{i=0}^{n} p_i r_i.$$

The Euclidean norm associated with it is:

$$\|P(s)\|^2 =< P(s), P(s) >= p_0^2 + p_1^2 + \cdots + p_n^2.$$

For any l and n we now denote by $\mathcal{P}_n^l$ the vector space

$$\underbrace{\mathcal{P}_n \times \mathcal{P}_n \times \cdots \times \mathcal{P}_n}_{l \text{ times}},$$

where $\times$ designates the Cartesian product. $\mathcal{P}_n^l$ is given the induced inner product defined as follows: if,

$$\underline{P} = (P_1(s), P_2(s), \cdots, P_l(s)), \quad \text{and} \quad \underline{R} = (R_1(s), R_2(s), \cdots, R_l(s)),$$

$$\text{then} \quad \ll \underline{P}, \underline{R} \gg = \sum_{i=1}^{l} < P_i(s), R_i(s) > = \sum_{i=1}^{l}\left(\sum_{j=0}^{n} p_{i,j} r_{i,j}\right). \tag{5.3}$$

The norm associated with this inner product still corresponds with the Euclidean norm:

$$[[\underline{P}]]^2 = \|P_1\|^2 + \|P_2\|^2 + \cdots + \|P_l\|^2. \tag{5.4}$$

We use the notation $[[\cdot]]$, and $\ll \cdot, \cdot \gg$ to clearly distinguish the two vector spaces $\mathcal{P}_n$ and $\mathcal{P}_n^l$.

The closed-loop characteristic polynomial is

$$\delta(s) = d^c(s)d^p(s) + n_m^c(s)n_m^p(s) + \cdots + n_1^c(s)n_1^p(s),$$

so that $\delta(s)$ belongs to $\mathcal{P}_n$, with $n = q + r$. This can also be viewed as a linear operator δ_X, which maps $\underline{P}$ into the characteristic polynomial $\delta(s)$:

$$\mathcal{P}_q^{m+1} \xrightarrow{\delta_X} \mathcal{P}_n = \mathcal{P}_{r+q}$$

$$\underline{P} = (n_1^p(s), \cdots, n_m^p(s), d^p(s)) \longrightarrow \delta(s) = \sum_{j=1}^{m} n_j^p(s) n_j^c(s) + d^p(s) d^c(s).$$

We now show how it is possible to compute the radius $\rho(\underline{P})$ of the largest stability hypersphere around $\underline{P}$. Define the following subspaces of $\mathcal{P}_n$: Δ_0, the subspace containing all polynomials with a root at the origin, Δ_n, the subspace of all elements of $\mathcal{P}_n$ which are of degree less than n, and finally Δ_ω, the subspace of all polynomials having $\pm j\omega$ among their roots. Since the application $\delta_X(\cdot)$ is a linear operator, we can define the following subspaces of $\mathcal{P}_q^{m+1}$:

$$\Pi_0 = \delta_X^{-1}(\Delta_0), \quad \Pi_n = \delta_X^{-1}(\Delta_n), \quad \Pi_\omega = \delta_X^{-1}(\Delta_\omega),$$

where $\delta_X^{-1}(\cdot)$ designates the inverse image with respect to the linear map $\delta_X(\cdot)$.

$\mathcal{P}_q^{m+1}$ is also a Euclidean space, so that we can use the projection theorem. We can thus define the distances from $\underline{P}$ to the subspaces Π_0, Π_n and Π_ω for $\omega \geq 0$, and denote them by d_0^p, d_n^p and d_ω^p respectively. Letting

$$d_{min}^p = \inf_{\omega \geq 0} d_\omega^p,$$

it can be shown that ([5],[6]):

$$\rho(\underline{P}) = min(d_0^p, d_n^p, d_{min}^p).$$

The expressions of d_0^p and d_n^p are easy to find, but d_ω^p and d_{min}^p are hard to calculate. Our main results which calculate these quantities are summarized in the following theorem. Before stating our theorem, we introduce some notation. For any polynomial

$$p(s) = p_0 + p_1 s + \cdots + p_n s^n,$$

we denote by $p_{even}(s)$ its even part and by $p_{odd}(s)$ its odd part. Also $p^e(\omega)$ and $p^o(\omega)$ are defined as follows:

$$p^e(\omega) = p_{even}(j\omega) = p_0 - p_2\omega^2 + p_4\omega^4 - \cdots$$

and

$$p^o(\omega) = \frac{p_{odd}(j\omega)}{j\omega} = p_1 - p_3\omega^2 + p_5\omega^4 - \cdots.$$

<u>Theorem 5.1</u>: Let $\underline{P} = (n_1^p(s), \cdots, n_m^p(s), d^p(s))$ be a plant of order q and let $C(s)$ be a stabilizing controller of order r determined by $\underline{X} = (n_1^c(s), \cdots, n_m^c(s), d^c(s))$. The distances d_ω^p, d_0^p and d_n^p from $\underline{P}$ to Π_ω, Π_0 and Π_n respectively are given by:
a)

$$d_\omega^{p\,2} = \frac{\lambda_1^2 [[\underline{Z}_1]]^2 + \lambda_2^2 [[\underline{Z}_2]]^2 - 2\lambda_1\lambda_2 \ll \underline{Z}_1, \underline{Z}_2 \gg}{[[\underline{Z}_1]]^2 [[\underline{Z}_2]]^2 - \ll \underline{Z}_1, \underline{Z}_2 \gg^2},$$

with

$$\lambda_1 = \sum_{i=1}^{m}\left(n_i^{ce}(\omega)n_i^{pe}(\omega) - \omega^2 n_i^{co}(\omega)n_i^{po}(\omega)\right) + d^{ce}(\omega)d^{pe}(\omega) - \omega^2 d^{co}(\omega)d^{po}(\omega),$$

$$\lambda_2 = \sum_{i=1}^{m}\left(n_i^{ce}(\omega)n_i^{po}(\omega) + n_i^{co}(\omega)n_i^{pe}(\omega)\right) + d^{ce}(\omega)d^{po}(\omega) + d^{co}(\omega)d^{pe}(\omega),$$

and

$$\underline{Z}_1 = \Big(n_1^{ce}(\omega)P_1(s) + n_1^{co}(\omega)P_2(s), \cdots, n_m^{ce}(\omega)P_1(s) + n_m^{co}(\omega)P_2(s),$$
$$d^{ce}(\omega)P_1(s) + d^{co}(\omega)P_2(s)\Big),$$

$$\underline{Z}_2 = \Big(n_1^{ce}(\omega)P_2(s) - \omega^2 n_1^{co}(\omega)P_1(s), \cdots, n_m^{ce}(\omega)P_2(s) - \omega^2 n_m^{co}(\omega)P_1(s),$$
$$d^{ce}(\omega)P_2(s) - \omega^2 d^{co}(\omega)P_1(s)\Big),$$

where $P_1(s), P_2(s)$ are defined as follows (depending on the plant order q):
i) $\underline{q = 2l}$

$$P_1(s) = \begin{cases} s - \omega^2 s^3 + \cdots\cdots + (-1)^{l-1}\omega^{2l-2}s^{2l-1} \text{ if } q \neq 0 \\ 0 \text{ if } q = 0, \end{cases}$$
$$P_2(s) = 1 - \omega^2 s^2 + \cdots\cdots + (-1)^l \omega^{2l} s^{2l}.$$

ii) $\underline{q = 2l + 1}$

$$P_1(s) = s - \omega^2 s^3 + \cdots\cdots + (-1)^l \omega^{2l} s^{2l+1},$$
$$P_2(s) = 1 - \omega^2 s^2 + \cdots\cdots + (-1)^l \omega^{2l} s^{2l}.$$

b)

$$d_0^{p\,2} = \frac{(\sum_{i=1}^{m} n_{i,0}^{p} n_{i,0}^{c} + d_0^p d_0^c)^2}{\sum_{i=1}^{m} n_{i,0}^{c\;2} + d_0^{c\,2}}.$$

c)

$$d_n^{p\,2} = \frac{(\sum_{i=1}^{m} n_{i,q}^{p} n_{i,r}^{c} + d_q^p d_r^c)^2}{\sum_{i=1}^{m} n_{i,r}^{c\;2} + d_r^{c\,2}}.$$

The proof of this theorem may be found in [4] and [7].

Example

Consider the following single input, single output plant of order $q = 3$,

$$G(s) = \frac{n^p(s)}{d^p(s)} = \frac{s}{1 - s + 4s^2 + s^3}.$$

A stabilizing controller for $G(s)$ is: $C(s) = \frac{n^c(s)}{d^c(s)} = \frac{3}{1+s}$, which is of order $r = 1$ and the resulting characteristic polynomial is

$$\delta(s) = n^c(s)n^p(s) + d^c(s)d^p(s) = 1 + 3s + 3s^2 + 5s^3 + s^4.$$

In this case we immediately have: $d_0^{p\,2} = \frac{1}{10}$ and $d_n^{p\,2} = 1$, and for $d_\omega^{p\,2}$, we compute

$$P_1(s) = s - \omega^2 s^3, \qquad \text{and} \qquad P_2(s) = 1 - \omega^2 s^2,$$

$$n^{ce}(\omega) = 3, \quad n^{co}(\omega) = 0, \quad d^{ce}(\omega) = 1, \quad d^{co}(\omega) = 1,$$

$$n^{pe}(\omega) = 0, \quad n^{po}(\omega) = 1, \quad d^{pe}(\omega) = 1 - 4\omega^2, \quad d^{po}(\omega) = -1 - \omega^2$$

and then, $\lambda_1 = \delta^e(\omega) = 1 - 3\omega^2 + \omega^4$, and $\lambda_2 = \delta^o(\omega) = 3 - 5\omega^2$,

$$\underline{Z}_1 = \left(3P_1(s), P_1(s) + P_2(s)\right) = \left(3s - 3\omega^2 s^3, 1 + s - \omega^2 s^2 - \omega^2 s^3\right),$$

and

$$\underline{Z}_2 = \left(3P_2(s), P_2(s) - \omega^2 P_1(s)\right) = \left(3 - 3\omega^2 s^2, 1 - \omega^2 s - \omega^2 s^2 + \omega^4 s^3\right),$$

so that

$$[[\underline{Z}_1]]^2 = 11 + 11\omega^4 = 11(1 + \omega^4),$$

$$[[\underline{Z}_2]]^2 = 10 + 11\omega^4 + \omega^8 = (10 + \omega^4)(1 + \omega^4),$$

and also

$$\ll \underline{Z}_1, \underline{Z}_2 \gg = 1 - \omega^2 + \omega^4 - \omega^6 = (1 - \omega^2)(1 + \omega^4).$$

Finally we get for d_ω^p,

$$d_\omega^{p\,2} = \frac{11(1-3\omega^2+\omega^4)^2 + (10+\omega^4)(3-5\omega^2)^2 - 2(1-\omega^2)(1-3\omega^2+\omega^4)(3-5\omega^2)}{(1+\omega^4)(109+2\omega^2+10\omega^4)}.$$

And the minimization of this function over $[0, +\infty)$ yields $d_{min}^{p\;2} \simeq 0.012678$.

Alternatively, $d_\omega^{p\,2}$ is a rational function in ω^2 and by letting $t = \omega^2$ we can write:

$$d_\omega^{p\,2}(t) = \frac{95 - 332t + 316t^2 - 50t^3 + 26t^4}{109 + 2t + 119t^2 + 2t^3 + 10t^4}.$$

The numerator of the derivative of this rational function has only one positive root at $t^* = 0.575544$, for which we get $d_\omega^{p\,2}(t^*) \simeq 0.012678$.

Remarks: It can be shown that the above minimization over an infinite range can be reduced to two similar minimizations on the finite range $[0, 1]$ in order to compute $d_{min}^p = \inf_{\omega \geq 0} d_\omega^p$. After one minimization, one operates the following permutations:

$$n_i^p(s), d^p(s) \text{ are replaced by } s^q n_i^p\left(\frac{1}{s}\right) \text{ and } s^q d^p\left(\frac{1}{s}\right) \text{ respectively,}$$

whereas,

$$n_i^c(s), d^c(s) \text{ are replaced by } s^r n_i^c\left(\frac{1}{s}\right), s^r d^c\left(\frac{1}{s}\right).$$

For example in the case that we treated above, one just replaces

$n^c(s) = 3$ by $n^{cr}(s) = 3s$, whereas $d^c(s)$ is unchanged,

and

$n^p(s) = s$ by $n^{pr}(s) = s^2$, and $d^p(s) = 1 - s + 4s^2 + s^3$ by $d^{pr}(s) = 1 + 4s - s^2 + s^3$.

6. SYNTHESIS OF ROBUST CONTROLLERS

The robust synthesis problem of interest to us is the following: given a plant whose parameters ares subject to perturbations within known ranges, find, if possible, a controller that is able to maintain a desired level of performance for all possible values of the parameters. Of course the basic requirement to be satisfied by the closed-loop system is that of stability and this is the problem we consider here. This problem can be viewed as a simultaneous stabilization problem. One version of this problem namely the question of simultaneously stabilizing a finite number n of plants has already been studied by Saeks, Murray [8] as well as Vidyasagar [9] and has proved to be quite complicated as soon as $n > 2$. In fact very little is known about the general problem that is formulated above and in the following sections we just present two available results that deal with special cases of the robust stabilization problem. The first result, which can be interpreted as a robust state-feedback stabilization problem, is the following. Given a family of interval polynomials $a_0 + a_1 s + \cdots + a_{n-1}s^{n-1} + s^n$, with $a_i \in [a_i^o - \frac{\Delta a_i}{2}, a_i^o + \frac{\Delta a_i}{2}], i = 0, 1, \cdots, n-1$, determine $k_i, i = 0, \cdots, n-1$, such that the interval polynomials $(a_0 + k_0) + (a_1 + k_1)s^{n-1} + \ldots + s^n$ are all stable. We show in the next section that this problem always has a solution for an arbitrary box in the space of a_i. This result is proved by first developing a lemma derived from the Hermite-Bieler theorem. The lemma shows how the degree of a stable polynomial can be increased without losing stability. This lemma, in conjunction with formulas for the stability hypersphere, and Kharitonov's theorem are used to calculate the gains k_i.

Our second result concerns the simultaneous stabilization of a compact (possibly infinite) family of minimum phase plants. In this case also the problem is shown to always have a solution and in fact the controller can be chosen to be itself stable. This is established in Section 8 of the paper.

7. ROBUST STATE-FEEDBACK STABILIZATION

Let us consider the following problem: Suppose that you are given a set of n nominal parameters $\{a_0^o, a_1^o, \cdots, a_{n-1}^o\}$, together with a set of prescribed uncertainty ranges: $\Delta a_0, \Delta a_1, \cdots, \Delta a_{n-1}$, and that you consider the family $\mathcal{F}_{\underline{0}}$ of monic polynomials,

$$\delta(s) = \delta_0 + \delta_1 s + \delta_2 s^2 + \cdots + \delta_{n-1}s^{n-1} + s^n,$$

where

$$\delta_0 \in [a_0^o - \frac{\Delta a_0}{2}, a_0^o + \frac{\Delta a_0}{2}], , \cdots, \delta_{n-1} \in [a_{n-1}^o - \frac{\Delta a_{n-1}}{2}, a_{n-1}^o + \frac{\Delta a_{n-1}}{2}].$$

We consider only the case of Hurwitz or left half plane stability here; the discrete case is analogous and is omitted. To avoid trivial cases assume that the family $\mathcal{F}_{\underline{0}}$ contains unstable polynomials.

Suppose now that you can use a vector of n free parameters $\underline{k} = (k_0, k_1, \cdots, k_{n-1})$, to transform the family $\mathcal{F}_{\underline{0}}$ into the family $\mathcal{F}_{\underline{k}}$ described by:

$$\delta(s) = (\delta_0 + k_0) + (\delta_1 + k_1)s + (\delta_2 + k_2)s^2 + \cdots + (\delta_{n-1} + k_{n-1})s^{n-1} + s^n.$$

The problem of interest, then, is the following: Given $\Delta a_0, \Delta a_1, \cdots, \Delta a_{n-1}$ the perturbation ranges fixed a priori, find, if possible a vector $\underline{k}$ so that the new family of polynomials $\mathcal{F}_{\underline{k}}$, is entirely stable. This problem arises, for example, when one applies a state-feedback control to a single input system where the matrices A, b are in controllable companion form, and the coefficients of the characteristic polynomial of A are subject to bounded perturbations. The answer to this problem is always affirmative and is precisely given in theorem 7.1. Before stating it, however, we need to prove the following lemma.

Lemma 7.1: Let n be a positive integer and let $P(s)$ be a stable polynomial of degree $n-1$:

$$P(s) = p_0 + p_1 s + \cdots + p_{n-1}s^{n-1}, \qquad \text{with all the } p_i > 0.$$

Then there exists $\alpha > 0$ such that:

$$Q(s) = P(s) + p_n s^n = p_0 + p_1 s + \cdots + p_{n-1}s^{n-1} + p_n s^n,$$

is stable if and only if: $\quad p_n \in [0, \alpha)$.

Proof: To be absolutely rigorous there should be four different proofs depending on whether n is of the form $4r$ or $4r+1$ or $4r+2$ or $4r+3$. We will give the proof of this lemma when n is of the form $4r$ and one can check that only slight changes are needed if n is of the form $4r+j$, $\quad j = 1, 2, 3$.

If $n = 4r$, $r > 0$, we can write

$$P(s) = p_0 + p_1 s + \cdots + p_{4r-1}s^{4r-1},$$

and the even and odd parts of $P(s)$ are given by:

$$P_{even}(s) = p_0 + p_2 s^2 + \cdots + p_{4r-2}s^{4r-2},$$

and

$$P_{odd}(s) = p_1 s + p_3 s^3 + \cdots + p_{4r-1}s^{4r-1}.$$

Let us also define

$$\begin{aligned} P^e(\omega) &:= P_{even}(j\omega) = p_0 - p_2\omega^2 + p_4\omega^4 - \cdots - p_{4r-2}\omega^{4r-2}, \\ P^o(\omega) &:= \frac{P_{odd}(j\omega)}{j\omega} = p_1 - p_3\omega^2 + p_5\omega^4 - \cdots - p_{4r-1}\omega^{4r-1}. \end{aligned} \tag{7.1}$$

$P(s)$ being stable, we know by the Hermite-Bieler theorem that $P^e(\omega)$ has precisely $2r-1$ positive roots $\omega_{e,1}, \omega_{e,2}, \cdots, \omega_{e,2r-1}$, that $P^o(\omega)$ has also $2r-1$ positive roots $\omega_{o,1}, \omega_{o,2}, \cdots, \omega_{o,2r-1}$, and that these roots interlace in the following manner:

$$0 < \omega_{e,1} < \omega_{o,1} < \omega_{e,2} < \omega_{o,2} < \cdots < \omega_{e,2r-1} < \omega_{o,2r-1}.$$

It can be also checked that,

$P^e(\omega_{o,j}) < 0$ if and only if j is odd, and $P^e(\omega_{o,j}) > 0$ if and only if j is even, that is,

$$P^e(\omega_{o,1}) < 0, P^e(\omega_{o,2}) > 0, P^e(\omega_{o,3}) < 0, \cdots, P^e(\omega_{o,2r-2}) > 0, P^e(\omega_{o,2r-1}) < 0. \tag{7.2}$$

Let us denote

$$\alpha = \min_{j\ odd} \left\{ \frac{-P^e(\omega_{o,j})}{(\omega_{o,j})^{4r}} \right\}. \tag{7.3}$$

By (7.2), we know that α is positive. We can now prove the following:

$$Q(s) = P(s) + p_{4r}s^{4r} \text{ is stable if and only if } \quad p_{4r} \in [0, \alpha).$$

$Q(s)$ is certainly stable when $p_{4r} = 0$. Let us now suppose that

$$0 < p_{4r} < \alpha. \tag{7.4}$$

$Q^o(\omega)$ and $Q^e(\omega)$ are given by

$$\begin{aligned} Q^o(\omega) &= P^o(\omega) = p_1 - p_3\omega^2 + p_5\omega^4 - \cdots - p_{4r-1}\omega^{4r-1}, \\ Q^e(\omega) &= P^e(\omega) + p_{4r}\omega^{4r} = p_0 - p_2\omega^2 + p_4\omega^4 - \cdots - p_{4r-2}\omega^{4r-2} + p_{4r}\omega^{4r}. \end{aligned} \tag{7.5}$$

We are going to show that $Q^e(\omega)$ and $Q^o(\omega)$ satisfy the Hermite-Bieler theorem provided that p_{4r} remains within the bounds defined by (7.4).
First we know the roots of $Q^o(\omega) = P^o(\omega)$. Then we have that $Q^e(0) = p_0 > 0$, and also,

$$Q^e(\omega_{o,1}) = P^e(\omega_{o,1}) + p_{4r}(\omega_{o,1})^{4r}.$$

But, by (7.3) and (7.4) we have

$$Q^e(\omega_{o,1}) < \underbrace{P^e(\omega_{o,1}) - \frac{P^e(\omega_{o,1})}{(\omega_{o,1})^{4r}}(\omega_{o,1})^{4r}}_{=0}.$$

Thus $Q^e(\omega_{o,1}) < 0$. Then we have

$$Q^e(\omega_{o,2}) = P^e(\omega_{o,2}) + p_{4r}(\omega_{o,2})^{4r}.$$

But by (7.2), we know that $P^e(\omega_{o,2}) > 0$, and therefore we also have

$$Q^e(\omega_{o,2}) > 0.$$

Pursuing the same reasonning we could prove in exactly the same way that the following inequalities hold

$$Q^e(0) > 0, Q^e(\omega_{o,1}) < 0, Q^e(\omega_{o,2}) > 0, \cdots, Q^e(\omega_{o,2r-2}) > 0, Q^e(\omega_{o,2r-1}) < 0. \tag{7.6}$$

From this we already conclude that $Q^e(\omega)$ has precisely $2r-1$ roots in the open interval $(0, \omega_{o,2r-1})$, namely

$$\omega'_{e,1}, \omega'_{e,2}, \cdots, \omega'_{e,2r-1},$$

and that these roots interlace with the roots of $Q^o(\omega)$,

$$0 < \omega'_{e,1} < \omega_{o,1} < \omega'_{e,2} < \omega_{o,2} < \cdots < \omega'_{e,2r-1} < \omega_{o,2r-1}. \tag{7.7}$$

Moreover, we see in (7.6) that

$$Q^e(\omega_{o,2r-1}) < 0,$$

and since $p_{4r} > 0$, we also obviously have

$$Q^e(+\infty) > 0.$$

Therefore $Q^e(\omega)$ has a final positive root $\omega'_{e,2r}$ which satisfies

$$\omega_{o,2r-1} < \omega'_{2r}. \tag{7.8}$$

From (7.7) and (7.8) we conclude that $Q^o(\omega)$ and $Q^e(\omega)$ satisfy the Hermite-Bieler theorem and therefore $Q(s)$ is stable.

To complete the proof of this lemma, notice that $Q(s)$ is obviously unstable if $p_{4r} < 0$ since we have assumed that all the p_i are positive. Moreover it can be shown by using (7.3) that for $p_{4r} = \alpha$, the polynomial $P(s) + \alpha s^{4r}$ has a pure imaginary root and therefore is unstable. Now, it is impossible that $P(s) + p_{4r}s^{4r}$ be stable for some $p_{4r} > \alpha$, because otherwise we could use Kharitonov's theorem and say,

$$P(s) + \frac{\alpha}{2}s^{4r} \text{ and } P(s) + p_{4r}s^{4r} \text{ both stable } \Longrightarrow P(s) + \alpha s^{4r} \text{ stable },$$

which would be a contradiction. This completes the proof of the theorem when $n = 4r$. ◇

For the sake of completeness, let us just make precise that in general we have,

$$\text{if } n = 4r, \quad \alpha = \min_{j \text{ odd}} \left\{ \frac{-P^e(\omega_{o,j})}{(\omega_{o,j})^{4r}} \right\},$$

$$\text{if } n = 4r+1, \quad \alpha = \min_{j \text{ even}} \left\{ \frac{-P^o(\omega_{e,j})}{(\omega_{o,j})^{4r+1}} \right\},$$

$$\text{if } n = 4r+2, \quad \alpha = \min_{j \text{ even}} \left\{ \frac{P^e(\omega_{o,j})}{(\omega_{o,j})^{4r+2}} \right\},$$

$$\text{if } n = 4r+3, \quad \alpha = \min_{j \text{ odd}} \left\{ \frac{P^o(\omega_{e,j})}{(\omega_{o,j})^{4r+3}} \right\}.$$

The details of the proof for the other cases are omitted. ◇

We can now enunciate the following theorem to answer the question raised at the beginning of this section.

Theorem 7.1: For any set of nominal parameters $\{a_0, a_1, \cdots, a_{n-1}\}$, and for any set of positive numbers $\Delta a_0, \Delta a_1, \cdots, \Delta a_{n-1}$, it is possible to find a vector $\underline{k}$ such that the entire family $\mathcal{F}_{\underline{k}}$ is stable.

Proof: The proof is constructive.
Step 1: Take any stable polynomial $R(s)$ of degree $n-1$. Let $\rho(R(\cdot))$ be the radius of the largest stability hypersphere around $R(s)$ [4]. For any positive real number λ, we have

$$\rho(\lambda R(\cdot)) = \lambda \rho(R(\cdot)).$$

Thus it is possible to find a positive real λ such that if $P(s) = \lambda R(s)$,

$$\rho(P(\cdot)) > \sqrt{\frac{{\Delta a_0}^2}{4} + \frac{{\Delta a_1}^2}{4} + \cdots + \frac{{\Delta a_{n-1}}^2}{4}}. \tag{7.9}$$

If we denote

$$P(s) = p_0 + p_1 s + p_2 s^2 + \cdots + p_{n-1} s^{n-1},$$

we conclude from (7.9) that the four following Kharitonov polynomials of degree $n-1$ are stable

$$\begin{aligned} P^1(s) &= (p_0 - \frac{\Delta a_0}{2}) + (p_1 - \frac{\Delta a_1}{2})s + (p_2 + \frac{\Delta a_2}{2})s^2 + \cdots, \\ P^2(s) &= (p_0 - \frac{\Delta a_0}{2}) + (p_1 + \frac{\Delta a_1}{2})s + (p_2 + \frac{\Delta a_2}{2})s^2 + \cdots, \\ P^3(s) &= (p_0 + \frac{\Delta a_0}{2}) + (p_1 - \frac{\Delta a_1}{2})s + (p_2 - \frac{\Delta a_2}{2})s^2 + \cdots, \\ P^4(s) &= (p_0 + \frac{\Delta a_0}{2}) + (p_1 + \frac{\Delta a_1}{2})s + (p_2 - \frac{\Delta a_2}{2})s^2 + \cdots. \end{aligned} \tag{7.10}$$

Step 2: Now, applying lemma 7.1, we know that we can find four positive numbers $\alpha_1, \alpha_2, \alpha_3, \alpha_4$, such that

$$P^j(s) + p_n s^n, \text{ is stable for } 0 \le p_n < \alpha_j, \quad j = 1, 2, 3, 4.$$

Let us select a single positive number α such that the polynomials,

$$P^j(s) + \alpha s^n, \tag{7.11}$$

are all stable. If α can be chosen to be equal to 1 (that is if the four α_j are greater than 1) then we do choose $\alpha = 1$; otherwise we multiply everything by $\frac{1}{\alpha}$ which is greater than 1 and we know from (7.11) that the four polynomials

$$K^j(s) = \frac{1}{\alpha} P^j(s) + s^n,$$

are stable. But the four polynomials $K^j(s)$ are nothing but the four Kharitonov polynomials associated with the family of polynomials

$$\delta(s) = \delta_0 + \delta_1 s + \cdots + \delta_{n-1} s^{n-1} + s^n,$$

where,

$$\delta_0 \in [\frac{1}{\alpha}p_0 - \frac{1}{\alpha}\frac{\Delta a_0}{2}, \frac{1}{\alpha}p_0 + \frac{1}{\alpha}\frac{\Delta a_0}{2}], \cdots\cdots$$

$$\cdots \delta_{n-1} \in [\frac{1}{\alpha}p_{n-1} - \frac{1}{\alpha}\frac{\Delta a_{n-1}}{2}, \frac{1}{\alpha}p_{n-1} + \frac{1}{\alpha}\frac{\Delta a_{n-1}}{2}],$$

and therefore this family is entirely stable.
Step 3: It suffices now to chose the vector $\underline{k}$ such that

$$k_i + a_i^o = \frac{1}{\alpha}p_i, \quad \text{for } i = 1, \cdots, n-1. \diamond$$

Remark: It is clear that in step 1 one can instead determine the largest box around $R(\cdot)$ with sides proportional to Δa_i. The dimensions of such a box are also enlarged by the factor λ when $R(\cdot)$ is replaced by $\lambda R(\cdot)$. This change does not affect the following steps.
Example: Suppose that our nominal polynomial is

$$s^6 - s^5 + 2s^4 - 3s^3 + 2s^2 + s + 1, \text{ that is,}$$

$$(a_0^o, a_1^o, a_2^o, a_3^o, a_4^o, a_5^o) = (1, 1, 2, -3, 2, -1).$$

And suppose that we want to handle the following set of uncertainty ranges:

$$\Delta a_0 = 3, \Delta a_1 = 5, \Delta a_2 = 2, \Delta a_3 = 1, \Delta a_4 = 7, \Delta a_5 = 5.$$

Step 1: Consider the following stable polynomial of order 5

$$R(s) = (s+1)^5 = 1 + 5s + 10s^2 + 10s^3 + 5s^4 + s^5.$$

The calculation of $\rho(R(\cdot))$ gives: $\rho(R(\cdot)) = 1$.
On the other hand we have

$$\sqrt{\frac{\Delta a_0{}^2}{4} + \frac{\Delta a_1{}^2}{4} + \cdots + \frac{\Delta a_{n-1}{}^2}{4}} = 5.31.$$

Taking therefore $\lambda = 6$, we have that

$$P(s) = 6 + 30s + 60s^2 + 60s^3 + 30s^4 + 6s^5,$$

has a radius $\rho(P(\cdot)) = 6$ that is greater than 5.31 .
And the four polynomials $P^j(s)$ are given by

$$P^1(s) = 4.5 + 27.5s + 61s^2 + 60.5s^3 + 26.5s^4 + 3.5s^5,$$

$$P^2(s) = 4.5 + 32.5s + 61s^2 + 59.5s^3 + 26.5s^4 + 8.5s^5,$$

$$P^3(s) = 7.5 + 27.5s + 59s^2 + 60.5s^3 + 33.5s^4 + 3.5s^5,$$

$$P^4(s) = 7.5 + 32.5s + 59s^2 + 59.5s^3 + 33.5s^4 + 8.5s^5.$$

Step 2: The application of lemma 2.1 gives the following values

$$\alpha_1 \simeq 1.360, \quad \alpha_2 \simeq 2.667, \quad \alpha_3 \simeq 1.784, \quad \alpha_4 \simeq 3.821,$$

and therefore we can chose $\alpha = 1$, so that the four polynomials

$$K^1(s) = 4.5 + 27.5s + 61s^2 + 60.5s^3 + 26.5s^4 + 3.5s^5 + s^6,$$
$$K^2(s) = 4.5 + 32.5s + 61s^2 + 59.5s^3 + 26.5s^4 + 8.5s^5 + s^6,$$
$$K^3(s) = 7.5 + 27.5s + 59s^2 + 60.5s^3 + 33.5s^4 + 3.5s^5 + s^6,$$
$$K^4(s) = 7.5 + 32.5s + 59s^2 + 59.5s^3 + 33.5s^4 + 8.5s^5 + s^6,$$

are stable.
Step 3: we just have to take,

$$k_0 = p_0 - a_0 = 5, \quad k_1 = p_1 - a_1 = 29, \quad k_2 = p_2 - a_2 = 58,$$
$$k_3 = p_3 - a_3 = 63, \quad k_4 = p_4 - a_4 = 28, \quad k_5 = p_5 - a_5 = 7.$$

We now turn to a more general result concerning the simultaneous stabilization of a compact family of minimum phase plants.

8. SIMULTANEOUS STRONG STABILIZATION In this section we show have an infinite family of single input single output (SISO) plants can be simultaneously stabilized by a single stable controller, provided mainly that each member in the family represent a minimum phase plant. Consider a standard unity feedback system, where the plant is a single input single output system described by the transfer function

$$G(s) = \frac{n(s)}{d(s)} = \frac{n_0 + n_1 s + \ldots + n_r s^r}{d_0 + d_1 s + \ldots + d_q s^q}.$$

Let $\mathcal{F}_n$ be a compact set of polynomials $n(s)$ satisfying the following three properties:

a.1) $\forall n(\cdot) \in \mathcal{F}_n,\ n(\cdot)$ is stable.

a.2) $\forall n(\cdot) \in \mathcal{F}_n,\ n(\cdot)$ is of degree r (fixed degree).

a.3) The sign of the highest coefficient of any polynomial $n(\cdot)$ in $\mathcal{F}_n$ is always the same, either always positive or always negative.

Let also $\mathcal{F}_d$ be a family of polynomials satisfying the following three properties:

b.1) $\forall d(\cdot) \in \mathcal{F}_d,\ d(\cdot)$ is of degree q (fixed degree).

b.2) $\mathcal{F}_d$ is bounded, that is there exists a constant B such that:

$$\forall d(\cdot) \in \mathcal{F}_d, \forall j \in [0, q],\ |d_j| \leq B.$$

b.3) The coefficient of order q of any polynomial $d(\cdot)$ in $\mathcal{F}_d$ is always of the same sign and bounded from below (or from above). That is,

$$\exists b > 0 \text{ such that } \forall d(\cdot) \in \mathcal{F}_d,\ d_q > b > 0,$$

or

$$\exists b > 0 \text{ such that } \forall d(\cdot) \in \mathcal{F}_d,\ d_q < b < 0.$$

Now, assuming that $r \leq q$, consider the family $\mathcal{P}$ of proper SISO plants described by their transfer functions,

$$G(s) = \frac{n(s)}{d(s)}, \text{ where} \begin{cases} n(s) \in \mathcal{F}_n \\ d(s) \in \mathcal{F}_d. \end{cases}$$

Then we have the following result.

Theorem 8.1

i) q=r: There exists a constant compensator that stabilizes the entire family of plants $\mathcal{P}$.

ii) q¿r: There exists a proper, stable and minimum phase compensator $C(s)$ of degree $q-r-1$ that stabilizes the entire family of plants $\mathcal{P}$.

First, we can assume without loss of generality that we have,

$$\forall n(\cdot) \in \mathcal{F}_n, \; n_r > 0, \tag{8.1}$$

and,

$$\forall d(\cdot) \in \mathcal{F}_d, \; d_q > 0. \tag{8.2}$$

Then we can also assume, still without loss of generality,that the family $\mathcal{F}_d$ is itself compact, otherwise it would be enough to replace $\mathcal{F}_d$ by the family of interval polynomials $\mathcal{F}_d'$ defined by:

$$d_0 \in [-B, B], d_1 \in [-B, B], \ldots, d_{q-1} \in [-B, B], d_q \in [b, B].$$

Given this, the proof of this result depends on some general properties of such compact stable families as $\mathcal{F}_n$, and of such compact families as $\mathcal{F}_d$.

Property 1: Obviously, since the family $\mathcal{F}_n$ contains only stable polynomials, and since they all satisfy property a.3) and (8.1), then any coefficient of any polynomial $n(\cdot)$ in $\mathcal{F}_n$ is positive. Moreover since the set $\mathcal{F}_n$ is compact it is always possible to find two constants a and A such that,

$$\forall n(\cdot) \in \mathcal{F}_n, \forall j \in [0, r], \; 0 < a \leq n_j \leq A. \tag{8.3}$$

Now, $\mathcal{F}_n$ being compact it is always possible to find a closed bounded curve $\mathcal{C}$ included in the left-half plane and that strictly contains all zeroes of any element in $\mathcal{F}_n$. For example it is well known that in view of equation (8.3), any zero z_n of element $n(\cdot)$ if $\mathcal{F}_n$ satisfies:

$$|z_n| \leq 1 + \frac{A}{a}. \tag{8.4}$$

Hence it is always possible to chose $\mathcal{C}$ as a semi circle or radius $1 + \frac{A}{a}$. Now, again by a compacity argument we can write:

$$\inf_{n(\cdot) \in \mathcal{F}_n} \left[\inf_{s \in \mathcal{C}} |n(s)| \right] = \alpha_n > 0. \tag{8.5}$$

Proof: by contradiction, if $\alpha_n = 0$, then it is possible to find a sequence of polynomials $n_k(s)$ in $\mathcal{F}_n$, such that for each $k > 0$,

$$\exists z_k \in \mathcal{C} \text{ such that } |n_k(z_k)| \leq \frac{1}{k}. \tag{8.6}$$

But, $\mathcal{C}$ being compact in the complex plane, it is possible to find a subsequence $z_{\phi(k)}$ that converges to $z_0 \in \mathcal{C}$. Moreover, $n_{\phi(k)}(\cdot)$ is now a sequence of elements of the compact set $\mathcal{F}_n$ and therefore it is possible to find a subsequence $n_{\phi(\psi(k))}(\cdot)$ that converges to $n_0(\cdot) \in \mathcal{F}_n$. Then we have by (8.6),

$$|n_{\phi(\psi(k))}(z_{\phi(\psi(k))})| \leq \frac{1}{\phi(\psi(k))}. \tag{8.7}$$

Passing to the limit as k goes to infinity in (8.7), one gets:

$$n_0(z_0) = 0.$$

But this is a contradiction because $\mathcal{C}$ is supposed to strictly enclose all the zeroes of any polynomial in $\mathcal{F}_n$.
Property 2: Now, the family $\mathcal{F}_d$ being bounded we have that for any $d(\cdot)$ in $\mathcal{F}_d$,

$$\forall s, \ |d(s)| \leq B(1 + |s| + \cdots + |s|^q) = \phi(s).$$

Let,

$$\beta_d = \sup_{s \in \mathcal{C}} \phi(s),$$

then β_d is obviously finite (because $\mathcal{C}$ is compact and $\phi(\cdot)$ is continuous) and we have that

$$\sup_{d(\cdot) \in \mathcal{F}_d} \left[\sup_{s \in \mathcal{C}} |d(s)| \right] \leq \beta_d. \tag{8.8}$$

We can now proceed and prove i) and ii).

Proof of i): Let $\mathcal{C}$ be a closed bounded curve enclosing every zero of each element in $\mathcal{F}_n$, and let α_n and β_d be defined as in (8.5) and (8.8).
Then, if we choose ϵ such that $0 < |\epsilon| < \frac{\alpha_n}{\beta_d}$,

$$\forall n(\cdot) \in \mathcal{F}_n, \text{ and } \forall d(\cdot) \in \mathcal{F}_d,$$

we have that

$$\forall s \in \mathcal{C}, \ |\epsilon d(s)| \leq |\epsilon| \beta_d < \alpha_n \leq |n(s)|. \tag{8.9}$$

Hence, by Rouché's theorem, we conclude from equation (8.9) that for this choice of ϵ, $n(s) + \epsilon d(s)$ has the same number of zeroes as $n(s)$ in $\mathcal{C}$, that is r. But since $n(s) + \epsilon d(s)$ is itself of degree r it is stable. ◇

N.B.: In this case one can notice that the property b.3) of the family $\mathcal{F}_d$ is not needed.

Proof of ii): Let us first suppose that $q = r + 1$.
Again let $\mathcal{C}$ be a closed bounded curve enclosing every zero of each element in $\mathcal{F}_n$, and let α_n and β_d be defined as in (8.5) and (8.8).
If we start by choosing ϵ_1 such that $0 < \epsilon_1 < \frac{\alpha_n}{\beta_d}$, and any μ such that $0 < \mu < \epsilon_1$, then

$$\forall \ n(\cdot) \in \mathcal{F}_n, \text{ and } \forall d(\cdot) \in \mathcal{F}_d,$$

we have

$$\forall s \in \mathcal{C}, \ |\mu d(s)| \leq \mu \beta_d < \alpha_n \leq |n(s)|. \tag{8.10}$$

Here again, we conclude by Rouché's theorem, that for any such μ, $n(s)+\mu d(s)$ has already r zeroes inside $\mathcal{C}$. Moreover it is also possible to find ϵ_2 such that for any μ satisfying $0 < \mu < \epsilon_2$, we have that every coefficient of $n(s)+\mu d(s)$ is positive.
If we now choose any ϵ such that $0 < \epsilon < min(\epsilon_1, \epsilon_2)$, we have that $n(s)+\epsilon d(s)$ is of degree less than or equal to $r+1$, has r stable roots, and all its coefficients are positive. But this implies that $n(s)+\epsilon d(s)$ is necessarily stable.
We now proceed by induction on $n = q-r$. Suppose that part ii) of the theorem is true when $q = r+p$, $p \geq 1$. Let $\mathcal{F}_n$ and $\mathcal{F}_d$ be two families of polynomials satisfying properties a.1),a.2),a.3), and b.1),b.2),b.3) respectively, and let us suppose that $q = r+p+1$.
Now consider the new family $\mathcal{F}'_n$ of polynomials $n'(s)$ of the form,

$$n'(s) = (s+1)n(s), \text{ where } n(s) \in \mathcal{F}_n.$$

Obviously $\mathcal{F}'_n$ is also a compact set and each element of $\mathcal{F}'_n$ satisfies properties a.1),a.2),a.3), but now with $r' = r+1$. Hence by the induction hypothesis it is possible to find a stable polynomial $n'_c(s)$ of degree less than or equal to $p-1$, and a stable polynomial $d'_c(s)$ of degree $p-1$ such that,

$$\forall n(\cdot) \in \mathcal{F}_n, \text{ and } \forall d(\cdot) \in \mathcal{F}_d,$$

we have that

$$n(s)(s+1)n'_c(s) + d(s)d'_c(s) \text{ is stable}. \tag{8.11}$$

Now, let $n_c(s) = (s+1)n'_c(s)$, and consider the new family of polynomials $\mathcal{F}'_n$ described by (8.11), that is consisting of all polynomials $n'(\cdot)$ of the form,

$$n'(s) = n(s)n_c(s) + d(s)d'_c(s) \text{ where} \begin{cases} n(s) \text{ arbitrary in } \mathcal{F}_n \\ d(s) \text{ arbitrary in } \mathcal{F}_d. \end{cases},$$

and the new family of polynomials $\mathcal{F}'_d$ consisting of all polynomials $d'(\cdot)$ of the form,

$$d'(s) = sd'_c(s)d(s), \text{ where } d(s) \text{ is an element of } \mathcal{F}_d.$$

Clearly the family $\mathcal{F}'_n$ is compact and satisfies properties a.1),a.2),a.3) with $r' = r+2p$, and $\mathcal{F}'_d$ is also a compact family of polynomials satisfying properties b.1),b.2),b.3) with $q' = r+2p+1$. Hence by applying our result when $n = 1$, we can find an $\epsilon > 0$ such that,

$$\forall n'(\cdot) \in \mathcal{F}'_n, \text{ and } \forall d'(\cdot) \in \mathcal{F}'_d,$$

$$n'(s) + \epsilon d'(s) \text{ is stable.}$$

But in particular this implies that,

$$\forall n(\cdot) \in \mathcal{F}_n, \text{ and } \forall d(\cdot) \in \mathcal{F}_d,$$

$$n(s)n_c(s) + d'_c(s)d(s) + \epsilon s d'_c(s)d(s) = n(s)n_c(s) + (\epsilon s+1)d'_c(s)d(s) \text{ is stable.}$$

Therefore the controller defined by,

$$c(s) = \frac{n_c(s)}{d_c(s)} = \frac{n_c(s)}{(\epsilon s+1)d'_c(s)},$$

is an answer to our problem and this ends the proof of theorem 8.1. ◊

9. CONCLUDING REMARKS: In this paper we focused on linear time invariant control systems containing an interval plant and described some new recent results on the robust stability analysis and synthesis problems for such systems. A significant generalization of Kharitonov's theorem, called the Box Theorem was described for dealing with robustness in the parameter space. New formulas for the computation of the radius of the largest stability hypersphere in the parameter space, centered around a give nominal plant were also given. The calculation of the stability margin for multiinput multioutput plants subject to structured perturbations and the problem of determining robust stabilizability need to be the subject of some future research.

A synthesis procedure for robust state feedback stabilization was developed. Also a procedure for robust output feedback stabilization for minimum phase plants was given results concerning the robust stability problem. These results are but two steps towards the solution to the general robust synthesis problem, but so little is known about this solution that every step is of interest. Many problems are still to be solved in this domain. For example it would be interesting to extend the robust state feedback stabilization of section 7 to the case when A, B are not in controllable companion form. Another open problem of particular interest is the following. For a Single-Input Single-Output interval plant find the necessary and sufficient conditions for the existence of a stabilizing controller. Moreover, if stabilization is possible, give a constructive method for finding the controller. Moreover, if stabilization is possible, give a constructive method for finding the controller. If the four Kharitonov polynomials associated with the numerator of the interval plant are stable then every plant in the family is minimum phase and the problem is reduced to that of section 8 of this paper and it is always possible to find a solution. On the other hand if these Kharitonov polynomials are not all stable, there will no always be a solution and the solution will certainly not be a 'high-gain' controller as in section 8.

10. NOTES AND REFERENCES

The results of Section 3 can be found in Chapellat and Bhattacharyya [3] and Chapellat [4]. The formulas of Section 4 are derived in Chapellat [4] and Chapellat and Bhattacharyya [7]; they improve upon the procedure for stability margin calculation give in Biernacki, Hwang and Bhattacharyya [5] and Bhattacharyya [6]. The results given in Section 8 are based on Chapellat and Bhattacharyya [10]. The problem treated in Section 8 has also been treated by Wei and Barmish [12]. The problem of simultaneous stabilization of a discrete set of plants has been considered by Vidyasagar and Viswanadham [8] and Saeks and Murray [9].

BIBLIOGRAPHY

[1] V. L. Kharitonov, "Asymptotic Stability of an Equilibrium Position of Family of Systems of Linear Differential Equations," *Differential. Uravnen.*, Vol. 14, pp. 2086-2088, 1978.

[2] A. C. Bartlett, C. V. Hollot and H. Lin, "Root Locations for a polytope of polynomials: It suffices to check the edges," *Mathematics of Controls, Signals and Systems*, Vol. 2, No. 1, pp. 611-71, 1988.

[3] Hervé Chapellat and S. P. Bhattacharyya, "A Generalization of Kharitonov's Theorem: Robust Stability of Interval Plants" to appear *IEEE Transactions on Automatic Control*, March 1989.

[4] Hervé Chapellat, *Geometric Conditions for Robust Stability*, M.S. Thesis, Department of Electrical Engineering, Texas A&M University, Nov. 1987.

[5] R. M. Biernacki, H. Hwang and S. P. Bhattacharyya, "Robust stability with structured real parameter perturbations," *IEEE Transactions on Automatic Control*, Vol. AC-32, No. 6, pp. 495-506, June 1987.

[6] S. P. Bhattacharyya, *Robust Stabilization Against Structured Perturbations*, Springer-Verlag, Lecture Notes in Control and Information Sciences, Vol. 99, 1987.

[7] Hervé Chapellat and S. P. Bhattacharyya, "Exact Calculation of Stability Margin With Respect to Transfer Function Coefficients" Dept. of Elect. Engr. TCSP Research Report 88-04, Texas A & M University, January 1988.

[8] R. Saeks and J. Murray, "Fractional Representation, Algebraic Geometry and the Simultaneous Stabilization Problem," *IEEE Transactions Automatic Control*, Vol. AC-27, pp. 895-903, Aug. 1982.

[9] M. Vidyasagar and N. Viswanadham, Algebraic Design Techniques for Reliable Stabilization," *IEEE Transactions on Automatic Control*, Vol. AC-27, pp. 1085-1095.

[10] Hervé Chapellat and S. P. Bhattacharyya "Simultaneous Strong Stabilization" Dept. of Elect. Engr., Texas A & M University TCSP Research Report 88-011, March 1988.

[11] K. H. Wei and B. R. Barmish, "Simultaneous Stabilizability of Single-input Single-output Systems," Proceedings of the 7th International Symposium on Mathematics of Networks and Systems, Stockholm, Sweden, 1985.

SHAPING CONDITIONS AND THE STABILITY OF SYSTEMS WITH PARAMETER UNCERTAINTY

T. E. Djaferis and C. V. Hollot

Electrical and Computer Engineering Department
University of Massachusetts
Amherst, Massachusetts 01003

ABSTRACT

Let $\phi(s,\underline{a}) = \phi_0(s) + a_1\phi_1(s) + a_2\phi_2(s) + \ldots + \phi_k(s) = \phi_0(s) + q(s,\underline{a})$ be a family of real polynomials in s, with coefficients that depend linearly on a_i which are confined in a k dimensional hypercube Ω_a. Let $\phi_0(s)$ be stable of degree n and the $\phi_i(s)$ polynomials ($i \geq 1$) of degree less than n. It follows from the Nyquist Theorem that the family $\phi(s,\underline{a})$ is stable if and only if the complex number $\phi_0(j\omega)$ lies outside the set of complex numbers $-q(j\omega,\Omega_a)$ for every real ω. In this paper we show that $-q(j\omega,\Omega_a)$, the so called "-q locus", is in general a 2k convex parpolygon - a convex polygon with an even number of sides (2k) in which opposite sides are equal and parallel. We then exploit this special structure and show that to test for stability only a finite number of frequency checks need to be done. The number of critical frequencies is shown to be polynomial in k, $O(k^3)$, and these frequencies correspond to the real nonnegative roots of some polynomials.

INTRODUCTION

In robustness problems one is frequently faced with the problem of determining the stability of an entire family of polynomials. It is therefore highly desirable to have simple stability tests. For a special polynomial family such a simple test has been shown to exist. The result by Kharitonov,[5] states that a "box" of polynomials is stable (has roots in the open left half plane) if and only if four vertex polynomials are stable. For the class of polynomials with coefficients which are linear in the uncertain parameters Barmish,[2] developed a test which required a "frequency sweep", and thus lacks the simplicity of Kharitonov's test. For the case of an entire polytope of polynomials Bartlett et al,[1] show that it suffices to check the stability of the edge polynomials. Such a test of course requires an exponential number of one dimensional sweeps.

This paper is also concerned with the stability of families of polynomials and our goal is to develop simple tests for stability. We will focus on the family of polynomials with coefficients which are linear in the uncertain parameters. In particular let

$$\phi(s,\underline{a}) = \phi_0(s) + a_1\phi_1(s) + a_2\phi_2(s) + \ldots + a_k\phi_k(s) = \phi_0(s) + q(s,\underline{a}) \qquad (1)$$

where $\phi_0(s)$ is monic, stable and of degree n and where the $\phi_i(s)$ are nonzero polynomials of degree less than n. The vector of parameters $\underline{a} = (a_1, a_2, \ldots, a_k)$ is confined to the hypercube Ω_a; $\Omega_a = \{\underline{a} \mid a_i^- \leq a_i \leq a_i^+$ $1 \leq i \leq k$, $a_i^- < 0$, $a_i^+ > 0\}$. Since $\phi_0(s)$ is stable as the a_i are allowed to change, a time comes when in general instability occurs. From the Nyquist Theorem this will occur when

$$\frac{q(j\omega,\underline{a})}{\phi_0(j\omega)} = -1$$

for some $\underline{a}$ and frequency $\omega\varepsilon[0,\infty)$. Actually due to the "finite bandwidth" of family (1), one need only consider a bounded interval of frequencies, say $[0,\Delta]$. Consider then the locus $-q(j\omega,\Omega_a)$. Instability would have occurred if the point $\phi_0(j\omega)$ was included in the $-q$ locus. This is equivalent to having the origin of the complex plane be included in the $\phi(j\omega,\Omega_a)$ locus. Therefore family (1) is stable if the point ϕ_0 lies outside the $-q$ locus at each frequency ω. Knowing the shape of this locus helps a great deal in carrying out this test. In the next section we show that for the parameter region Ω_a the $-q$ locus is in general a 2k convex parpolygon.

Our next priority is to exploit the structure of 2k convex parpolygons and show that ϕ_0-location tests need not be done at each frequency. Indeed we will show that this test need only be performed at a finite number of frequencies. Moreover the number of these critical frequencies is polynomial in k, $O(k^3)$, and the frequencies themselves correspond to real nonnegative roots of some easily constructed polynomials. These results lead to the most computationally efficient algorithm presently available for deducing whether the polynomial family in (1) is stable.

<u>Notation</u>: Let $g(s,\underline{a}) = g_0(s) + g_1(\underline{a})s + \ldots + g_n s^n$ be a real polynomial in n. Then $g(s,\underline{a}) = E_g(s) + sO_g(s)$ where $E_g(s) = g_0(\underline{a}) + g_2(\underline{a})s^2 + \ldots$, $O_g(s) = g_1(\underline{a}) + g_3(\underline{a})\ g_3(\underline{a})s^2 + \ldots$, are the even and odd parts of the polynomial g. Furthermore we denote by $Re(\cdot)$ and $Im(\cdot)$ the real and imaginary parts of a complex expression.

<u>Definition</u>

Let $\phi_i(s)$, $\phi_j(s)$ be components of $\phi(s,\underline{a})$ in (1). We say that $\phi_i(s)$ and $\phi_j(s)$ satisfy the <u>shaping condition</u> if any only if $E_{\phi_i}(j\omega)\,O_{\phi_j}(j\omega) - E_{\phi_j}(j\omega)\,O_{\phi_i}(j\omega) = 0$ identically.

THE -q LOCUS IS A 2k CONVEX PARPOLYGON

In this section we prove that at each frequency ω, the -q locus is in general a 2k convex parpolygon. We shall first assume that none of the ϕ_i, ϕ_j in (1) satisfy the shaping condition. If there had been a pair of ϕ_i,ϕ_j which did satisfy the shaping condition one can show,[3] that in essence one uncertain parameter can be "eliminated" and the problem is reduced to a k-1 dimensional one.

Let $\mathrm{Re}(-q(j\omega,\underline{a})) = x = -E_{\phi_1}a_1 - E_{\phi_2}a_2 - \ldots - E_{\phi_k}a_k$,

$\mathrm{Im}(-q(j\omega,\underline{a})) = y = -\omega O_{\phi_1}a_1 - \omega O_{\phi_2}a_2 - \ldots - \omega O_{\phi_k}a_k$,

which in matrix form is:

$$\begin{bmatrix} x \\ \\ y \end{bmatrix} = \underbrace{\begin{bmatrix} -E_{\phi_1} & -E_{\phi_2} & \cdots & -E_{\phi_k} \\ \\ -\omega O_{\phi_1} & -\omega O_{\phi_2} & \cdots & -\omega O_{\phi_k} \end{bmatrix}}_{T} \begin{bmatrix} a_1 \\ a_2 \\ \vdots \\ a_k \end{bmatrix} . \tag{2}$$

Clearly at each frequency the map $(a_1,a_2,\ldots,a_k) \to (x,y)$ is linear and thus the -q locus (the image of Ω_a under T) is a polytope. The shape of this polytope depends on T, e.g., if T is rank 2, it will be a 2-dimensional set. If T has rank 1 this polytope degenerates to a straight line segment and if T happens to be zero then the -q locus is the zero point. More can be said about this polytope. In particular one can identify 2k of its exposed edges. This can be easily seen if in (2) one eliminates the a_i parameters one at a time. For instance if a_1 is eliminated (with $\gamma_{uv} = O_{\phi_u}E_{\phi_v} - E_{\phi_u}O_{\phi_v}$, $1 \leq u, v \leq k$, $u \neq v$, and

$E_{\phi_1}(j\omega) \neq 0$)

$$y = \underbrace{\frac{\omega O_{\phi_1}}{E_{\phi_1}}}_{\lambda_1(\omega)} x + \underbrace{\frac{\omega(\gamma_{12}a_2 + \gamma_{13}a_3 + \ldots + \gamma_{1k}a_k)}{E_{\phi_1}}}_{y_1(\omega,a_2,a_3,\ldots,a_k)} \tag{3}$$

$\to \; y = \lambda_1(\omega)\, x + y_1(\omega,a_2,\ldots,a_k)$.

Let

$y_{1max} = \max\limits_{a_2,\ldots,a_k} y_1(\omega,a_2,\ldots,a_k)$ attained at $\bar{a}_2,\bar{a}_3,\ldots,\bar{a}_k$

$y_{1min} = \min\limits_{a_2,\ldots,a_k} y_1(\omega,a_2,\ldots,a_k)$ attained at $\underline{a}_2,\underline{a}_3,\ldots,\underline{a}_k$

Two exposed edges are:

$$\ell_{11}: y_e = \lambda_1(\omega)x_e + y_{1max} \quad \min_{a_1} x(\omega,a_1,\bar{a}_2,\ldots,\bar{a}_k) \le x_e \le \max_{a_1} x(\omega,a_1,\bar{a}_2,\ldots,\bar{a}_k)$$

$$\ell_{12}: y_e = \lambda_1(\omega)x_e + y_{1min} \quad \min_{a_1} x(\omega,a_1,\underline{a}_2,\ldots,\underline{a}_k) \le x_e \le \max_{a_1} x(\omega,a_1,\underline{a}_2,\ldots,\underline{a}_k)$$

Proceeding in a similar fashion eliminating in turn $a_2, a_3, \ldots, a_k$ in (2) one can generate line segments

$$\ell_{i1} : y_e = \lambda_i(\omega)x_e + y_{imax} \quad 2 \le i \le k$$

$$\ell_{i2} : y_e = \lambda_i(\omega)x_e + y_{imin} \tag{4}$$

This means that 2k exposed edges of the -q locus can be identified. As a matter of fact these are all the exposed edges as the next result proves.

Theorem 1

Let $\phi(s,a)$ be as in (1). Let all pairs of columns of T be linearly independent at some frequency ω. The line segments ℓ_{i1}, ℓ_{i2} $1 \le i \le k$ are the exposed edges of the -q polytope. It is thus a 2k convex parpolygon.

proof

At any frequency $\omega \neq 0$, the mapping $(a_1,a_2,\ldots,a_k) \to (x,y)$ can be viewed as being accomplished by first fixing $a_2, a_3, \ldots a_4$ and then allowing a_1 to vary. All these are straight lines parallel to ℓ_{11}, ℓ_{12}. We know that ℓ_{11}, ℓ_{12} are both on the -q polytope. The point 0 must lie in between them by construction (or perhaps lie on one of them). No point of the -q locus can lie "outside" the space between these two parallel lines. Suppose it did. then it would lie on one such parallel line, which had a y intercept greater than y_{1max} or y_{1min}. But this is a contradiction. Furthermore no point of the -q polytope can lie outside the line segment as again a contradiction would follow. These arguments can be repeated for all other line segments ℓ_{i1}, ℓ_{i2}. Let $\vec{i}_j$ be the unit vector in the complex plane parallel to line ℓ_{j1}, $1 \le j \le k$. From the assumption that all pairs of columns in T are linearly independent at this frequency $\gamma_{uv}(\omega) \neq 0$ for all $u \neq v$. All line segments ℓ_{i1}, ℓ_{i2} will be exposed edges with ℓ_{i1}, ℓ_{j1} not parallel to each other for $i \neq j$. We have therefore identified 2k exposed edges. Our claim is that these are all the exposed edges of the -q polytope. To show this we shall generate the polytope in the following manner: Let S_i be the subset of Ω_a where $a_{i+1} = a_{i+2} = \ldots = a_k = 0$ and $a_1,a_2,\ldots,a_i$ are allowed to vary. Let $T(S_i)$ denote its image under T. Clearly $T(S_1)$ is a line segment in the direction $\vec{i}_1$. $T(S_2)$ is obtained by translating $T(S_1)$ in the direction $\vec{i}_2$ as a_2 is allowed to vary. $T(S_2)$ is thus a parallelogram since $\vec{i}_1 \neq \vec{i}_2$. $T(S_3)$ is obtained by translating $T(S_2)$ in the direction i_3 as a_3 is allowed to vary. $T(S_3)$ is thus a polygon with 6 exposed edges since $\vec{i}_2 \neq \vec{i}_3$, $\vec{i}_1 \neq \vec{i}_3$. Assume that $T(S_i)$ is such a polygon with 2i sides for $2 \le i \le m$. The image of $T(S_{m+1})$ is obtained by translating $T(S_m)$ in the direction $\vec{i}_{m+1}$ as a_{m+1} is allowed to vary. Since $\vec{i}_{m+1}$ is different than all previous direction vectors this will add two additional exposed edges. The number of exposed edges in $T(S_{m+1})$ is $2(m+1)$. The induction proof is complete and therefore the -q locus has 2k exposed edges. Q.E.D.

NUMBER OF FREQUENCY CHECKS IS POLYNOMIAL IN K

The -q locus has been shown to be a 2k-convex parpolygon at each frequency and equations for its 2k edge lines are given in (4). In order to simplify the exposition we first consider the case when k = 2. The four edge lines are:

$$\{(x,y): E_{\phi_1} y - \omega O_{\phi_1} x - \omega\gamma_{12} a_2^+ = 0\}; \quad \{(x,y): E_{\phi_1} y - \omega O_{\phi} x - \omega\gamma_{12} a_2^- = 0\};$$

$$\{(x,y): E_{\phi_2} y - \omega O_{\phi_2} x + \omega\gamma_{12} a_1^+ = 0\}; \quad \{(x,y): E_{\phi_2} y - \omega O_{\phi} x + \omega\gamma_{12} a_1^- = 0\}. \quad (5)$$

These are valid expressions as long as $E_{\phi_1}(j\omega)$, $E_{\phi_2}(j\omega)$, $O_{\phi_1}(j\omega)$ $O_{\phi_2}(j\omega)$ are not zero for some ω.

Since the polynomial family $\phi(s,\Omega_a)$ contains at least one stable polynomial, then it contains only stable polynomials if and only if the point $\phi_0(j\omega)$ (which corresponds to the nominal portion of $\phi(s,\Omega_a)$) lies outside the -q locus at each frequency. Suppose that ϕ_0 is outside the -q locus at some frequency. Given that the -q locus has a boundary described by the edge lines (5), ϕ_0 "enters" the -q locus only if it crosses one of these lines at some frequency. Evaluating each of these lines at the point $(x,y) = (E_{\phi_0}(j\omega), \omega O_{\phi_0}(j\omega))$ gives the four polynomials.

$$g_1(\omega) \triangleq \omega E_{\phi_1} O_{\phi_0} - \omega O_{\phi_1} E_{\phi_0} - \omega\gamma_{12}\, a_2^+ \qquad g_2(\omega) \triangleq \omega E_{\phi_1} O_{\phi_0} - \omega O_{\phi_1} E_{\phi_0} - \omega\gamma_{12}\, a_2^-$$

$$g_3(\omega) \triangleq \omega E_{\phi_2} O_{\phi_0} - \omega O_{\phi_2} E_{\phi_0} + \omega\gamma_{12}\, a_1^+ \qquad g_4(\omega) \triangleq \omega E_{\phi_2} O_{\phi_0} - \omega O_{\phi_2} E_{\phi_0} + \omega\gamma_{12}\, a_1^-.$$

Let $\tilde{g}_i(\omega)$, $i = 1,2,\ldots, k \leq 4$ be those $g_i(\omega)$ which are not identically zero and define $\tilde{g}_0(\omega) = \omega(E_{\phi_1} O_{\phi_0} - O_{\phi_1} E_{\phi_0})$.

Let $W_1 = \{\omega \mid \omega = 0$, or a real positive zero of $\tilde{g}_i$ $1 \leq i \leq k$, $E_{\phi_1}, E_{\phi_2}, O_{\phi_1}, O_{\phi_2}, \gamma_{12}\}$.

Let $W_2 = \{\omega \mid \omega = 0$, or a real positive zero of $\tilde{g}_0$, $E_{\phi_1}, O_{\phi_1}, E_{\phi_2}, O_{\phi_2}\}$.

Theorem 2

Let $E_{\phi_1}, E_{\phi_2}, O_{\phi_1}, O_{\phi_2}$ be nonzero polynomials. The family $\phi(s,\Omega_a)$ contains only stable polynomials if and only if $\phi_0(j\omega)$ lies outside the -q locus at the following frequencies:

(i) when $\gamma_{12} \neq 0$, for all $\omega \in W_1$, (ii) when $\gamma_{12} = 0$, for all $\omega \in W_2$.

proof

Let us first consider the case when $\gamma_{12} \neq 0$. Now if ϕ_0 is outside the $-q$ locus at some frequency (say $\omega = 0$) it can only enter the $-q$ locus through an edge. This implies that the point ϕ_0 must lie on one of these exposed edge lines at some frequency. Specifically we must have

$$g_1(\omega) = 0 \text{ or } g_2(\omega) = 0 \text{ or } g_3(\omega) = 0 \text{ or } g_4(\omega) = 0 \qquad (6)$$

These are valid at all frequencies except the zeros of $E_{\phi_1}(j\omega)$, $E_{\phi_2}(j\omega)$, $0_{\phi_1}(j\omega)$, $0_{\phi_2}(j\omega)$.

Suppose that none of the g_i polynomials are identically zero, and let W_1 be the set defined above. It is then clear that ϕ_0 will be outside the $-q$ locus for all frequencies iff ϕ_0 is outside the $-q$ locus at this finite set of frequencies W_1. The set W_1 contains the potentially troublesome "critical frequencies", that need to be checked.

Suppose that exactly one of the polynomials in (6) is identically zero. This implies that the point ϕ_0 lies on an exposed edge line of the $-q$ locus for all frequencies. Then ϕ_0 will be outside the $-q$ locus for all frequencies iff it is outside the $-q$ locus at frequencies in W_1. This is true because the only way the ϕ_0 point can enter is through a different exposed edge (one other than that corresponding to the identically zero g_i).

If more than one $g_i = 0$, then either $\gamma_{12} = 0$ (a contradiction to our assumption) or the frequencies in W_1 are adequate to determine location.

When $\gamma_{12} = 0$ we have the following simplification. In this case the $-q$ locus reduces to a line segment since

$$x = -E_{\phi_1}\underbrace{\left(a_1 + \frac{E_{\phi_2}}{E_{\phi_1}} a_2\right)}_{A_1} = -E_{\phi_1} A_1 \qquad y = -\omega 0_{\phi_1}\left(a_1 + \frac{0_{\phi_2}}{0_{\phi_1}} a_2\right) = -\omega 0_{\phi_1} A_1$$

therefore

$$y = \frac{\omega 0_{\phi_1}}{E_{\phi_1}} x.$$

Then ϕ_0 will be on this line iff $\tilde{g}_0(\omega) = \omega(E_{\phi_1} 0_{\phi_0} - 0_{\phi_1} E_{\phi_0}) = 0$.

Now $\tilde{g}_0(\omega)$ cannot be the zero polynomial because then ϕ_1, ϕ_0 would satisfy a shaping condition. From,[4] we know that this would imply

$$\phi_1(s) = g(s)e_1(s) \qquad \phi_0(s) = g(s)e_2(s)$$

where g is arbitrary and e_1, e_2 are even polynomials. Since ϕ_0 is stable e_2 must be equal to a nonzero constant otherwise ϕ_0 would have at least one root in the right half plane. But then g(s) would be of degree n. But ϕ_1 can have degree up to n-1. The set of critical frequencies is thus W_2.

Q.E.D.

Remark

In the Theorem we have assumed that the $E_{\phi_i}, 0_{\phi_i}$ are not identically zero. The Theorem holds in these cases as well as we now demonstrate. Let $\gamma_{12} \neq 0$, $E_{\phi_1} = 0$ and E_{ϕ_2}, 0_{ϕ_1}, 0_{ϕ_2} nonzero. The g_i polynomials in this case are:

$$g_1(\omega) = E_{\phi_0} + E_{\phi_2} a_2^+ \qquad g_2(\omega) = E_{\phi_0} + E_{\phi_2} a_2^-$$

$$g_3(\omega) = \omega(E_{\phi_2} 0_{\phi_0} - 0_{\phi_2} E_{\phi_0} + 0_{\phi_1} E_{\phi_2} a_2^+) \qquad g_4(\omega) = \omega(E_{\phi_2} 0_{\phi_0} - 0_{\phi_2} E_{\phi_0} + 0_{\phi_1} E_{\phi_2} a_1^-)$$

If none of these are identically zero the set of critical frequencies becomes:

$$W_1' = \{\omega | \omega = 0 \text{ or a real positive root of } g_i, E_{\phi_2}, 0_{\phi_1}, 0_{\phi_2}\}.$$

Similarly if $E_{\phi_2} = 0$, or $0_{\phi_1} = 0$, or $0_{\phi_2} = 0$. If say $E_{\phi_1} = 0$ and $0_{\phi_2} = 0$ then $x = -E_{\phi_2} a_2$ $y = -\omega 0_{\phi_1} a_1$, and the g_i polynomials are:

$$g_1(\omega) = E_{\phi_0} + E_{\phi_2} a_2^+ \qquad g_2(\omega) = E_{\phi_0} + E_{\phi_2} a_2^-$$

$$g_3(\omega) = \omega 0_{\phi_0} + \omega 0_{\phi_1} a_1^+ \qquad g_4(\omega) = \omega 0_{\phi_0} + \omega 0_{\phi_1} a_1^-$$

generating a corresponding set of potentially troublesome frequencies W. Appropriate modifications in W should be made if some of the g_i are identically zero.

Now if $\gamma_{12} = 0$ and $E_{\phi_1} = 0$, then we must also have either $0_{\phi_1} = 0$ or $E_{\phi_2} = 0$. If $0_{\phi_1} = 0$ then parameter a_1 does not appear in ϕ and we have a single parameter (trivial case). If $E_{\phi_2} = 0$ then the -q locus lives always on the imaginary axis and thus we need only check frequencies which make $E_{\phi_0} = 0$, (a finite number).

Let us now turn our attention to the k-parameter case.

Theorem 3

Let E_{ϕ_i}, 0_{ϕ_i} $1 \leq i \leq k$ be nonzero polynomials. The family $\phi(s, \Omega_a)$ contains only stable polynomials iff ϕ_0 lies outside the -q locus at a finite number of frequencies which are given as the real nonnegative zeros of real polynomials in the single variable ω.

proof

First consider the case when no shaping conditions are satisfied, i.e., ($\gamma_{uv} \neq 0$ $1 \leq u \leq k$, $1 \leq v \leq k$, $u \neq v$).

Let $V_1 = \{\omega | \omega \text{ real positive root of some } \gamma_{1v}\ 2 \leq v \leq k \text{ in the interval } \Delta.\}$
$= \{\omega_1 \omega_2, \ldots, \omega_{z_1 - 1}\}$.

These roots partition the interval Δ into open intervals $\Delta_{11}, \Delta_{12}, \ldots, \Delta_{1z_1}$.

In each of these intervals the sign of the γ_{1v}'s remains the same. In particular assume that $\gamma_{12}, \gamma_{14}, \gamma_{1k}$ are positive whereas the rest are negative in Δ_{11}. Then it is clear that for $\omega \epsilon \Delta_{11}$

$$c_{1max}(\omega) \triangleq \max_{a_2,\ldots,a_k} (\gamma_{12}a_2+\ldots+\gamma_{1k}a_k)=\gamma_{12}a_2^+ + \gamma_{13}a_3^- + \gamma_{14}a_4^+ + \gamma_{15}a_5^- + \ldots + \gamma_{1k}a_k^+$$

$$c_{1min}(\omega) \triangleq \min_{a_2,\ldots,a_k} (\gamma_{12}a_2+\ldots+\gamma_{1k}a_k)=\gamma_{12}a_2^- + \gamma_{13}a_3^+ + \gamma_{14}a_4^- + \gamma_{15}a_5^+ + \ldots + \gamma_{1k}a_k^-$$

This implies that at frequencies in Δ_{11} (which are not zeros of E_{ϕ_1}, O_{ϕ_1}) the two exposed edge lines are:

$$E_{\phi_1}y - \omega O_{\phi_1}x = \omega(\gamma_{12}a_2^+ + \gamma_{13}a_3^- + \gamma_{14}a_4^+, + \ldots + \gamma_{1k}a_k^+)$$

$$E_{\phi_1}y - \omega O_{\phi_1}x = \omega(\gamma_{12}a_2^- + \gamma_{13}a_3^+ + \gamma_{14}a_4^-, + \ldots + \gamma_{1k}a_k^-).$$

This procedure can be repeated for all other parameters as well (i.e., $a_2, a_3, \ldots, a_k$). Specifically for polynomials γ_{uv} $2 < u \leq k$, $v \neq u$ let

$V_u = \{\omega | \omega$ real positive root of some γ_{uv} $1 \leq v \leq k$ $u \neq v$ in the interval $\Delta.\}$

Let $V = V_1 \cup V_2 \ldots \cup V_k$. It is then evident that these frequencies will partition the interval Δ into open intervals $\Delta_1, \Delta_2, \Delta_3, \ldots, \Delta_z$. The number z is computable as it represents the number of real positive roots of a finite number of polynomials. Since the roots of γ_{uv} and γ_{vu}, $u \neq v$ are the same we will have at most $\frac{(k-1)}{2}k$ such polynomials each of degree at most n. Then we must have:

$$z \leq n\frac{(k-1)}{2}k + 1.$$

What we now have is that within each interval Δ_i the 2k edge lines are

$$E_{\phi_1}y - \omega O_{\phi_1}x = \omega\, c_{1imax} \qquad E_{\phi_1}y - \omega O_{\phi_1}x = \omega\, c_{1imin}$$

$$E_{\phi_2}y - \omega O_{\phi_2}x = \omega\, c_{2imax} \qquad E_{\phi_2}y - \omega O_{\phi_2}x = \omega\, c_{2imin}$$

$$\vdots$$

$$E_{\phi_k}y - \omega O_{\phi_k}x = \omega\, c_{kimax} \qquad E_{\phi_k}y - \omega O_{\phi_k}x = \omega\, c_{kimin}$$

where the c_{jimax}, c_{jimin} are solely functions of frequency. It is then clear that the point ϕ_0 will be on any one of these lines for $\omega \epsilon \Delta_i$ if any one of the 2k polynomials

$$g_{1i}(\omega) = \omega((E_{\phi_1}0_{\phi_0} - 0_{\phi_1}E_{\phi_0}) - c_{1imax})$$
$$g_{2i}(\omega) = \omega((E_{\phi_1}0_{\phi_0} - 0_{\phi_1}E_{\phi_0}) - c_{1imin})$$
$$\vdots$$
$$g_{2k-1i}(\omega) = \omega((E_{\phi_k}0_{\phi_0} - 0_{\phi_k}E_{\phi_0}) - c_{kimax})$$
$$g_{2ki}(\omega) = \omega((E_{\phi_k}0_{\phi_0} - 0_{\phi_k}E_{\phi_0}) - c_{kimin})$$

has a real positive root in Δ_i. Assuming that none of the g_{ti} are zero polynomials define:

$U_i = \{\omega | \omega$ is a real positive root of any one of the g_{ti} $1 \leq t \leq 2k$ in $\Delta_i\}$ and $U = U_1 \cup U_2 \cup \ldots \cup U_z$.

Let us now define the set of "critical frequencies":

$$W_1 = U \cup V \cup \{\omega = 0, \text{ real positive root of } E_{\phi_i}, 0_{\phi_i}\}$$

This is clearly a finite set of frequencies. It contains all the frequencies that are potentially troublesome in the sense that it is at one of these that the ϕ_0 point has a chance of entering the -q locus. If then ϕ_0 lies outside the -q locus at these frequencies it must be outside the -q locus for all ω.

Suppose that some (not all) of the $g_{ti} = 0$. Since by assumption $\gamma_{uv} \neq 0$ for all u,v. This will correspond to the situation where ϕ_0 lies on one or more of the g_{ti} for all frequencies. Now if the -q locus continues to be of dimension 2 for most frequencies (except perhaps at positive real roots of the γ_{uv}) and ϕ_0 lies outside the -q locus for some ω (say $\omega = 0$) it can only enter through a different exposed edge. We now modify the sets U_i and U by excluding these zero polynomials. Specifically let $\bar{U}_i = \{\omega | \omega$ is a real positive root of any one of the <u>nonzero</u> g_{ti} $1 \leq t \leq 2k$ in $\Delta_i\}$ and $\bar{U} = \bar{U}_1 \cup \bar{U}_2 \cup \ldots \cup \bar{U}_z$. The set of critical frequencies then becomes

$$W_2 = V \cup \bar{U} \cup \{\omega = 0, \text{ real positive root of } E_{\phi_i}, 0_{\phi_i}\}.$$

Now suppose that some shaping conditions are satisfied. The consequence of this fact will be the following: Suppose that $\phi_1, \phi_2, \ldots, \phi_{j_1}$ satisfy the shaping condition (i.e., $\gamma_{uv} = 0$ for $1 \leq u \leq j_1$, $1 < v < j_1$ $u \neq v$). When we then eliminate a_1 from (2) we also eliminate $a_2, a_3, \ldots a_{j_1}$. This will result in a -q locus with fewer than 2k exposed edges. Specifically if k' such groups of a_i parameters are formed then the -q locus will have at most 2k' edges at any frequency. This will in essence reduce the problem to one of "size" k' rather than k. If all $\gamma_{uv} = 0$ $1 \leq u \leq k$, $1 < v \leq k$ $u \neq v$, then the -q locus will lie on a straight line and be of dimension less than 2 for all frequencies.

In the case we are currently considering (not all $\gamma_{uv} = 0$) we have $k' > 1$. The required modifications to the set of critical frequencies are:

First define for $1 \leq u \leq k$,

$\bar{V}_u = \{\omega | \omega$ is a real positive root of some <u>nonzero</u> γ_{uv}, $1 \leq v \leq k$, $u \neq v\}$

$$\bar{V} = \bar{V}_1 \cup \bar{V}_2 \cup \dots \cup \bar{V}_k.$$

The frequency range Δ will be partitioned by these frequencies into open intervals $\bar{\Delta}_1, \dots \bar{\Delta}_{\bar{z}}$. Equations for the $2k'$ exposed edges can again be given as in (9) and polynomials $\bar{g}_{ti}$ defined, $2k'$ in each interval $\bar{\Delta}_i$. The sets $\bar{U}_i$ and $\bar{U}$ are modified accordingly, $\bar{U}$ becomes $\bar{\bar{U}}$ and in the case when the $\bar{g}_{ti}$ are nonzero the set of critical frequencies becomes:

$$W_3 = \bar{V} \cup \bar{\bar{U}} \cup \{\omega = 0, \text{ real positive root of } E_{\phi_i}, O_{\phi_i}\}$$

If some of the $\bar{g}_{ti}$ now become zero the set of critical frequencies should be suitably modified (as in the 2-parameter case) and set equal to W_4.

Let us now direct attention to the situation when all $\gamma_{uv} = 0$, but ϕ_0 does not lie on the $-q$ locus for all frequencies.

The $-q$ locus is a straight line segment given by: $y = \dfrac{\omega O_{\phi_1}}{E_{\phi_1}} x$

where $\quad x = -E_{\phi_1} a_1 - E_{\phi_2} a_2 - \dots - E_{\phi_k} a_k \qquad a_i^- \leq a_i \leq a_i^+.$

Clearly ϕ_0 will be on this line if $\tilde{g}_0(\omega) = \omega(E_{\phi_1} O_{\phi_0} - O_{\phi_1} E_{\phi_0}) = 0.$

The set of critical frequencies now is:

$$W_5 = \{\omega | \omega = 0, \text{ real positive zero of } g_1(\omega) \text{ or } E_{\phi_i}, O_{\phi_i}\}.$$

As we saw in the 2-parameter case it is impossible for $\tilde{g}_0$ to be the zero polynomial. Q.E.D.

Modifications will be necessary in the set of critical frequencies W in the case when some O_{ϕ_i}, E_{ϕ_i} are zero, as we saw in the 2-parameter case. Even though no attempt has been made to compute the "minimal" W sets, one can see that for the parameter set Ω_a, the number of frequencies that need to be checked is <u>polynomial</u> in k, specifically $O(k^3)$.

REFERENCES

1. A. C. Bartlett, C. V. Hollot and L. Huang, "Root Locations for an Entire Polytope of Polynomials: It Suffices to Check the Edges," Mathematics of Control, Signals and Systems, Vol. 1, pp. 61-71, 1987.

2. B. R. Barmish, "A Generalization of Kharitonov's Four Polynomial Concept for Robust Stability Problems with Linearly Dependent Coefficient Perturbations," Technical Report #ECE-87-18, Department of Electrical and Computer Engineering, University of Wisconsin-Madison, Madison, Wisconsin, November 1987.

3. T. E. Djaferis, C. V. Hollot, "Parameter Partitioning Via Shaping Conditions for the Stability of Families of Polynomials," to appear IEEE Trans. on AC.

4. T. E. Djaferis, "Shaping Conditions for the Robust Stability of Polynomials with Multilinear Parameter Uncertainty,", Proceedings 27th IEEE CDC, Austin, Texas, December 1988.

5. V. L. Kharitonov, "Asymptotic Stability of an Equilibrium Position of a Family of Systems of Linear Differential Equations," Differential'nye Uravneniya, Vol. 14, pp. 2086-2088, 1978.

STRUCTURED AND SIMULTANEOUS LYAPUNOV FUNCTIONS FOR SYSTEM STABILITY PROBLEMS

Stephen Boyd and Qinping Yang[1]

Electrical Engineering Department
Stanford University
Stanford, CA 94305

abstract

It is shown that many system stability and robustness problems can be reduced to the question of when there is a quadratic Lyapunov function of a certain structure which establishes stability of $\dot{x} = Ax$ for some appropriate A. The existence of such a Lyapunov function can be determined by solving a convex program. We present several numerical methods for these optimization problems. A simple numerical example is given. Proofs can be found in Boyd and Yang [BY88].

1 Notation and preliminaries

$\mathbb{R}$ ($\mathbb{R}_+$) will denote the set of real numbers (nonnegative real numbers). The set of $m \times n$ matrices will be denoted $\mathbb{R}^{m\times n}$. I_k will denote the $k \times k$ identity matrix (we will sometimes drop the subscript k if it can be determined from context). $\mathbb{R}I_k$ will denote all multiples of I_k. If $G_i \in \mathbb{R}^{k_i\times k_i}$, $i = 1, \dots, m$, then $\bigoplus_{i=1}^m G_i = G_1 \oplus \cdots \oplus G_m$ will denote the block diagonal matrix with diagonal blocks $G_1, \dots, G_m$. We extend this notation to sets of matrices, so that for example $\bigoplus_{i=1}^3 \mathbb{R}$ is the set of diagonal 3×3 matrices, and

$$\mathbb{R}^{2\times 2} \oplus \mathbb{R}I_2 = \left\{ \begin{bmatrix} a_1 & a_2 & 0 & 0 \\ a_3 & a_4 & 0 & 0 \\ 0 & 0 & a_5 & 0 \\ 0 & 0 & 0 & a_5 \end{bmatrix} \middle| \; a_1, \dots, a_5 \in \mathbb{R} \right\}.$$

Many of our results will pertain to the basic feedback system (shown in figure 1),

$$\begin{aligned} \dot{x} &= Ax + Bu \\ y &= Cx + Du \end{aligned} \tag{1}$$

$$u = \Delta(y) \tag{2}$$

where $x(t) \in \mathbb{R}^n$, $u(t)$, $y(t) \in \mathbb{R}^k$, and Δ is a (possibly nonlinear) causal operator mapping $\left[\mathrm{L}^2_{loc}(\mathbb{R}_+)\right]^k$ into itself (see Desoer and Vidyasagar [DV75] for a complete definition of causality and more background). Throughout this paper we will assume that the linear system (1) is minimal, that is, controllable and observable. We will say that the system (1-2) is *stable* if for all solutions, $x(t)$ is bounded for $t \geq 0$.

[1]Research sponsored in part by ONR under N00014-86-K-0112, NSF under ECS-85-52465, an IBM faculty development award, and Bell Communications Research.

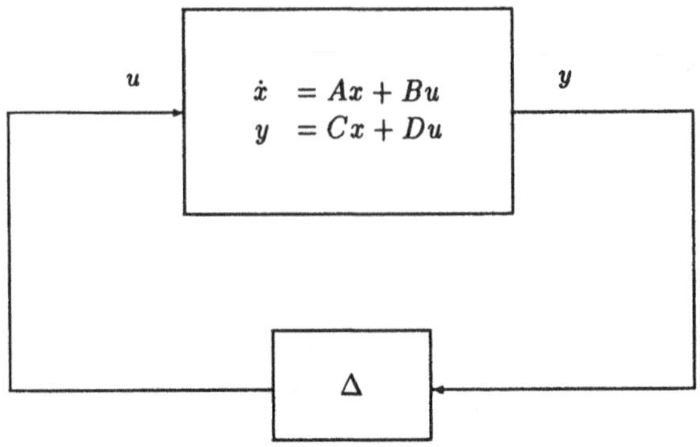

Figure 1. Basic feedback system.

Sometimes the operator Δ can be decomposed into a number of smaller operators in parallel, as shown in figure 2. More precisely, suppose u and y can be partitioned as $u^T = \left[u_1^T \cdots u_m^T\right]$, $y^T = \left[y_1^T \cdots y_m^T\right]$, $u_i(t),\ y_i(t) \in \mathbb{R}^{k_i}$, such that (2) can be expressed as

$$u_i = \Delta_i(y_i), \quad i = 1, \ldots, m. \tag{3}$$

In this case we say the operator Δ has the *block structure* $[k_1, \ldots, k_m]$. If Δ has block structure $[1, \ldots, 1]$, we say Δ is a *diagonal* operator.

The term 'block structure' and the symbol Δ follow Doyle's usage[Doy82].

If Δ has block structure $[k_1, \ldots, k_m]$ and $a_1, \ldots, a_m$ are nonzero constants, we can perform the block structure preserving scaling transformation $\bar{u}_i = a_i u_i$, $\bar{y}_i = a_i y_i$, so that (1-2) can be expressed

$$\begin{aligned} \dot{x} &= Ax + BF^{-1}\bar{u} \\ \bar{y} &= FCx + FDF^{-1}\bar{u} \end{aligned} \tag{4}$$

$$\bar{u} = \bar{\Delta}(\bar{y}) \tag{5}$$

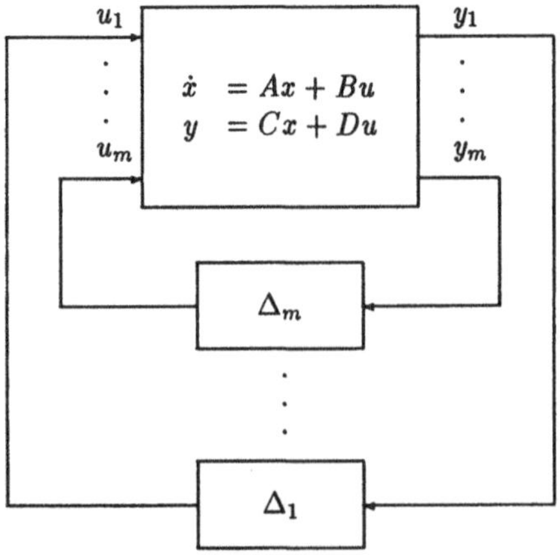

Figure 2. Basic feedback system with block structured feedback.

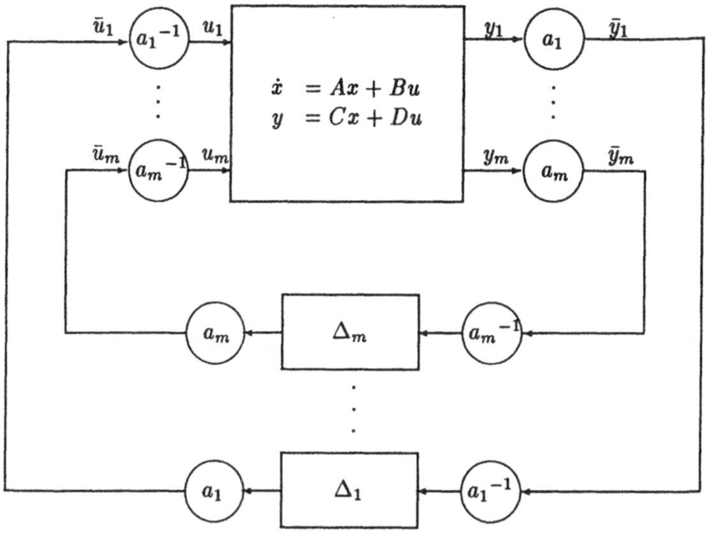

Figure 3. Basic feedback system with block structured feedback, showing the 'block structure preserving scaling transformation'.

where $F = \bigoplus_{i=1}^{m} a_i I_{k_i}$ and $\bar{\Delta}$ is the operator defined by $\bar{u}_i = a_i \Delta_i(a_i^{-1}\bar{y}_i)$. A block diagram of this scaling transformation is shown in figure 3. We note for future reference that $\bar{\Delta}$ also has block structure $[k_1, \ldots, k_m]$ and the transfer matrix of the scaled linear system (4) is $FH(s)F^{-1}$, where $H(s) = C(sI - A)^{-1}B + D$ is the transfer matrix of the original linear system (1).

2 Structured Lyapunov functions

We say $A \in \mathbb{R}^{n \times n}$ is *stable* if all solutions of $\dot{x} = Ax$ are bounded for $t \geq 0$, or equivalently, all eigenvalues of A have nonpositive real parts, and the pure imaginary eigenvalues are simple zeros of the minimal polynomial of A.[2] A famous result of Lyapunov theory states that A is stable if and only if there is a $P = P^T > 0$ such that $A^T P + PA \leq 0$. In this case we say the 'Lyapunov function' $V(x) = x^T P x$ establishes stability of the differential equation $\dot{x} = Ax$, since V is positive definite and $\dot{V}(x) = -2x^T PAx$ is negative semidefinite.

The topic of this paper is the following question: given A, is there a P of a certain structure, for example, block diagonal, for which the Lyapunov function $V(x) = x^T P x$ establishes stability of $\dot{x} = Ax$? We call this the *structured Lyapunov problem* for A. We will show that (a) several problems involving stability of the basic feedback system (1-2) can be answered by solving a structured Lyapunov problem for a certain structure and matrix A, and (b) practical (numerical) solution of the structured Lyapunov problem involves a convex minimization problem. The implication of (b) is that there are *effective* algorithms for solving the structured Lyapunov problem.

Definition 1 *Let* S *be a subspace of* $\mathbb{R}^{n \times n}$. $A \in \mathbb{R}^{n \times n}$ *is* S-structured Lyapunov stable *(*S*-SLS or just SLS if* S *is understood) if there is a* $P \in$ S *such that* $P = P^T > 0$ *and* $A^T P + PA \leq 0$.

We will refer to S as a *structure*, and V an S-structured Lyapunov function (S-SLF) for

[2]This is often called *marginal stability* in the linear systems literature.

A. The structures we will encounter will be very simple, usually consisting of block diagonal matrices, perhaps with some blocks repeated.

Note the distinction between a 'block structure' $[k_1, \ldots, k_m]$ (an attribute of an operator), and a 'structure' S (a subset of $\mathbb{R}^{n \times n}$).

If $\mathbf{S} = \mathbb{R}^{n \times n}$, then by Lyapunov's theorem, A is SLS if and only if A is stable (this could be called unstructured Lyapunov stability); but in general the condition that A is S-SLS is stronger than mere stability of A. At the other extreme, if $\mathbf{S} = \mathbb{R}I_n$, then A is SLS if and only if $A + A^T \leq 0$, which is sometimes referred to as *dissipative dynamics*. This is precisely the condition under which all solutions of $\dot{x} = Ax$ are not only bounded, but in addition $\|x\| = \sqrt{x^T x}$ is nonincreasing. For intermediate structures, the condition that A be SLS will fall between these two extremes: stability, and dissipative dynamics.

A very important special case of the structured Lyapunov problem is the following:

$$\mathbf{S} = \{\, P \oplus \cdots \oplus P \mid P \in \mathbb{R}^{n \times n} \}, \tag{6}$$

$$A = A_1 \oplus \cdots \oplus A_k, \quad A_i \in \mathbb{R}^{n \times n} \tag{7}$$

In this case, A is S-SLS if and only if there is a *single Lyapunov function* $V(x) = x^T P x$ (no structure requirement on P) which establishes the stability of the matrices $A_1, \ldots, A_k$. If the matrix A in (7) is S-SLS, then we say the set of matrices $\{A_1, \ldots, A_k\}$ is *simultaneously Lyapunov stable* (SILS), and the Lyapunov function V is a *simultaneous Lyapunov function* (SILF) for the set.

Several nontrivial cases of the structured Lyapunov problem have been investigated, notably for the case where P is diagonal. This problem is considered in Araki [Ara76], Barker, Berman, and Plemmons [BBP78], Moylan and Hill [MH78], Khalil and Kokotovic [KK79], Khalil [Kha82], and others; their applications range from stability of large interconnected systems to multi-parameter singular perturbations. Matrices which are diagonal-SLS or satisfy a very similar condition (for example, $A^T P + PA > 0$) are sometimes called D-stable or diagonally stable. In the papers cited above various relations (often, sufficient conditions for D-stability) have been found between such matrices and M-matrices, so called quasi-dominant matrices, and P_0-matrices. We refer the reader to the papers mentioned above and the references therein. We mention that a structured Lyapunov stability problem with a *block-diagonal* structure is briefly mentioned in Khalil and Kokotovic [KK79].

The simultaneous Lyapunov problem has also been investigated, more or less directly in Horisberger and Belanger [HB76], and also in connection with the absolute stability problem (see §4) in, for example, Kamenetskii [Kam83] and Pyatnitskii and Skorodinskii [PS83].

In the next two sections (§3 and §4) we show how the important system theoretic notions of passivity and nonexpansivity are easily characterized in terms of SLS problems. The Kalman Yacubovich Popov lemma establishes the equivalence between these important system theoretic notions and the existence of quadratic Lyapunov functions which establish the stability of the basic feedback system for appropriate classes of Δ's (passive and nonexpansive, respectively).

More importantly, we show that the questions of whether a linear system can be scaled so as to be passive or nonexpansive are also readily cast as SLS problems. These conditions are weaker than passivity or nonexpansivity, and we show that the conditions are related to the existence of a quadratic Lyapunov function establishing the stability of the basic feedback system for appropriate classes of *block diagonal* Δ's.

In §5 we show how the general (multiple nonlinearity, nonzero D) absolute stability problem can be attacked as a SILS problem, extending the results of Kamenetskii [Kam83], Pyatnitskii and Skorodinskii [PS83], and Horisberger and Belanger [HB76].

In §6 we show how the results of the previous sections can be combined to yield SLS problems which can determine the existence of a quadratic Lyapunov function establishing the stability of a complex system containing sector bounded memoryless nonlinearities and nonexpansive Δ_i.

In §7 we discuss numerical methods for determining whether a given A is S-SLS for some given structure S. We establish that this question can be cast as a nondifferentiable convex programming problem, a fact which has been noted for several special cases by several authors (see §7). We give some basic results for this optimization problem, such as optimality conditions and descriptions of subgradients and descent directions. We describe several algorithms appropriate for these convex programs.

In §8 we present a numerical example which demonstrates some of the results of this paper.

3 Passivity and scaled passivity

Recall that the linear system (1) is *passive* if every solution of (1) with $x(0) = 0$ satisfies

$$\int_0^T u(t)^T y(t)dt \geq 0 \tag{8}$$

for all $T \geq 0$. This implies that A is stable.[3] Passivity is equivalent to the transfer matrix $H(s) = C(sI - A)^{-1}B + D$ being *positive real* (PR) (see e.g. [DV75]), meaning,

$$H(s) + H(s)^* \geq 0 \quad \text{for} \quad \Re s > 0. \tag{9}$$

Theorem 3.1 *Let* $\mathbf{S} = \mathbb{R}^{n\times n} \oplus \mathbb{R}I_k$. *Then the matrix*

$$\begin{bmatrix} A & B \\ -C & -D \end{bmatrix} \tag{10}$$

is S*-stable if and only if the linear system (1) is passive.*

This theorem is really a restatement of the Kalman Yacubovich Popov (KYP) lemma (see e.g. Anderson [And67, p179]), which states that the linear system (1) is passive if and only if there is a symmetric positive definite matrix P and matrices L and W such that

$$A^T P + PA = -LL^T \tag{11}$$

$$PB = C^T - LW \tag{12}$$

$$W^T W = D + D^T. \tag{13}$$

The only property of P important for us, and indeed in any application, is that the function $V(x) = x^T Px$ satisfies the inequality (see e.g. [Wil71a, Wil72])

$$\frac{1}{2}\frac{d}{dt}V(x) = u^T y - \frac{1}{2}(L^T x + Wu)^T(L^T x + Wu) \leq u^T y \tag{14}$$

for any solution of (1),[4] or equivalently,

$$x^T P(Ax + Bu) \leq u^T(Cx + Du) \quad \text{for all} \quad x,\ u. \tag{15}$$

In the single-input single-output strictly proper case, we can recast the structured Lyapunov stability condition in theorem 3.1 as a simultaneous Lyapunov stability condition.

Corollary 3.2 *The single-input, single-output, strictly proper system* $\dot{x} = Ax + bu$, $y = cx$, *is passive if and only if the matrices* A *and* $-bc$ *are simultaneously Lyapunov stable.*

[3] We remind the reader of the minimality assumption in force, and our use of the term stable.

[4] Equation (14) has the following simple interpretation: the time rate of increase of the Lyapunov function V does not exceed the power input ($u^T y$) to the system.

Passivity is an important tool in stability analysis. The *passivity theorem* (e.g. [DV75]) can be used to establish stability of the feedback system (1-2). It states that if the linear system (1) is passive and $-\Delta$ is a passive operator, meaning for any signal z and $T \geq 0$,

$$\int_0^T z(t)^T(-\Delta(z)(t))dt \geq 0, \tag{16}$$

then the feedback system (1-2) is stable. This conclusion is immediate from (14) and (16), since integration yields

$$V(x(T)) \leq V(x(0)) + \int_0^T u(t)^T y(t)dt \leq V(x(0))$$

and thus x is bounded for $t \geq 0$.

If $-\Delta$ is not only passive but has block structure $[k_1, \dots, k_m]$, then it can be advantageous to apply a block structure preserving transformation to the system before applying the passivity theorem. Such a transformation does not affect the passivity of the feedback, that is, $-\tilde{\Delta}$ is also passive. This results in the following less conservative condition for stability: if there exists an invertible matrix $F \in \bigoplus_{i=1}^m \mathbb{R}I_{k_i}$ such that $FH(s)F^{-1}$ is PR, where H is the transfer matrix of the system (1), then the feedback system (1-2) is stable. This block structure preserving scaled passivity condition is also readily cast as a SLS problem.

Theorem 3.3 *Let* $\mathbf{S} = \mathbb{R}^{n\times n} \oplus \bigoplus_{i=1}^m \mathbb{R}I_{k_i}$. *Then the matrix (10) is* $\mathbf{S}$*-stable if and only if there exists an invertible* $F \in \bigoplus_{i=1}^m \mathbb{R}I_{k_i}$ *such that* $FH(s)F^{-1}$ *is PR. Under this condition, the feedback system (1-2) is stable whenever* $-\Delta$ *is passive and* Δ *has block structure* $[k_1, \dots, k_m]$.

Just as in corollary 3.2, we can recast the structured Lyapunov stability condition appearing in theorem 3.3 as a simultaneous Lyapunov stability condition when the linear system is strictly proper and the structure is diagonal.

Corollary 3.4 *Suppose that* $D = 0$, $b_i \neq 0$, *and* $c_i \neq 0$, $i = 1, \dots, k$, *where* b_i (c_i) *is the ith column (row) of* B (C). *Then there exists a diagonal invertible* F *such that* FHF^{-1} *is PR if and only if* $\{A, -b_1c_1, \dots, -b_kc_k\}$ *is simultaneously Lyapunov stable.*

We can give a more intuitive statement of theorem 3.3, which moreover provides an interpretation of the SLF of theorem 3.3.

Theorem 3.5 *There exists an invertible* $F \in \bigoplus_{i=1}^m \mathbb{R}I_{k_i}$ *such that* $FH(s)F^{-1}$ *is PR if and only if there is a symmetric positive definite* $P_0 \in \mathbb{R}^{n\times n}$ *and positive constants* $\lambda_1, \dots, \lambda_m$ *such that for all solutions of (1), with* $V(x) = x^T P_0 x$, *we have*

$$\frac{d}{dt} V(x(t)) \leq \sum_{i=1}^m \lambda_i u_i(t)^T y_i(t). \tag{17}$$

Like (14), (17) has a simple and obvious interpretation. We note that this theorem provides an immediate proof of the last assertion of theorem 3.3, since if (17) and (16) hold, integration yields

$$V(x(T)) \leq V(x(0)) + \sum_{i=1}^m \lambda_i \int_0^T u_i(t)^T y_i(t)dt \leq V(x(0)) \tag{18}$$

and hence stability of the feedback system.

We also note that theorem 3.5 shows that the structured Lyapunov condition of theorem 3.3 is very nearly the most general condition under which a quadratic Lyapunov function exists which establishes stability of the feedback system (1-2) for arbitrary Δ with block structure $[k_1, \dots k_m]$ and $-\Delta$ passive. The gap is simply this: the quadratic Lyapunov function V would still establish stability if it satisfied (18), but with some of the λ_i *zero*, as opposed to positive.

4 Nonexpansivity and scaled nonexpansivity

We now turn to the important notion of *nonexpansivity.* The linear system (1) is nonexpansive if every solution with $x(0) = 0$ satisfies

$$\int_0^T y(t)^T y(t)dt \leq \int_0^T u(t)^T u(t)dt, \quad \forall T \geq 0. \tag{19}$$

Nonexpansivity also implies that A is stable. In terms of the transfer matrix $H(s) = C(sI - A)^{-1}B + D$, nonexpansivity is equivalent to

$$\|H\|_\infty = \sup_{\Re s>0} \sigma_{max}(H(s)) \leq 1 \tag{20}$$

where $\sigma_{max}(\cdot)$ denotes the maximum singular value.

If the linear system (1) is nonexpansive, then the feedback system (1-2) is stable for any nonexpansive Δ, meaning

$$\int_0^T \Delta(z)^T \Delta(z)dt \leq \int_0^T z^T z dt \quad \forall\, z,\, T \geq 0. \tag{21}$$

A simple proof of this follows from a nonexpansivity form of the KYP lemma which states that the linear system (1) is nonexpansive if and only if there exists a symmetric positive definite $P \in \mathbb{R}^{n\times n}$ such that with $V(x) = x^T Px$, we have

$$\frac{d}{dt} V(x(t)) \leq u(t)^T u(t) - y(t)^T y(t) \tag{22}$$

for any solution of (1).[5] Integration of (22), along with (21) yields $V(x(T)) \leq V(x(0))$ for all $T \geq 0$.

By means of the Cayley transformation, the results on passivity in the previous section can be made to apply to nonexpansivity. If S is a complex $k \times k$ matrix with $\det(I+S) \neq 0$, we define its Cayley transform to be $Z = (I-S)(I+S)^{-1}$. It can be shown that $\sigma_{max}(S) \leq 1$ if and only if $Z + Z^* \geq 0$. Let us now apply the Cayley transform to the transfer matrix $H = C(sI - A)^{-1}B + D$. If $\det(I + D) \neq 0$, the transfer matrix $H = C(sI - A)^{-1}B + D$ satisfies $\|H\|_\infty \leq 1$ if and only if $G = (I - H)(I + H)^{-1}$ is PR. A state space realization of G can be derived: $G = C_c(sI - A_c)^{-1}B_c + D_c$, where

$$\begin{aligned} A_c &= A - B(I+D)^{-1}C \\ B_c &= B(I+D)^{-1} \\ C_c &= -2(I+D)^{-1}C \\ D_c &= (I-D)(I+D)^{-1}. \end{aligned} \tag{23}$$

Theorem 4.1 *Let* $\mathbf{S} = \mathbb{R}^{n\times n} \oplus \bigoplus_{i=1}^m \mathbb{R} I_{k_i}$, *and suppose that* $\det(I + D) \neq 0$. *Then the matrix*

$$\begin{bmatrix} A_c & B_c \\ -C_c & -D_c \end{bmatrix} \tag{24}$$

is $\mathbf{S}$*-stable if and only if there exists an invertible* $F \in \bigoplus_{i=1}^m \mathbb{R} I_{k_i}$ *such that* $\|FHF^{-1}\|_\infty \leq 1$. *If this condition holds, then the feedback system (1-2) is stable for any nonexpansive* Δ *with block structure* $[k_1, \ldots, k_m]$.

Remark

To apply theorem (4.1) when $\det(I + D) = 0$, we simply pick a sign matrix S such that $\det(I + DS) \neq 0$ and apply the theorem to the modified linear system $\{A, BS, C, DS\}$.

[5] Equation (22) has exactly the same interpretation as (14), if we think of u and y as *scattering variables,* since then $u^T u - y^T y$ represents the power input to the system (1).

Let us justify this. The modified linear system has transfer matrix HS. Since F above is diagonal, it commutes with any sign matrix, so that $F(HS)F^{-1} = FHF^{-1}S$, and thus $\|F(HS)F^{-1}\|_\infty = \|FHF^{-1}S\|_\infty = \|FHF^{-1}\|_\infty$.

Now let us show that we can always pick a sign matrix S such that $\det(I + DS) \neq 0$. Let $S = s_1 \oplus \cdots \oplus s_k$, where $s_i \in \{-1, 1\}$. By elementary properties of determinants, we have e.g.

$$\det(I + D(1 \oplus s_2 \oplus \cdots \oplus s_k)) + \det(I + D(-1 \oplus s_2 \oplus \cdots \oplus s_k))$$
$$= 2\det(I + D(0 \oplus s_2 \oplus \cdots \oplus s_k))$$

and thus we have

$$\sum_{s_i \in \{-1,1\}} \det(I + DS) = 2^k.$$

Since the sum of these 2^k numbers is 2^k, at least one of them is nonzero, and that is precisely what we wanted to show.

Block diagonal scaled nonexpansivity can be restated in a 'KYP' form, that is, in terms of the existence of a quadratic Lyapunov function with certain properties:

Theorem 4.2 *There exists an invertible $F \in \bigoplus_{i=1}^m \mathbb{R}I_{k_i}$ such that $\|FHF^{-1}\| \leq 1$ if and only if there is a symmetric positive definite $P \in \mathbb{R}^{n\times n}$ and positive constants $\lambda_1, \ldots, \lambda_m$ such that for all solutions of (1), with $V(x) = x^TPx$, we have*

$$\frac{d}{dt}V(x(t)) \leq \sum_{i=1}^m \lambda_i \left(u_i(t)^T u_i(t) - y_i(t)^T y_i(t)\right). \tag{25}$$

This can be proved by applying a Cayley transform and theorem 3.5.

Remark

Doyle [Doy82] has studied the feedback system (1-2) for the case when Δ is nonexpansive, has block structure $[k_1, \ldots, k_m]$, and in addition Δ *is a linear time-invariant system.* He shows that necessary and sufficient conditions for stability of the feedback system for all such Δ are that

$$\mu(H(j\omega)) \leq 1 \quad \forall\, \omega \in \mathbb{R} \tag{26}$$

where μ denotes the ($[k_1, \ldots, k_m]$-) *structured singular value* of a matrix.

Doyle demonstrates that for any matrix G and any invertible $F \in \bigoplus_{i=1}^m \mathbb{R}I_{k_i}$, we have $\mu(G) \leq \sigma_{max}(FGF^{-1})$ (and indeed if the right hand side is minimized over F, the result is thought to be an excellent approximation to $\mu(G)$). Thus the condition $\|FHF^{-1}\|_\infty \leq 1$ appearing in theorem 4.1 immediately implies Doyle's condition (26). Alternatively, we may note that $\|FHF^{-1}\|_\infty \leq 1$ is sufficient to guarantee stability of the feedback system for all (nonlinear, time-varying) nonexpansive Δ with block structure $[k_1, \ldots, k_m]$, and hence in particular for those Δ which are in addition linear and time-invariant. Since Doyle's condition (26) is necessary for stability of the feedback system for all nonexpansive linear time-invariant block structured Δ, it must be implied by $\|FHF^{-1}\|_\infty \leq 1$.

Remark

Theorem 4.1 yields an effective algorithm for computing

$$\bar{\mu}^{-1} = \inf\left\{ \|FHF^{-1}\|_\infty \;\middle|\; F \in \bigoplus_{i=1}^m \mathbb{R}I_{k_i},\ \det F \neq 0 \right\}. \tag{27}$$

$\bar{\mu}$ has the following interpretation: the feedback system (1-2) is stable for all Δ with block structure $[k_1, \ldots, k_m]$ and $\mathbf{L}^2$-gain at most $\bar{\mu}$, that is,

$$\int_0^T \Delta(z)^T \Delta(z)dt \leq \bar{\mu}^2 \int_0^T z^T z dt \quad \forall\, z,\, T \geq 0. \tag{28}$$

Thus $\bar{\mu}$ could be considered an upper bound on a *nonlinear* version of Doyle's structured singular value.

5 The absolute stability problem

We now consider the system (1-2) with Δ diagonal and *memoryless*, meaning

$$u_i(t) = (\Delta_i(y_i))(t) = f_i(y_i(t), t), \tag{29}$$

where the f_i are functions from $\mathbb{R} \times \mathbb{R}_+$ into $\mathbb{R}$, in sector $[\alpha_i, \beta_i]$, meaning, for all $a \in \mathbb{R}$ and $t \geq 0$,

$$\alpha_i a^2 \leq a f_i(a, t) \leq \beta_i a^2. \tag{30}$$

The *absolute stability problem* is to find conditions under which all trajectories of the system (1, 29) are bounded for $t \geq 0$, for all f_i satisfying (30). It is well known that we do not change the absolute stability problem by restricting the f_i to be time-varying linear gains, since the set of trajectories $x(t)$ satisfying (1), (29) for some f_i's satisfying (30) is identical with the set of trajectories satisfying the equations (1) and

$$u_i(t) = k_i(t) y_i(t) \tag{31}$$

for some $k_i(t)$ which satisfy

$$\alpha_i \leq k_i(t) \leq \beta_i. \tag{32}$$

Since the time-varying linear gains (31) satisfy the sector conditions (30), it is clear that if x satisfies (1) and (31) for some k_i's satisfying (32), then x satisfies (1) and (29) for some f_i satisfying the sector conditions (30). Conversely, suppose x is a trajectory of (1),(29). Then $x(t)$ is also a trajectory of the linear time-varying system (1),(31), where

$$k_i(t) = \begin{cases} \frac{f_i(y_i(t),t)}{y_i(t)} & y_i(t) \neq 0 \\ \alpha_i & y_i(t) = 0 \end{cases} \tag{33}$$

(note that the k_i defined in (33) depends on the particular trajectory $x(t)$). Of course, the k_i defined in (33) satisfy $\alpha_i \leq k_i(t) \leq \beta_i$.

A Lyapunov method can be used to establish absolute stability of the feedback system. The feedback system is absolutely stable if there is a symmetric positive definite $P \in \mathbb{R}^{n \times n}$ such that for any trajectory $x(t)$ satisfying (1) and (29), or equivalently, (1) and (31), $x(t)^T P x(t)$ is nonincreasing. In this case we say that the (quadratic) Lyapunov function $V(x) = x^T P x$ establishes the absolute stability of the feedback system (1, 29).

In this section we will show that the quadratic Lyapunov function V establishes absolute stability of the feedback system if and only if V is a simultaneous Lyapunov function for the 2^m linear systems resulting when the linear time-varying gains k_i are constant and set to every combination of their extreme values. For the $D = 0$ case, which is considerably simpler, this result appears in Kamenetskii [Kam83] and is implicit in the work of Pyatnitskii and Skorodinskii [PS83]. We note that sufficiency of the simultaneous Lyapunov stability condition for the $D = 0$ case follows from Theorem 1 of Horisberger and Belanger [HB76].

We will prove this main result after examining a more fundamental question.

5.1 Wellposedness

We first consider the question of when the feedback system is *well posed* for any nonlinearities satisfying the sector condition (30). By this we mean simply that equations (29) and

$$y = Cx + Du \tag{34}$$

should determine u as a function of x, for any f_i's satisfying (30). Of course if $D = 0$ the system is well posed, since then $u_i(t) = f_i(c_i x(t), t)$, where c_i is the ith row of C.

In view of the equivalence discussed above, the system will be well posed if and only if equations (31) and (34) determine u as a function of x whenever (32) holds. This is the case if and only if

$$\det\{I - D(k_1 \oplus \cdots \oplus k_m)\} \neq 0 \quad \forall\, k_i \in [\alpha_i, \beta_i]. \tag{35}$$

Let $\phi(k_1, \ldots, k_m)$ denote the left hand side of (35).

Theorem 5.1 *Necessary and sufficient conditions for (35) are that the* 2^m *numbers*

$$\phi(k_1, \ldots, k_m), \quad k_i \in \{\alpha_i, \beta_i\}, \tag{36}$$

all have the same nonzero sign.

Remark

When the intervals $[\alpha_i, \beta_i]$ are replaced by $(0, \infty)$, the condition (35) is the definition of D being a 'P_0-matrix', and there is a similar necessary and sufficient condition for D to be a 'P_0-matrix' [FP62, FP66].

5.2 Existence of quadratic Lyapunov function

We suppose now that the wellposedness condition is satisfied, so that $V(x) = x^T P x$, $P = P^T > 0$, establishes absolute stability of the feedback system if and only if every trajectory x of the linear time-varying system

$$\dot{x} = \left(A + BK(t)\,(I - DK(t))^{-1}C\right) x \tag{37}$$

has $V(x(t))$ nonincreasing for arbitrary $K(t) \in \bigoplus_{i=1}^{k} [\alpha_i, \beta_i]$. Of course this is equivalent to

$$\left(A + BK(I - DK)^{-1}C\right)^T P + P\left(A + BK(I - DK)^{-1}C\right) \leq 0 \tag{38}$$

for all $K \in \mathcal{K}$.

We note that the set of matrices

$$\mathcal{A} = \left\{A + BK(I - DK)^{-1}C \;\middle|\; K \in \mathcal{K}\right\} \tag{39}$$

is not in general a polytope of matrices, although in fact $\mathcal{A}$ is contained in the convex hull of the images of the vertices of $\mathcal{K}$, that is,

$$\mathcal{A} \subseteq \mathrm{Co}\left\{A + B\tilde{K}(I - D\tilde{K})^{-1}C \;\middle|\; \tilde{K} \text{ a vertex of } \mathcal{K}\right\}. \tag{40}$$

We now state the main result of this section.

Theorem 5.2 *There exists a positive definite quadratic Lyapunov function which establishes absolute stability of the system (1, 29) if and only if the set of* 2^m *matrices*

$$\left\{A + BK(I - DK)^{-1}C \;\middle|\; K \textit{ a vertex of } \mathcal{K}\right\} \tag{41}$$

is simultaneously Lyapunov stable.

5.3 Brayton-Tong and Safonov results

For the absolute stability problem there are two very nice results available.

Brayton and Tong [BT79, BT80] have derived *necessary and sufficient conditions* for absolute stability: simply, the existence of a *convex* Lyapunov function which (simultaneously) establishes stability of the 2^m matrices (41). They give an effective algorithm for constructing such a Lyapunov function or determining that none exists (in which case the system is not absolutely stable). Note that theorem 5.2 only determines conditions for the existence of a *quadratic* Lyapunov function establishing absolute stability.

Safonov [SW87] has studied a variation on the absolute stability problem: Δ is single-input, single-output, memoryless, time-invariant, and incrementally sector bounded. He has shown that stability of the system for all such Δ can be determined by solving an (infinite dimensional) convex program, and gives a simple algorithm for solving it. Thus for this variation of the absolute stability problem, Safonov has developed an effective algorithm for determining absolute stability.

6 Comparison and hybrid results

Let us compare theorem 4.1, which pertains to the feedback system with Δ diagonal and nonexpansive, with theorem 5.2 with the sector conditions $\alpha_i = -1$, $\beta_i = 1$, which pertains to the feedback system with Δ diagonal, nonexpansive, and memoryless. As mentioned above, theorem 4.1 essentially determines the conditions under which a quadratic Lyapunov function establishes stability of the feedback system for all diagonal nonexpansive Δ, whereas theorem 5.2 determines the conditions under which a quadratic Lyapunov function establishes stability of the feedback system for all diagonal nonexpansive *memoryless* Δ, a weaker condition (on A, B, C, D). Doyle's condition (26) is also weaker (as a condition on A, B, C, D) than that of theorem 3.3; it determines the precise conditions under which the feedback system is stable for all diagonal nonexpansive *linear time-invariant* Δ. Doyle's condition (26) and the absolute stability condition of theorem 5.2 are not comparable, that is, neither is a weaker condition on A, B, C, D.

In terms of Lyapunov functions, the difference between theorem 4.1 and theorem 5.2 with sector $[-1, 1]$ nonlinearities can be stated as follows. These theorems determine conditions under which there exists a symmetric positive definite $P \in \mathbb{R}^{n\times n}$ such that $V(x) = x^T P x$ satisfies:

(theorem 4.1; Δ diagonal and nonexpansive):

$$\frac{d}{dt} V(x(t)) \leq \sum \lambda_i (u_i(t)^2 - y_i(t)^2), \qquad \lambda_i > 0, \tag{42}$$

(theorem 5.2; Δ diagonal, nonexpansive, and memoryless):

$$\frac{d}{dt} V(x(t)) \leq 0 \qquad \text{whenever } |u_i| \leq |y_i|. \tag{43}$$

It is clear that (42) implies (43).

This last observation suggests that the two theorems can be combined. Consider the case where Δ is nonexpansive with block structure $[k_1, \ldots, k_m]$, with $k_1 = \cdots = k_s = 1$ and $\Delta_1, \ldots, \Delta_s$ memoryless (figure 4).

We will assume that this system is well posed, meaning that the absolute stability problem resulting by considering only the memoryless operators $\Delta_1, \ldots, \Delta_s$ is well posed.

A quadratic Lyapunov function $V = x^T P x$ would establish stability of the feedback system (1-2) for all such Δ if there are positive $\lambda_{s+1}, \ldots, \lambda_m$ such that

$$\frac{d}{dt} V(x(t)) \leq \sum_{i=s+1}^{m} \lambda_i (u_i^T u_i - y_i^T y_i) \quad \text{whenever } |u_i| \leq |y_i|,\ i = 1, \ldots, s. \tag{44}$$

Note that this combines the conditions (42) and (43).

We will see that the condition (44) can also be cast as a structured Lyapunov stability question. As in the absolute stability problem, we may consider the case where the memoryless nonlinearities are linear time-varying gains, that is, $u_i = k_i(t) y_i$, $i = 1, \ldots, s$. Let us eliminate $u_1, \ldots, u_s$ from (1) to yield:

$$\dot{x} = A^{(k)} x + B^{(k)} \begin{bmatrix} u_{s+1} \\ \vdots \\ u_m \end{bmatrix} \tag{45}$$

$$\begin{bmatrix} y_{s+1} \\ \vdots \\ y_m \end{bmatrix} = C^{(k)} x + D^{(k)} \begin{bmatrix} u_{s+1} \\ \vdots \\ u_m \end{bmatrix} \tag{46}$$

We will spare the reader the formulas for $A^{(k)}, B^{(k)}, C^{(k)}, D^{(k)}$, only noting that they are linear fractional in the k_i's. Let $A_c^{(k)}, B_c^{(k)}, C_c^{(k)}, D_c^{(k)}$ denote the state space Cayley transform

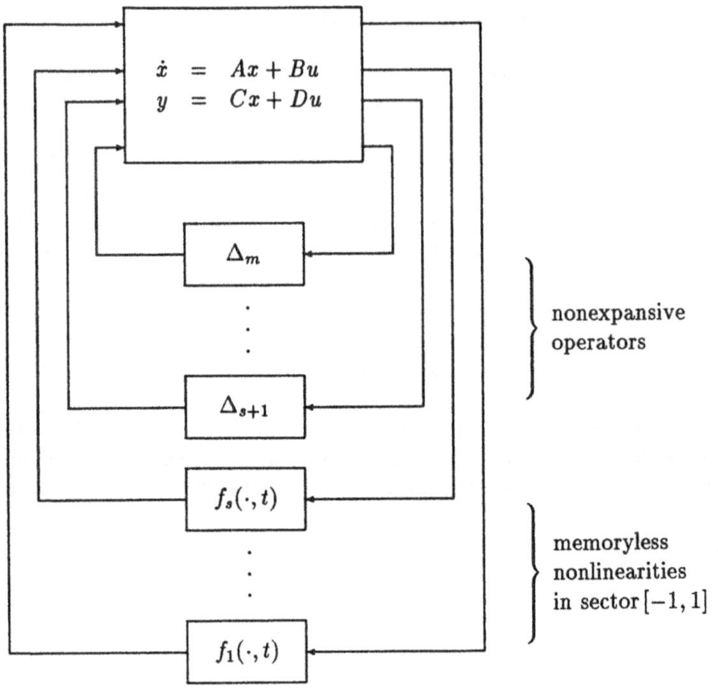

Figure 4. Basic feedback system with block structured nonexpansive Δ, with $\Delta_1, \ldots, \Delta_s$ memoryless.

of the system (45-46) (formulas (23); we assume that $\det(I + D^{(k)}) \neq 0$). We can now state our result.

Theorem 6.1 *There exists a symmetric positive definite $P \in \mathbb{R}^{n \times n}$ and positive $\lambda_{s+1}, \ldots, \lambda_m$ such that for all solutions of (1), with $V(x) = x^T P x$, (44) holds,* if and only if *there is a symmetric positive definite matrix in $\mathbb{R}^{n \times n} \oplus \bigoplus_{i=s+1}^{m} \mathbb{R} I_{k_i}$ which establishes stability of the 2^s matrices*

$$\begin{bmatrix} A_c^{(k)} & B_c^{(k)} \\ -C_c^{(k)} & -D_c^{(k)} \end{bmatrix} \tag{47}$$

where the linear gains $k_i(t)$ are constant and set to their extreme values, ± 1. In this case, the feedback system (1-2) is stable for all nonexpansive block structured Δ with $\Delta_1, \ldots, \Delta_s$ memoryless.

7 Numerical methods for the SLS problem

In this section we consider the problem of actually determining whether A is S-SLS, given A and S. Our first observation is that A is S-SLS if and only if the set

$$\mathcal{P} = \left\{ P \,\middle|\, P = P^T > 0,\ P \in \mathrm{S},\ A^T P + PA \leq 0 \right\} \tag{48}$$

is nonempty. Since $\mathcal{P}$ is convex, we see that the question of whether A is S-SLS is really a *convex feasibility program,* that is, a (nondifferentiable) convex optimization problem.

Similar observations can be found in Horisberger and Belanger [HB76], Khalil [Kha82], Kamenetskii and Pyatnitskii [KP87], and Pyatnitskii and Skorodinskii [PS83]. Of course this means that there are effective algorithms for determining whether a given A is **S**-SLS.

Although it is possible to use numerical methods to determine whether $\mathcal{P}$ is empty, there are several reasons why in practice we should prefer to check the slightly stronger condition that $\mathcal{P}$ have nonempty interior. In terms of A, this stronger condition, which we will call *strict* SLS or SSLS, is the existence of a symmetric positive definite $P \in \mathbf{S}$ such that $A^TP + PA < 0$ (note the strict inequality here).

First, small perturbations in A (e.g. roundoff error) do not destroy the SSLS property; the same cannot be said of the SLS property. In other words, the set of A which are **S**-SSLS for some **S** is always open, whereas the set of A which are **S**-SLS need not be. Second, when the strict SLS property is determined, it allows us to conclude *asymptotic stability* ($x(t) \to 0$) of the system under study, as opposed to mere stability ($x(t)$ bounded). In the remainder of this section we will consider numerical methods for determining whether A is SSLS.

Let $Z_1, \ldots, Z_r$ be a basis for the subspace $\left\{Z \,\middle|\, Z = Z^T \in \mathbf{S}\right\}$. Then A is SSLS if and only if there exist $a_1, \ldots, a_r$ such that $Q = \sum_{i=1}^r a_iQ_i < 0$, where $Q_i = -Z_i \oplus \left(A^TZ_i + Z_iA\right)$. Let us define

$$\Phi(a) = \Phi(a_1, \ldots, a_r) = \lambda_{max}\left(\sum_{i=1}^r a_iQ_i\right).$$

Since Φ is positive homogeneous ($\Phi(\alpha a) = \alpha\Phi(a)$ for all positive α), and thus A is SSLS if and only if $\Phi^* < 0$, where

$$\Phi^* = \min_{|a_i| \le 1} \Phi(a). \tag{49}$$

If A is SSLS, then from the positive homogeneity of Φ we conclude that the optimum a^* always occurs on a boundary of the constraint set, that is, there is at least one i with $|a_i^*| = 1$. Note that A is not SSLS if and only if $a = 0$ is optimal for (49).

Before turning to numerical algorithms appropriate for the convex program (49), let us comment on the significance of the bounds $|a_i| \le 1$. Suppose the matrices Z_i and A are scaled so that their largest elements are on the order of one, $\Phi^* = \Phi(a^*) < 0$, and $P = \sum_{i=1}^r a_i^*Z_i$. Then not only is $P \oplus -A^TP - PA$ positive definite, but its condition number is at most on the order of $1/|\Phi^*|$. Thus if we test whether the minimum value Φ^* of (49) is less than, say, -10^{-4}, we are really testing whether there is a P such that $P \oplus -A^TP - PA$ is positive definite and has condition number under approximately 10^4.

7.1 Descent directions, subgradients, and optimality conditions

A vector $\delta a \in \mathbb{R}^n$ is said to be a *descent direction* for Φ at a if for small positive h, $\Phi(a + h\delta a) < \Phi(a)$. Note that the existence of a descent direction at $a = 0$ is equivalent to A being SSLS; it will be useful for us to also consider descent directions at other, nonzero a. The conditions for δa to be a descent direction at a are readily determined from perturbation theory for symmetric matrices [Kat84]. Let $\Phi(a) = \lambda$, and let t denote the multiplicity of the eigenvalue λ of $\sum_{i=1}^r a_iQ_i$. Let the columns of $U \in \mathbb{R}^{n\times t}$ be an orthonormal basis for the nullspace of

$$\lambda I - \sum_{i=1}^r a_iQ_i. \tag{50}$$

Then δa is a descent direction if and only if

$$\delta a_1U^TQ_1U + \cdots + \delta a_rU^TQ_rU = G < 0 \tag{51}$$

and in fact

$$\lim_{h\searrow 0} \frac{\Phi(a + h\delta a) - \Phi(a)}{h} = \lambda_{max}(G).$$

Thus if the eigenvalue λ has multiplicity one, so that U is a single column, one choice of descent direction is $\delta a_i = -U^T Q_i U$. Indeed this is precisely the condition (i.e. $t = 1$) under which Φ is differentiable at a, and this δa is simply $-\nabla\Phi(a)$.

Whenever $t > 1$, (e.g. when $a = 0$, we have $t = n$) determining a descent direction (or that none exists) is much harder. One general method uses the notion of the *subgradient* $\partial\Phi(a)$ of a convex function Φ at $a \in \mathbb{R}^r$, defined as [Roc72, Cla83]

$$\partial\Phi(a) = \left\{ g \in \mathbb{R}^r \,\middle|\, \Phi(\tilde{a}) - \Phi(a) \geq g^T(\tilde{a} - a),\ \forall\, \tilde{a} \in \mathbb{R}^r \right\}. \tag{52}$$

$\partial\Phi(a)$ can be shown to be nonempty, compact, and convex, and moreover δa is a descent direction at a if and only

$$\delta a^T g < 0 \quad \forall\, g \in \partial\Phi(a), \tag{53}$$

so that descent directions correspond precisely to hyperplanes through the origin with the subgradient in the negative half-space. Thus we have the standard conclusion that there exists a descent direction at a if and only if $0 \notin \partial\Phi(a)$, and indeed in this case we may take as 'explicit' descent direction the negative of the element of $\partial\Phi(a)$ of least norm. In particular we have: A is SSLS if and only if $0 \notin \partial\Phi(0)$.

Polak and Wardi [PW82] have shown that for our particular Φ,

$$\partial\Phi(a) = \mathrm{Co}\left\{ g \in \mathbb{R}^r \,\middle|\, g_i = z^T U^T Q_i U z,\ \ z \in \mathbb{R}^t,\ z^T z = 1 \right\}. \tag{54}$$

In particular if u is *any* unit eigenvector of (50) corresponding to the maximum eigenvalue $\Phi(a)$ of the matrix (50), then $g_i = u^T Q_i u$ yields $g \in \partial\Phi(a)$. So it is very easy to find elements of the set $\partial\Phi(a)$.

From Polak and Wardi's characterization of the subgradient we can readily derive conditions for $a = 0$ to be optimal. These conditions can be found in Overton [Ove87, OW87], but with a completely different proof.

Theorem 7.1 *A is not SSLS, or equivalently, 0 is a global minimizer of Φ,* if and only if *there is a nonzero $R = R^T \geq 0$ such that $\mathrm{Tr} Q_i R = 0$, $i = 1, \ldots, r$.*

The algorithm we have found most effective for solving (49) is Kelley's cutting-plane algorithm [Kel60]. The algorithm requires only the ability to evaluate the function (i.e. compute $\Phi(a)$) and find an element in the subgradient at a point (i.e. compute a $g \in \partial\Phi(a)$), which we have already explained how to do. Suppose that $a^{(1)}, \ldots, a^{(s)}$ are the first s iterates with $g^{(i)} \in \partial\Phi(a^{(i)})$. Then from the definition of subgradient we have

$$\Phi(z) \geq \max_{i=1,\ldots,s} \Phi(a^{(i)}) + g^{(i)T}(z - a^{(i)})$$

for all z and thus

$$\Phi^* \geq = \Phi_{LB}^{(s)} = \min_{|z_i| \leq 1} \max_{i=1,\ldots,s} \Phi(a^{(i)}) + g^{(i)T}(z - a^{(i)}). \tag{55}$$

The right hand side of (55) is readily solved via linear programming, and we take $a^{(s+1)}$ to be the argument which minimizes the right hand side of (55), that is, $a^{(s+1)}$ is chosen such that

$$\Phi_{LB}^{(s)} = \max_{i=1,\ldots,s} \Phi(a^{(i)}) + g^{(i)T}(a^{(s+1)} - a^{(i)}).$$

Of course $\Phi_{LB}^{(s)}$ is a lower bound for Φ^*, which is extremely useful in devising stopping criteria—for example, we may stop when $\Phi_{LB}^{(s)}$ exceeds some threshold, say, -10^{-4}, or when the difference $\Phi(a^{(s)}) - \Phi_{LB}^{(s)}$ is smaller than some specified tolerance.

Although the number of constraints in the linear program which must be solved at each iteration grows with iteration number, if these linear programs are initialized at the last iterate it usually takes only a very few iterations to converge.

The great advantage of the cutting-plane algorithm is that at all times a lower bound $\Phi_{LB}^{(s)}$ and upper bound $\Phi_{UB}^{(s)}$ ($= \min_{i \le s} \Phi(a^{(i)})$) on Φ^* are maintained. Of course it is readily shown that $\Phi_{UB}^{(s)} - \Phi_{LB}^{(s)} \to 0$ as $s \to \infty$, so the cutting-plane algorithm is therefore completely effective—it cannot fail to unambiguously determine in a finite number of steps whether or not $\Phi^* < -\epsilon$.[6] The disadvantage is that the computation per iteration can be prohibitive for very large systems. In the next two subsections we describe two other algorithms for (49) which involve less computation per iteration, and thus may be appropriate for large systems.

7.2 Subgradient methods

Shor [Sho85] has introduced a method for solving nondifferentiable convex programs such as (49), the *subgradient algorithm*. In appearance it is quite similar to a descent method for a differentiable convex function. Shor's algorithm generates $a^{(s+1)}$ as

$$a^{(s+1)} = a^{(s)} + h_s \delta a^{(s)} \tag{56}$$

where $\delta a^{(s)}$ is the *direction* and h_s the *step-size* of the sth iteration. In a descent method, $\delta a^{(s)}$ would be a descent direction for Φ at $a^{(s)}$, and then h_s might be chosen to minimize or approximately minimize $\Phi(a^{(s)} + h_s \delta a^{(s)})$. In Shor's subgradient methods, the direction $\delta a^{(s)}$ is allowed to be the negative of *any* element of the subgradient $\partial\Phi(a^{(s)})$, and usually the step size h_s depends only on the iteration number s. One possible choice is:

$$-\delta a^{(s)} \in \partial\Phi(a^{(s)}), \qquad h_s = \frac{\alpha}{s\|\delta a^{(s)}\|} \tag{57}$$

where α is the largest number under one which ensures $|a_i^{(s+1)}| \le 1$.

Thus the subgradient method requires at each iteration the computation of *any* element of the subgradient, as opposed to a descent direction. As we have already noted, finding an element of the subgradient $\partial\Phi(a)$ is straightforward, essentially involving the computation of the largest eigenvalue of the symmetric matrix Q and a vector in its associated eigenspace. This computation can be very efficiently done, even for large systems [Par80].

If the subgradient $\partial\Phi(a^{(s)})$ subtends an angle exceeding $\pi/2$ from the origin, then it is possible that $\delta a^{(s)}$ is *not* a descent direction, and indeed it (often) occurs that $\Phi(a^{(s+1)}) > \Phi(a^{(s)})$. Nevertheless it can be proved that the algorithm (56-57) has guaranteed global convergence, that is,

$$\lim_{s \to \infty} \Phi(a^{(s)}) = \Phi^*. \tag{58}$$

Thus if A is SSLS, so that $\Phi^* < 0$, then the subgradient algorithm (56-57) will find an a with $\Phi(a) < 0$ in a finite number of iterations. These assertions follow immediately from the results in Shor [Sho85] or Demyanov and Vasilev [DV85].

This algorithm involves much less computation per iteration than the cutting-plane method described above, especially for large systems. It has two disadvantages: First, if A is SSLS, it may take a large number of subgradient iterations to produce a SLF. Second, and more important, if A is *not* SSLS, there is no good method to know when to stop—no good lower bounds on Φ^* are available. In other words, the subgradient method cannot unambiguously determine that A is not SSLS—it will simply fail to produce a SLF in a large number of iterations. Even if it appears that the a's are converging to zero, as they must if A is not SSLS, there is no way to be certain of this after only a finite number of iterations.

[6] As mentioned above, $1/\epsilon$ can be interpreted as a maximum allowable condition number for $P \oplus -A^T P - PA$.

7.3 Kamenetskii-Pyatnitskii saddle point method

Kamenetskii and Pyatnitskii [KP87] have developed an algorithm for (49) which involves even less computation per iteration than the subgradient method, and thus may be useful for very large systems. Kamenetskii and Pyatnitskii consider the function

$$F(a,x) = x^T(\sum_{i=1}^{r} a_i Q_i)x. \tag{59}$$

Recall that $\tilde{a}$, $\tilde{x}$ is said to be a *saddle point* of F [AHU58, Roc72] if

$$F(\tilde{a},x) \le F(\tilde{a},\tilde{x}) \le F(a,\tilde{x}) \qquad \forall\, a,\ x.$$

It is easy to see that $\tilde{a}$, $\tilde{x}$ is a saddle point of F if and only if $\Phi(a) \le 0$ and $Q_i\tilde{x} = 0$, $i = 0,\ldots,r$, which we assume without loss of generality occurs only if $\tilde{x} = 0$ (otherwise A is clearly not SSLS). This is theorem 2 of [KP87].

The Kamenetskii-Pyatnitskii algorithm is just the gradient method for finding saddle points of functions, most simply expressed as a differential equation for a and x:

$$\begin{array}{rcccl} \dot{x} & = & \partial F/\partial x & = & 2\sum_{i=1}^{r} a_i Q_i x, \\ \dot{a}_i & = & -\partial F/\partial a_i & = & -x^T Q_i x. \end{array} \tag{60}$$

It can be shown that if F were strictly concave in x for each a (which is not true for our F (59)) and convex in a for each x, then all solutions of the differential equation (60) would converge to saddle points of F [AHU58]. Despite the fact that (59) is not concave in x for each a, Kamenetskii and Pyatnitskii prove the remarkable fact that if A is SSLS, then for arbitrary initial conditions the solutions of DE (60) converge to saddle points of F as $t \to \infty$. Thus $x \to 0$ and $a \to \tilde{a}$, where $\Phi(\tilde{a}) \le 0$. They show moreover that for almost all initial conditions (zero is one of the exceptions), $\Phi(\tilde{a}) < 0$. Thus if A is SSLS, then the gradient method will find a SLF (for almost all initial x and a).

Of course in practice a suitable discretization of the differential equation (60) is solved (see [KP87]).

Compared to the cutting-plane or subgradient method, this algorithm is extremely simple, requiring no maximum eigenvalue/eigenvector computations. On the other hand, we have found extremely slow convergence of a to $\tilde{a}$, and of course this method shares with the subgradient method the disadvantage of not being able to establish that A is *not* SSLS.

8 An example

In this section we demonstrate some of the results of this paper on the simple two-input two-output control system shown in figure 5. The plant is modeled as a nominal LTI plant with transfer matrix

$$P_{nom}(s) = \frac{1}{s+1}\begin{bmatrix} 1 & 2 \\ -.2 & 1 \end{bmatrix}$$

and an *output 'multiplicative' perturbation* which consists of a nonexpansive but unknown two-input, two-output, (possibly nonlinear) operator Δ followed by a LTI weighting filter with transfer matrix

$$W(s) = 1.5\,\frac{s+1}{s+10}\,I_2.$$

Very roughly speaking, this means that our nominal plant is moderately accurate (about 15%) at low frequencies (say, $\omega < 0.5$), less accurate in the range $0.5 < \omega < 3$, and quite inaccurate for $\omega > 3$.

The two memoryless nonlinearities f_1 and f_2 represent actuator nonlinearities, and are assumed to be in sector $[0.7, 1.3]$.

The controller is a simple proportional plus integral (PI) controller with transfer matrix

$$C(s) = -\left(K_P + \frac{K_I}{s}\right)\begin{bmatrix} .7 & -1.4 \\ 0 & .7 \end{bmatrix}.$$

We set $K_P = 2\alpha - 1$ and $K_I = 2\alpha^2$, which with the nominal plant without actuator nonlinearity would yield closed loop eigenvalues at approximately $-\alpha \pm j\alpha$. Thus the parameter α approximately determines the closed-loop system bandwidth.

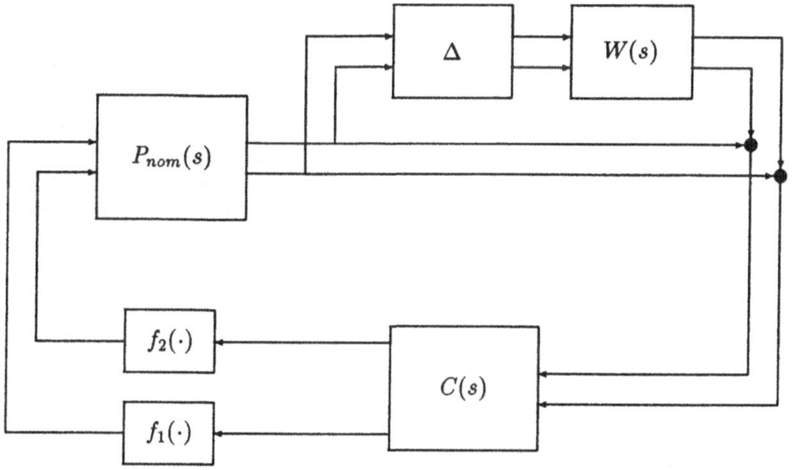

Figure 5. A simple control system. Δ is a nonexpansive operator representing unknown nonlinear dynamic plant perturbation; the memoryless nonlinearities $f_1(\cdot)$ and $f_2(\cdot)$ represent actuator nonlinearity.

The system can be put into the hybrid system form of figure 4 and thus the question of whether there exists a quadratic Lyapunov function which establishes stability of this control system can be formulated as a SLS problem (see theorem 6.1). For this example, the appropriate structure is $\mathbf{S} = \mathbb{R}^{6\times 6} \oplus \mathbb{R}I_2$. When formulated as a convex optimization problem as described in section 7, we find $r = 22$ (i.e. there are 22 variables in the optimization problem), and the matrices Q_i are 40×40, in fact block diagonal, with five 8×8 blocks. Thus to generate a subgradient involves roughly five 8×8 symmetric matrix eigenvalue computations.

Taking $\epsilon = 10^{-4}$ (see §7), which we remind the reader corresponds to an approximate limit of 10^4 on the condition number of acceptable $P \oplus -A^TP - PA$, we find that when $.5 \le \alpha < 1.2$, A is S-SSLS, and when $\alpha > 1.2$, A is not S-SSLS. Thus for $\alpha < 1.2$, we can find a quadratic Lyapunov function which establishes (asymptotic) stability of the control system, and for $\alpha \ge 1.2$, there exists no quadratic Lyapunov function establishing stability of our control system.

To give some idea of the performance of the algorithms discussed in §7 we will consider two cases: $\alpha = 1$ (A is S-SSLS in this case), and $\alpha = 2$ (A is not S-SSLS in this case).

For $\alpha = 1$, the cutting-plane method takes 109 iterations to find out that the system is S-SSLS ($\Phi_{UB} < -\epsilon$), and another 133 iterations to determine that $\Phi^* = -.0031$ within at most 10% (stopping criterion: $\Phi_{UB} - \Phi_{LB} < .1|\Phi_{LB}|$). The condition number of the corresponding $P \oplus -A^T P - PA$ is 382.

For $\alpha = 1$, the subgradient method takes 5507 iterations to determine that the system is S-SSLS ($\Phi_{UB} < 0$).

When $\alpha = 2$, the cutting-plane method takes 113 iterations to determine that A is not S-SSLS ($\Phi_{LB} > -\epsilon$). Of course the subgradient method simply fails to find a SLF for A; after a very large number of iterations we may suspect that A is not S-SSLS, but we cannot be sure.

9 Conclusion

We have introduced the simple notion of structured Lyapunov stability, and shown how several important system theoretic problems involving block diagonally scaled passivity and nonexpansivity can be recast as SLS problems. We have shown (theorem 6.1) how it can be used to determine conditions which guarantee stability of the feedback system (1-2) for all Δ of a specified class, for example of a certain block structure, with some blocks memoryless with sector constraints and other blocks nonexpansive (but possibly nonlinear and dynamic).

A very important fact is that the structured Lyapunov stability problem is equivalent to a convex optimization problem, and can therefore be effectively solved, for example using the methods described in §7.

References

[AHU58] K. J. Arrow, L. Hurwicz, and H. Uzawa. *Studies in Linear and Nonlinear Programming.* Stanford University Press, Stanford, California, 1958.

[And67] B. D. O. Anderson. A system theory criterion for positive real matrices. *SIAM J. Control*, 5:171–182, 1967.

[Ara76] M. Araki. Input-output stability of composite feedback sytems. *IEEE Trans. Aut. Control*, AC-21:254–259, 1976.

[BBP78] G. P. Barker, A. Berman, and R. J. Plemmons. Positive diagonal solutions to the Lyapunov equations. *Linear and Multilinear Algebra*, 5:249–256, 1978.

[BT79] R. K. Brayton and C. H. Tong. Stability of dynamical systems: a constructive approach. *IEEE Trans. Circuits Syst.*, CAS-26(4):224–234, 1979.

[BT80] R. K. Brayton and C. H. Tong. Constructive stability and asymptotic stability of dynamical systems. *IEEE Trans. Circuits Syst.*, CAS-27(11):1121–1130, 1980.

[BW65] R. W. Brockett and J. L. Willems. Frequency domain stability criteria. *IEEE Trans. Aut. Control*, AC-10:255–261, 401–413, 1965.

[BY88] S. Boyd and Q. Yang. Structured and simultaneous Lyapunov functions for system stability problems. *Int. J. Control*, to appear 1988.

[Cla83] F. H. Clarke. *Optimization and Nonsmooth Analysis. Canadian Mathematical Society Series*, Wiley, New York, 1983.

[Doy82] J. C. Doyle. Analysis of feedback systems with structured uncertainties. *IEE Proc.*, 129(6), November 1982.

[DV75] C. A. Desoer and M. Vidyasagar. *Feedback Systems: Input-Output Properties.* Academic Press, New York, 1975.

[DV85] V. F. Demyanov and L. V. Vasilev. *Nondifferentiable Optimization.* Optimization Software (Springer-Verlag), New York, 1985.

[FP62] M. Fiedler and V. Ptak. On matrices with non-positive off-diagonal elements and positive principal minors. *Czechoslovak Mathematical Journal,* 87:382–400, 1962.

[FP66] M. Fiedler and V. Ptak. Some generalizations of positive definiteness and monotonicity. *Numerische Mathematik,* 9:163–172, 1966.

[HB76] H. P. Horisberger and P. R. Belanger. Regulators for linear, time invariant plants with uncertain parameters. *IEEE Trans. Aut. Control,* AC-21:705–708, 1976.

[Hu87] Hui Hu. An algorithm for rescaling a matrix positive definite. *Linear Algerbra and Its Applications,* 96:131–147, 1987.

[Kam83] V. A. Kamenetskii. Absolute stability and absolute instability of control systems with several nonlinear nonstationary elements. *Automation and Remote Control, a translation of Automatika i Telemekhnika,* (12):1543–1552, 1983.

[Kat84] T. Kato. *Perturbation Theory for Linear Operators.* Springer-Verlag, New York (second edition), 1984.

[Kel60] J. E. Kelley. The cutting-plane method for solving convex programs. *J. Soc. Indust. Appl. Math,* 8(4):703–712, December 1960.

[Kha82] H. K. Khalil. On the existence of positive diagonal P such that $PA + A^T P < 0$. *IEEE Trans. Aut. Control,* AC-27:181–184, 1982.

[KK79] H. K. Khalil and P. V. Kokotovic. D-stability and multiparameter singular perturbation. *SIAM J. Contr. Optimiz.,* 17:56–65, 1979.

[KP87] V. A. Kamenetskii and E. S. Pyatnitskii. Gradient method of constructing Lyapunov functions in problems of absolute stability. *Automation and Remote Control, a translation of Automatika i Telemekhnika,* (1):1–9, 1987.

[MH78] P. J. Moylan and D. J. Hill. Stability criteria for large-scale systems. *IEEE Trans. Aut. Control,* AC-23:143–149, 1978.

[Ove87] M. L. Overton. *On Minimizing the Maximum Eigenvalue of a Symmetric Matrix.* Technical Report, Center for Mathematical Analysis, Australian National University, 1987. to appear, Linear Algebra in Signals, Systems and Control (SIAM, Philadelphia, 1987).

[OW87] M. L. Overton and R. S. Wormley. *On minimizing the spectral radius of a nonsymmetric matrix function—optimality conditions and duality theory.* Technical Report, Center for Mathematical Analysis, Australian National University, 1987.

[Par80] B. N. Parlett. *The Symmetric Eigenvalue Problem.* Prentice-Hall, 1980.

[PS83] E. S. Pyatnitskii and V. I. Skorodinskii. Numerical method of construction of Lyapunov functions and absolute stability criteria in the form of numerical procedures. *Automation and Remote Control, a translation of Automatika i Telemekhnika,* (11):1427–1437, 1983.

[PW82] E. Polak and Y. Wardi. A nondifferentiable optimization algorithm for the design of control systems subject to singular value inequalities over a frequency range. *Automatica,* 18(3):267–283, 1982.

[Roc72] R. T. Rockafellar. *Convex Analysis.* Princeton University Press, Princeton, second edition, 1972.

[Sho85] N. Z. Shor. *Minimization Methods for Non-differentiable Functions. Springer Series in Computational Mathematics*, Springer-Verlag, Berlin, 1985.

[SW87] M. G. Safonov and G. Wyetzner. Computer-aided stability criterion renders Popov criterion obsolete. *IEEE Trans. Aut. Control*, AC-32(12):1128–1131, december 1987.

[Wil71a] J. C. Willems. The construction of Lyapunov functions for input-output stable systems. *SIAM J. Control*, 9:105–134, 1971.

[Wil71b] J. C. Willems. Least squares stationary optimal control and the algebraic Riccati equation. *IEEE Trans. Automatic Control*, AC-16:621–634, 1971.

[Wil72] J. C. Willems. Dissipative dynamical systems I: General theory. II: Linear systems with quadratic supply rates. *Archive for Rational Mechanics and Analysis*, 45:321–343, 1972.

ROBUST STABILITY OF POLYNOMIALS WITH MULTILINEAR PARAMETER DEPENDENCE

F.J. Kraus and M. Mansour

Institute of Automatic Control and Industrial Electronics
Swiss Federal Institute of Technolog, Zurich (Switzerland)

B.D.O. Anderson

Department of Systems Engineering, Australian National University
Canberra ACT 2601, Australia
(The work of the author was predominantly performed at the Swiss Federal Institute of Technology, Zurich)

ABSTRACT

The problem is studied of testing for stability a class of real polynomials in which the coefficients depend on a number of variable parameters in a multilinear way. We show that the testing for real unstable roots can be achieved by examining the stability of a finite number of corner polynomials (obtained by setting parameters at their extreme values), while checking for unstable complex roots normally involves examining the real solutions of up to m+1 simultaneous polynomial equations, where m is the number of parameters. When m=2, this is an especially simple task.

1. INTRODUCTION

This paper is concerned with a robust stability problem. More specifically, we consider monic n-th degree polynomials $f(s; \gamma_1,...,\gamma_m)$ with real coefficients which depend in a multilinear fashion on the quantities γ_i. The parameters γ_i are contained in intervals $[\underline{\gamma}_i, \overline{\gamma}_i]$, and we seek a test for the stability of all f(s), where by the term stability, we mean that f(s) has all its roots in a prescribed region, e.g. Re[s] < 0, |s| < 1, etc. For the most part in this paper, we focus on the case Re[s] < 0; the ideas however with little variation will carry over to most other regions of interest. Stability inside the unit circle is easily covered for example by bilinear transformation.

To illustrate the occurrence of such problems we note that many physical systems described by linear differential equations in which parameters such as friction constants, mass, capacitance, etc. vary have associated transfer functions in which these variable parameters appear multilinearly in both numerator and denominator. Also, when a controller defined by a rational transfer function is connected, the characteristic polynomial of the closed-loop system is (apart from limited exceptions) necessarily multilinear in the parameters of the plant and controller transfer functions, see e.g. Section 9.17 of Zadeh and Desoer (1963), and Dasgupta and Anderson (1987).

In the following, two examples are given:

Example 1:
Let us consider the electrical circuit depicted in Figure 1:

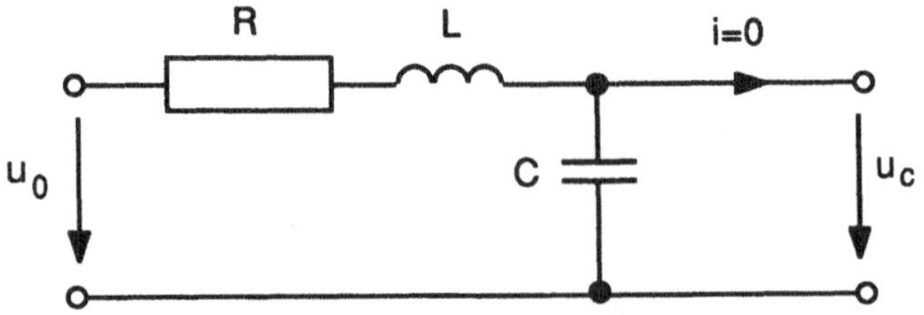

Fig. 1. Electrical circuit

The transfer function from u_0 to u_c is given by

$$G(s) = \frac{1}{s^2LC + sRC + 1}$$

The parameters of the characteristic polynomial depend bilinearly on the physical parameters R, L, C which can vary slowly, for example because of temperature variations or ageing.

Example 2:
Assume that $G_1(s) = B_1(s)/A_1(s)$ and $G_2(s) = B_2(s)/A_2(s)$ in the SISO control system of Figure 2, and that certain coefficients of Ai, Bi, i = 1,2, depend linearly on some parameters, different for each of the four polynomials.

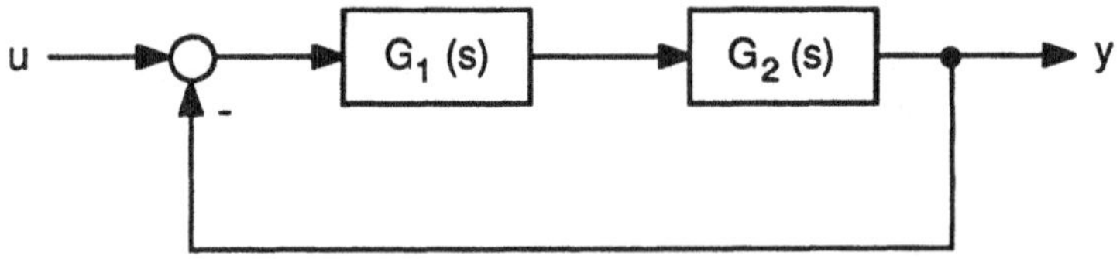

Fig. 2. SISO control system

Then the characteristic polynomial

$$N(s) = A_1(s)A_2(s) + B_1(s)B_2(s)$$

depends bilinearly on the coefficients of A_1 and A_2, and B_1 and B_2, respectively, and in turn bilinearly on the underlying parameters. This situation is significant in practical applications, because we often need to build control systems from different parts. The parameters of the parts can differ from the nominal values. But the stability of the closed loop should be preserved for all such parts.

Before proceeding further, we must define some terms. We work in three different spaces, which are parameter space, coefficient space and root space. The parameters γ_i are contained in closed intervals $[\underline{\gamma}_i, \overline{\gamma}_i]$. The endpoints of such intervals are denoted by $\{\underline{\gamma}_i, \overline{\gamma}_i\}$. Open parameter intervals are given by $(\underline{\gamma}_i, \overline{\gamma}_i)$. Corner points and corner polynomials in parameter and coefficient space are defined by taking $\gamma_i \in \{\underline{\gamma}_i, \overline{\gamma}_i\}$. Edges in parameter and coefficient space and edge polynomials are defined by taking $\gamma_i \in \{\underline{\gamma}_i, \overline{\gamma}_i\}$ for all but one value of i, say i_1, and $\gamma_{i1} \in [\underline{\gamma}_{i1}, \overline{\gamma}_{i1}]$. Notice that edges in both parameter and coefficient space are straight lines. Faces in parameter and coefficient space and face polynomials are defined by taking $\gamma_i \in \{\underline{\gamma}_i, \overline{\gamma}_i\}$ for all but two values of i, say i_1 and i_2, and $\gamma_{i1} \in [\underline{\gamma}_{i1}, \overline{\gamma}_{i1}]$ and $\gamma_{i2} \in [\underline{\gamma}_{i2}, \overline{\gamma}_{i2}]$.

In parameter space, faces are flat while in coefficient space, faces are two-dimensional curved surfaces, but in general not planar. Coefficient space faces are however ruled surfaces, i.e. through every point on the face there passes in general two straight lines of the surface defined by γ_{i1} = constant and γ_{i2} = constant.

In a search for necessary and sufficient conditions for stability, the general aim is naturally to avoid testing at all possible values of the parameters, i.e. one wants theorems which establish stability for all values given that stability holds for some restricted set of values. A Kharitonov-like theorem (Kharitonov (1979)) would be one which requires testing at just corner points, i.e. $\gamma_i \in \{\underline{\gamma}_i, \overline{\gamma}_i\}$. However, it is quickly seen that such a result is extremely unlikely; Kharitonov's theorem is valid for a region in coefficient space bounded by hyperplanes parallel to the coordinate axes, and only then for stability in the region Re(s) < 0 (counterexamples exist for the region $|s| < 1$, see Hollot and Bartlett (1986)).

The next possibility is to examine stability at the corners and along the edges. Such an idea is suggested by the work of Bartlett, Hollot and Lin (1988); these authors show that if the coefficients of a polynomials depend in an **affine** way on a collection of parameters, each of which lies in an interval, so that in coefficient space the collection of polynomials under test is a polytope, then it suffices to check the edges for stability. More precisely, the authors prove the following:

(a) if s_0 is a real root of any polynomial in the set under test, it is a root of at least one edge polynomial;
(b) if s_0 is a complex root of any polynomial in the set under test, it is a root of at least one face polynomial;
(c) if s_0 is at the boundary of the set of roots of all face polynomials, then it is also a root of at least one edge polynomial;
(d) if D is a simply connected domain, then the roots of all polynomials lie in D if and only if the roots of all polynomials defined by all edges lie in D. This is a consequence of (a), (b) and (c).

When we seek to carry over these ideas to our problem, where the coefficients depend multilinearly on the parameters, it turns out that only (a) remains valid. The following counterexample to (b) was supplied to us by C.V. Hollot. The polynomial

$$f(s) = s^5 + (-\gamma_1)s^4 + (-\gamma_1-\gamma_3+1)s^3 + \gamma_2 s^2 + (\gamma_2+\gamma_1\gamma_2+\gamma_2\gamma_3+\gamma_3\gamma_1)s + (-\gamma_3+\gamma_1\gamma_2\gamma_3)$$

with $|\gamma_i| \leq 1$ has the property that $\pm j$ is a root when $\gamma_1 = \gamma_2 = \gamma_3 = 0$. It is not, however, a root of any face polynomial.

What other approaches exist? In de Gaston and Safonov (1988), appeal is made to the fact that the set of all Nyquist diagrams of all polynomials in the set has a key property. For each ω, $f(j\omega;\gamma_1...\gamma_m)$ lies in the convex hull of the 2^m complex points obtained by setting the γ_i to their extreme value, a property pointed out in Zadeh and Desoer (1963) with the name Mapping Theorem. This idea is exploited to tackle the robust stability problem with a type of extension of Nyquist's theorem.

These ideas have something in common with those of Saeki (1986), which consider a roughly equivalent problem, but one in which the γ_i, in effect, are allowed to be complex. It turns out that in many ways, this simplifies the problem. Yet another possibility is to make special assumptions on the polynomials f(s), which have the aim of making the problem equivalent to, or very like, the problem considered in Bartlett, Hollot and Lin (1988). For example, Panier, Fan and Tits (1987) postulate uncoupled perturbations in the coefficients of even and odd powers of f(s), while Djaferis and Hollot (1988) and Djaferis (1988) impose restrictions which ensure that the image for $f(j\omega;\gamma_1,\gamma_2...\gamma_m)$ for each ω and variable γ_i is a polytopic set. This allows again an extension of Nyquist's theorem to be applied. The difficulty with this type of result is that it is highly non-generic.

Rather than working up from results such as Kharitonov's theorem and the edge theorem, another approach is to work down from the very general Tarski-Seidenberg decision algebra theorem described in textbooks such as Bose (1982) and Jacobson (1964). This theorem implies that the robust stability problem we have posed can always be solved using a finite number of rational calculations (in the sense that for a given polynomial dependent on $\gamma_1,\gamma_2...\gamma_m$ a yes/no answer to the robust stability question can be obtained). The number of calculations may be prohibitive, and the real interest then lies in finding shortcuts so that the number of calculations becomes acceptable.

A variant on the Tarski-Seidenberg theorem was suggested in Anderson and Scott (1977), who showed that an alternative approach for any decision algebra problem could be found which involved the construction and solutions of q polynomials equations in q unknowns, q being an integer determined by the problem statement. When this procedure is followed, much of the interest lies in ensuring that q is as small as possible. This actually will be the approach followed in two later sections of the paper, where we shall have $q = m+1$. Note that there exist systematic methods for solving such equations based on resultants, see Bose (1982). Also, software is increasingly becoming available, see (Watson et al., 1987).

When the γ_i correspond to physical parameters, in many cases the value of m will be quite small, say 2, 3 or 4. Under these circumstances, there is a good possibility that the computational burdens will not prove excessive.

The layout of the paper is as follows: In the next section, we show that the set of real roots of all polynomials is identical with the set of real roots of the edge polynomials. In section 3, we study faces, and explain a procedure whereby the faces may be checked for stability. In section 4, this is generalized to explain how stability inside the entire prescribed region of parameter space may be examined. (Several special cases yielding considerable simplifications are also covered in these sections.) In section 5, we show how differing necessary and sufficient conditions for robust stability can be derived, and we discuss how such conditions can be sharpened. Section 6 contains concluding remarks.

2. SIGNIFICANCE OF THE EDGES FOR REAL ROOTS

As mentioned before, we shall first establish the following result:

Theorem 2.1: Let $f(s;\gamma_1,...,\gamma_m)$ be an n-th degree monic polynomial, with real coefficient dependent multilinearly on the γ_i where γ_i is contained in an interval $\gamma_i \in [\underline{\gamma}_i, \overline{\gamma}_i]$, $i = 1...m$. Let s_0 be a real root of some such polynomial. Then s_0 is also a real root of an edge polynomial.

Proof: The proof of this result is by induction. Let s_0 be a real root of the polynomial f for some given $\tilde{\gamma}_i \in [\underline{\gamma}_i,\overline{\gamma}_i]$, $i = 1...m$. Suppose that for s_0, $f(s_0;\hat{\gamma}_1,...,\hat{\gamma}_r,\tilde{\gamma}_{r+1},...,\tilde{\gamma}_m) = 0$ for $\hat{\gamma}_1 \in \{\underline{\gamma}_1,\overline{\gamma}_1\},...,\hat{\gamma}_r \in \{\underline{\gamma}_r,\overline{\gamma}_r\}$ and to avoid trivial cases $\tilde{\gamma}_{r+1} \in (\underline{\gamma}_{r+1},\overline{\gamma}_{r+1}),...,\tilde{\gamma}_m \in (\underline{\gamma}_m,\overline{\gamma}_m)$, for some $r < m-1$.

We shall show that we can adjust either $\tilde{\gamma}_{r+1}$ to $\hat{\gamma}_{r+1} \in \{\underline{\gamma}_{r+1},\bar{\gamma}_{r+1}\}$ with $f(s_0, \hat{\gamma}_1\ldots\hat{\gamma}_r, \hat{\gamma}_{r+1},\tilde{\gamma}_{r+2},\ldots\tilde{\gamma}_m) = 0$, or $\tilde{\gamma}_{r+2}$ to $\hat{\gamma}_{r+2} \in \{\underline{\gamma}_{r+2},\bar{\gamma}_{r+2}\}$ with $f(s_0, \hat{\gamma}_1\ldots\hat{\gamma}_r, \tilde{\gamma}_{r+1}, \hat{\gamma}_{r+2}, \tilde{\gamma}_{r+3}, \ldots, \tilde{\gamma}_m) = 0$.

To verify this claim, set $\delta_{r+1} = \gamma_{r+1} - \tilde{\gamma}_{r+1}$, $\delta_{r+2} = \gamma_{r+2} - \tilde{\gamma}_{r+2}$; then we may write

$$\begin{aligned}
&f(s;\hat{\gamma}_1,\ldots,\hat{\gamma}_r,\gamma_{r+1},\gamma_{r+2},\tilde{\gamma}_{r+3},\ldots,\tilde{\gamma}_m)\\
&= f(s;\hat{\gamma}_1,\ldots,\hat{\gamma}_r,\tilde{\gamma}_{r+1}+\delta_{r+1},\tilde{\gamma}_{r+2}+\delta_{r+2},\tilde{\gamma}_{r+3},\ldots,\tilde{\gamma}_m)\\
&= g_0(s;\hat{\gamma}_1,\ldots,\hat{\gamma}_r,\tilde{\gamma}_{r+1},\tilde{\gamma}_{r+2},\ldots,\tilde{\gamma}_m) + \delta_{r+1}g_1(s;\hat{\gamma}_1,\ldots,\hat{\gamma}_r,\tilde{\gamma}_{r+2},\ldots,\tilde{\gamma}_m)\\
&\quad + \delta_{r+2}g_2(s;\hat{\gamma}_1,\ldots,\hat{\gamma}_r,\tilde{\gamma}_{r+1},\tilde{\gamma}_{r+3},\ldots,\tilde{\gamma}_m) + \delta_{r+1}\delta_{r+2}g_3(s;\hat{\gamma}_1,\ldots,\hat{\gamma}_r,\tilde{\gamma}_{r+3}\ldots,\tilde{\gamma}_m)
\end{aligned}$$

or in abbreviated notation

$$f(s) = g_0(s) + \delta_{r+1}g_1(s) + \delta_{r+2}g_2(s) + \delta_{r+1}\delta_{r+2}g_3(s) \ .$$

The $g_i(s)$ are multilinear in the parameters on which they depend. Also, $g_0(s_0) = 0$. Now if $g_1(s_0) = 0$, set $\delta_{r+2} = 0$ and choose δ_{r+1} to correspond to an extreme value [$\delta_{r+1} = \bar{\gamma}_{r+1} - \tilde{\gamma}_{r+1}$ is the upper boundary for δ_{r+1} for example]. Thus, $\hat{\gamma}_{r+1} \in \{\underline{\gamma}_{r+1},\bar{\gamma}_{r+1}\}$, and also $f(s_0; \hat{\gamma}_1,\ldots,\hat{\gamma}_r,\hat{\gamma}_{r+1},\tilde{\gamma}_{r+2},\tilde{\gamma}_{r+3},\ldots,\tilde{\gamma}_m) = 0$. Similarly, if $g_2(s_0) = 0$, set $\delta_{r+1} = 0$ and δ_{r+2} at an extreme value. If neither $g_1(s_0)$ nor $g_2(s_0)$ are zero, plot in the δ_{r+1}, δ_{r+2} plane the straight line or hyperbola defined by

$$\delta_{r+1}g_1(s_0) + \delta_{r+2}g_2(s_0) + \delta_{r+1}\delta_{r+2}g_3(s_0) = 0$$

[The straight line is encountered precisely when $g_3(s_0) = 0$]. This hyperbola necessarily intersects at least one of the four lines in the δ_{r+1}, δ_{r+2} plane which define the boundaries of the allowed parameter values. We choose one of the intersection points. At this intersection point, one of the associated γ_{r+1}, γ_{r+2} has an extreme value, say $\gamma_{r+2} = \hat{\gamma}_{r+2} \in \{\underline{\gamma}_{r+2},\bar{\gamma}_{r+2}\}$. So we have obviously

$$f(s_0;\hat{\gamma}_1,\ldots,\hat{\gamma}_r,\tilde{\gamma}_{r+1},\hat{\gamma}_{r+2},\tilde{\gamma}_{r+3},\ldots,\tilde{\gamma}_m) = 0$$

and therefore the induction step r+1 is proved. This proves the theorem.

Obviously, the theorem states that the set of all real roots of all polynomials is given by the set of all real roots of all edge polynomials. If one is interested in knowing whether or not there are unstable real roots, it is actually unnecesary to examine all edge polynomials, and it suffices, as we now argue, to consider corner polynomials only. We are indebted to J. Ackermann for this derivation. Suppose all corner polynomials are stable. This means that $f(s_0;\hat{\gamma}_1,\ldots\hat{\gamma}_m) > 0$ for all real non-negative s_0 and $\gamma_i \in \{\underline{\gamma}_i,\bar{\gamma}_i\}$ for all i.

[When $s_0 \to \infty$ the monic character of f ensures that $f(s_0) \to \infty$ and if $f(s_0;\hat{\gamma}_1,\ldots,\hat{\gamma}_m) \le 0$ for some non-negative s_0, then by continuity, there would exist $\bar{s}_0 \ge 0$ such that $f(\bar{s}_0;\hat{\gamma}_1,\ldots,\hat{\gamma}_m) = 0$.]

Now the inequality $f(s_0;\hat{\gamma}_1,\ldots\hat{\gamma}_m) > 0$ ensures that $f(s_0;\hat{\gamma}_1,\ldots,\hat{\gamma}_{i-1},\gamma_i,\hat{\gamma}_{i+1},\ldots,\hat{\gamma}_m) > 0$ for all $\gamma_i \in [\underline{\gamma}_i,\bar{\gamma}_i]$ since f is affine in γ_i alone, so that $f(s_0;\hat{\gamma}_1,\ldots,\hat{\gamma}_{i-1},\gamma_i,\hat{\gamma}_{i+1},\ldots,\hat{\gamma}_m)$ is a convex combination of the two values obtained by identifying γ_i with $\underline{\gamma}_i$ and $\bar{\gamma}_i$.

It is highly probable that one or more edges does need to be tested for stability, to rule out the possibility of either real or complex roots.

Edge tests are the most straightforward; basically, root locus procedures can be used. Actually, it is only necessary to use rational calculation. Suppose that the polynomial $f(s;\gamma_1) = g_0(s) + \gamma_1 g_1(s)$, $\gamma_1 \in (\underline{\gamma}_1,\bar{\gamma}_1)$. Stability is achieved by requiring all Hurwitz determinants to be positive; as functions of γ_1, these determinants are polynomials. So stability is equivalent to certain polynomials in γ_1 being positive $\forall\ \gamma_1 \in [\underline{\gamma}_1,\overline{\gamma}_1]$. This can be checked by Sturm's theorem. Actually, two simplifications are possible. One can use the Liénard-Chipart form of stability conditions, and one only needs to check that all stability conditions are satisfied for one value of γ_1 and the (n-1)-th Hurwitz determinant is positive $\forall\ \gamma_1 \in [\underline{\gamma}_1,\overline{\gamma}_1]$. Alternatively, a result given in Ackermann and Barmish (1987) using Hurwitz matrices at the corners can be used to test the edges. Another method is given in Zeheb (1987), which requires evaluating the roots of a single polynomial.

3. SIGNIFICANCE OF THE FACES FOR COMPLEX ROOTS

In the previous section we have shown that if s_0 is a real root of any real polynomial, it is a real root of an edge polynomial. Now even when $f(s;\gamma_1,\dots,\gamma_m)$ is linear in the γ_i, the same result, with real replaced by complex, is not true. Rather, any point on the boundary of the complex root set of all polynomials is necessarily a root of an edge polynomial (Bartlett, Hollott and Lin (1987)). It is thus natural to seek to extend this idea to the structures where $f(\cdot)$ is multilinear in the γ_i.

In general such an extension is impossible.

Example: Consider the polynomial

$$\begin{aligned} f(s;\gamma_1,\gamma_2) &= s^2 + (-\gamma_1-\gamma_2)s + (\gamma_1\gamma_2+4) \\ &= s^2 + a_1(\gamma_1,\gamma_2)s + a_2(\gamma_1,\gamma_2) \end{aligned}$$

with $\gamma_1 \in [-1,1]$ and $\gamma_2 \in [-3,2]$. In Figure 3, we have drawn the associated regions of parameter space and coefficient space. Points A_i and B_i correspond, the straight line A_5A_6 corresponds to the curve B_5B_6 (actually part of a parabola) and the two points A_7,A'_7 both correspond to B_7. Notice that each of A_1A_2, A_2A_3, A_3A_4 and A_4A_1 maps into a straight line, but these straight lines do *not* bound the image of the rectangle $A_1A_2A_3A_4$.

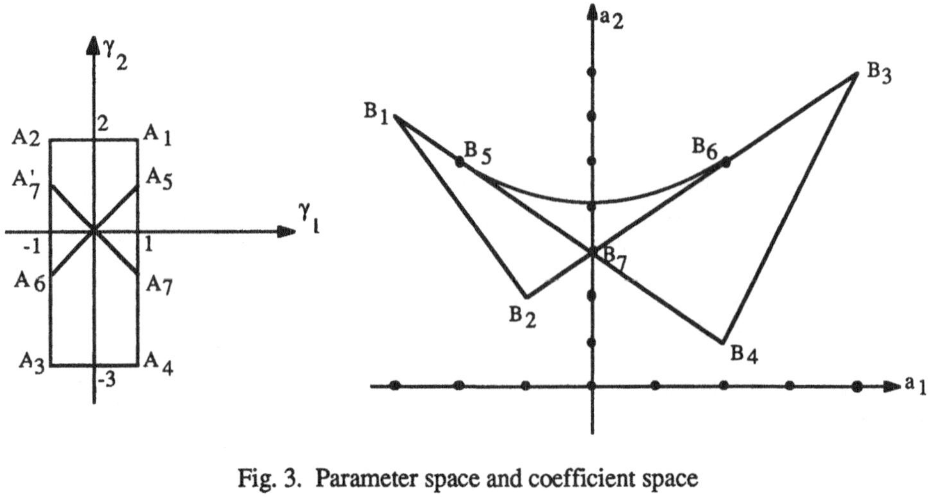

Fig. 3. Parameter space and coefficient space

Now consider the point $\gamma_1 = \gamma_2 = -1/2$. This corresponds to a point on the curve B_5B_6, viz. $a_1 = 1$, $a_2 = 17/4$. There do not exist variations $\Delta\gamma_1$, $\Delta\gamma_2$ around $\gamma_1 = \gamma_2 = -1/2$ which allow perturbations Δa_1, Δa_2 in an arbitrary direction — moving "above" B_5B_6 is impossible. Consequently, since $\gamma_1 = \gamma_2 = -1/2$ corresponds to a point on the boundary in coefficient space, and we are working with second order polynomials, it also corresponds to a point on the boundary in root space. Obviously, the root is complex. It is easy to see that there is no edge polynomial with the same complex root pair, for there is no point on any one of the straight lines B_1B_2, B_2B_3, B_3B_4, B_4B_1 (which define all the edge polynomials) that corresponds to the polynomial $s^2 + s + 17/4$.

This example illustrates a further point, which is that the boundary in coefficient space need not correspond with the boundary in parameter space; of course, for this two-dimensional example, this is almost the same statement as that concerning the roots. But it is non-trivially different for higher degree polynomials.

In this example, the problem arises because within the region of parameter space of interest to us, the Jacobian determinant

$$\frac{\partial(a_1,a_2)}{\partial(\gamma_1,\gamma_2)} = \gamma_2 - \gamma_1$$

can take zero values. Were this not the case, then the boundary of the parameter region would map into the boundary of the coefficient region. As we shall see below, the Jacobian determinant is of critical importance in a more general treatment.

We shall now explain how stability on faces can be checked. This is equivalent to checking stability when there are only two variable parameters. Without loss of generality, let these two parameters be γ_1, γ_2, and let us suppress mention of the other parameters, if any.

The idea is as follows. Suppose it has been established that all edges are stable. Suppose also that for some γ_1, γ_2 there exist unstable roots of $f(s;\gamma_1,\gamma_2)$, then by continuity, there exists a value or values of γ_1, γ_2 for which $f(s;\gamma_1,\gamma_2)$ has a purely imaginary root, and indeed a purely imaginary root on the boundary of the root set. We shall show how such roots can be determined; if none exist, this means that $f(s;\gamma_1,\gamma_2)$ has no roots in $\mathrm{Re}(s) \geq 0$ over the entire face.

Let $\sigma + j\omega$ be a complex root of $f(s;\gamma_1,\gamma_2)$ and consider the Jacobian determinant

$$\frac{\partial(\sigma,\omega)}{\partial(\gamma_1,\gamma_2)} = \frac{\partial(\sigma,\omega)}{\partial(\mathrm{Re}f,\mathrm{Im}f)} \frac{\partial(\mathrm{Re}f,\mathrm{Im}f)}{\partial(\gamma_1,\gamma_2)}$$

$$= \left[\frac{\partial(\mathrm{Re}f,\mathrm{Im}f)}{\partial(\sigma,\omega)}\right]^{-1} \frac{\partial(\mathrm{Re}f,\mathrm{Im}f)}{\partial(\gamma_1,\gamma_2)} \qquad (3.1)$$

Certainly,

$$\frac{\partial(\mathrm{Re}f,\mathrm{Im}f)}{\partial(\sigma,\omega)}$$

can never be infinite, being the 2×2 determinant of a matrix with entries polynomial in σ and ω. Hence,

$$\frac{\partial(\sigma,\omega)}{\partial(\gamma_1,\gamma_2)} \text{ can only be zero if } \frac{\partial(\mathrm{Re}f,\mathrm{Im}f)}{\partial(\gamma_1,\gamma_2)} \text{ is zero}.$$

So we must recognize the possibility that boundary values in the root set of all roots of $f(s;\gamma_1,\gamma_2)$, $\gamma_1 \in (\underline{\gamma}_1,\overline{\gamma}_1)$, $\gamma_2 \in (\underline{\gamma}_2,\overline{\gamma}_2)$ *could* only be achieved where

$$f(s;\gamma_1,\gamma_2) = 0 \tag{3.2a}$$

and

$$\frac{\partial(\mathrm{Re}f,\mathrm{Im}f)}{\partial(\gamma_1,\gamma_2)} = 0 \tag{3.2b}$$

Now the root set of all polynomials $f(s;\gamma_1,\gamma_2)$ with $\gamma_1 \in [\underline{\gamma}_1,\overline{\gamma}_1]$, $\gamma_2 \in [\underline{\gamma}_2,\overline{\gamma}_2]$ is a union of a finite number of closed connected sets $R_1,\dots,R_\alpha$, and is bounded. If all edge polynomials are stable, and if $f(s;\gamma_1,\gamma_2)$ has an unstable complex root pair for some γ_1,γ_2, it follows that the boundary of one of the sets R_i intersects the imaginary axis. Then we have proved the "only if" part of the following proposition. The "if" part is trivial.

Proposition 3.1: Consider $f(s;\gamma_1,\gamma_2)$ with $\gamma_1 \in [\underline{\gamma}_1,\overline{\gamma}_1]$, $\gamma_2 \in [\underline{\gamma}_2,\overline{\gamma}_2]$, a monic n-th degree polynomial bilinear in γ_1 and γ_2. Suppose that all edge polynomials are stable. Then at least one polynomial fails to be stable if and only if for some $s = j\omega$, ω real, (3.2) are satisfied.

We shall now show that the question of whether (3.2) are satisfied for some $s = j\omega$ is an easily answered question, via a procedure which we now indicate.

Let us set

$$\mathrm{Re}f(j\omega) = g_0(\omega) + \gamma_1 g_1(\omega) + \gamma_2 g_2(\omega) + \gamma_1\gamma_2 g_3(\omega) \tag{3.3a}$$

$$\mathrm{Im}f(j\omega) = h_0(\omega) + \gamma_1 h_1(\omega) + \gamma_2 h_2(\omega) + \gamma_1\gamma_2 h_3(\omega) \tag{3.3b}$$

Each of the g_i,h_i takes real values for real ω. Observe then that

$$\frac{\partial(\mathrm{Re}f,\mathrm{Im}f)}{\partial(\gamma_1,\gamma_2)} = \det\begin{bmatrix} g_1(\omega)+\gamma_2 g_3(\omega) & g_2(\omega)+\gamma_1 g_3(\omega) \\ h_1(\omega)+\gamma_2 h_3(\omega) & h_2(\omega)+\gamma_1 h_3(\omega)\end{bmatrix}$$

$$= (g_1h_2-g_2h_1) + \gamma_1(g_1h_3-g_3h_1) + \gamma_2(g_3h_2-g_2h_3) = 0 \tag{3.4a}$$

Now (3.2a) implies

$$g_0 + \gamma_1 g_1 + \gamma_2 g_2 + \gamma_1\gamma_2 g_3 = 0 \tag{3.4b}$$

$$h_0 + \gamma_1 h_1 + \gamma_2 h_2 + \gamma_1\gamma_2 h_3 = 0 \tag{3.4c}$$

From (3.4b) and (3.4c), there follows

$$(g_0h_3-h_0g_3) + \gamma_1(g_1h_3-g_3h_1) + \gamma_2(g_2h_3-g_3h_2) = 0 \tag{3.5}$$

Together, (3.4a) and (3.5) allow γ_1,γ_2 to be expressed in terms of the g_i,h_j. Their expressions can then be substituted into (3.4b) to obtain a *single* polynomial equations in ω. It may have no nonzero real solution. If it does, each solution determines values for γ_1,γ_2, via (3.4a) and (3.5). If these values lie inside the allowed region $[\underline{\gamma}_1,\overline{\gamma}_1] \times [\underline{\gamma}_2,\overline{\gamma}_2]$, then instability is proved.

Several other remarks should be made. First, in case $f(\cdot)$ is only linear rather than bilinear in γ_1,γ_2 (which is the situation considered in Bartlett, Hollot and Lin (1988), equations (3.4) become

$$g_1h_2 - h_2g_1 = 0 \tag{3.6a}$$

$$g_0 + \gamma_1 g_1 + \gamma_2 g_2 = 0 \tag{3.6b}$$

$$h_0 + \gamma_1 h_1 + \gamma_2 h_2 = 0 \tag{3.6c}$$

If there exists a real ω for which (3.6a) is zero, then (3.6b) and (3.6c) can only both be satisfied in cases g_0h_2-g_2h_0 is also zero at this frequency. In this case, the (γ_1,γ_2) pairs satisfying (3.6b) and (3.6c) lie on a straight line, and consequently, there exist edge values of either γ_1 or γ_2 which cause satisfaction for the same ω, i.e. there exists a pair satisfying (3.6) of one of the forms $(\overline{\gamma}_1,\gamma_2)$, $(\underline{\gamma}_1,\gamma_2)$, $(\gamma_1,\overline{\gamma}_2)$ or $(\gamma_1,\underline{\gamma}_2)$. Consequently, any root of a face polynomial on the boundary of the root set is a root of an edge polynomial. Then one never has to explicitly study face polynomials. This is the conclusion of Bartlett, Hollot and Lin (1988).

Second, decision algebra provides a tool for checking stability across a face which should not be too demanding, see Bose (1982). The Hurwitz determinants depend on two parameters γ_1,γ_2 and have to be checked for positivity inside a rectangle. Algorithms are available for this task, as set out in Bose (1982). These algorithms involve a finite number of rational calculations. The method we have suggested here, which introduces the need for polynomial factorization is an example of a general approach to decision algebra problems involving the setting up of q polynomial equations in q unknowns.

Third, bilinearity with respect to γ_1,γ_2 has not played a central role here, although it has played a helpful role. The derivation of a single equation in ω through the elimination of γ_1,γ_2 from (3.3) and (3.4a) is more complicated when the dependence of f on γ_1,γ_2 is polynomial rather than multilinear.

Fourth, the paper of Djaferis (1988) is entirely concerned with the case when a so-called shaping condition is fulfilled, namely $g_3h_2-h_3g_2 \equiv 0$. Clearly, this makes $\frac{\partial(\text{Re } f,\text{Im } f)}{\partial(\gamma_1,\gamma_2)}$ independent of γ_2. It is also easy to check that when this condition holds and also $\frac{\partial(\text{Re } f,\text{Im } f)}{\partial(\gamma_1,\gamma_2)}$ is zero, then Re f(jω) and Im f(jω) are independent of γ_2. Consequently, if $j\omega_0$ is on the boundary of the root set, $j\omega_0$ remains a root on the root set boundary when γ_2 varies. In particular, when γ_2 is set equal to an edge value $\underline{\gamma}_2,\overline{\gamma}_2$ it remains true that $j\omega_0$ is a root. Hence all purely imaginary roots on the root set boundary are roots of edge polynomials, which means that under the condition $g_3h_2-h_3g_2 \equiv 0$ only edge polynomials need to be tested. Obviously, the same holds true if $g_1h_3-h_1g_3 \equiv 0$.

Example (J. Ackermann, 1988):

Consider $f(s;\gamma_1,\gamma_2) = s^3 + (\gamma_1+\gamma_2+1)s^2 + (\gamma_1+\gamma_2+3)s + (2\gamma_1\gamma_2+6\gamma_1+6\gamma_2+1.25)$ with $\gamma_1 \in [0.3;2.5]$ and $\gamma_2 \in [0;1.7]$. It turns out (and can be established with the aid of for example the Hurwitz test) that the parameter values giving unstable f are defined by the shaded regions in Figure 4. The boundaries of the regions are given by $2\gamma_1\gamma_2+6(\gamma_1+\gamma_2) + 1.25 = 0$ and $(\gamma_1-1)^2 + (\gamma_2-1)^2 - 0.5^2 = 0$. These points are noted in order to allow comparison with the methods of this paper.

First, edge stability must be verified. Let us see how this can be done for one edge, say the edge $\gamma_2 = 0$. The Hurwitz conditions are

$$0 < \det\begin{bmatrix} \gamma_1+1 & 6\gamma_1+1.25 \\ 1 & \gamma_1+3 \end{bmatrix} = \gamma_1^2 - 2\gamma_1 + 1.75$$

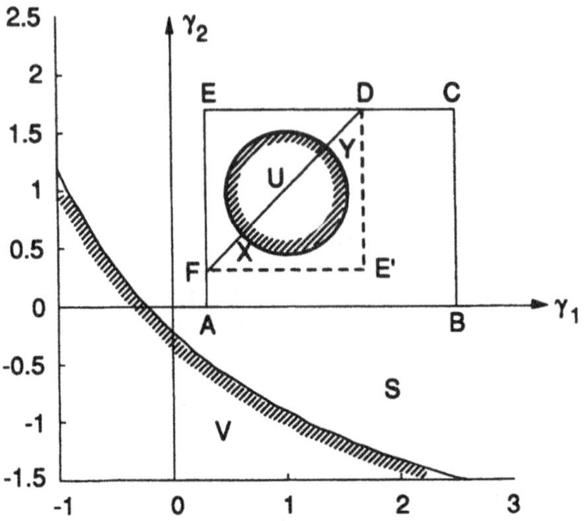

Fig. 4. Parameter space and stability region. s ... stable; u ... unstable

and

$$\begin{aligned} \gamma_1+1 &> 0 \\ \gamma_1+3 &> 0 \\ 6\gamma_1+1.25 &> 0 \end{aligned}$$

It is clear that these inequalities are all satisfied for $\gamma_1 \in [0.3, 2.5]$.

Next, we must look for points in the interior of the parameter region corresponding to purely imaginary roots on the boundary of the root set. These are determined from $\mathrm{Re}\, f(j\omega;\gamma_1,\gamma_2) = 0$, $\mathrm{Im}\, f(j\omega;\gamma_1,\gamma_2) = 0$, and $\frac{\partial(\mathrm{Re}\, f,\mathrm{Im}\, f)}{\partial(\gamma_1,\gamma_2)} = 0$. The relevant equations are

$$-(\gamma_1+\gamma_2+1)\omega^2 + (2\gamma_1\gamma_2+6\gamma_1+6\gamma_2+1.25) = 0$$

$$-\omega^2 + (\gamma_1+\gamma_2+3) = 0$$

$$2(\gamma_1-\gamma_2) = 0$$

It is readily verified, that these equations are satisfied by

$$\gamma_1 = \gamma_2 = 1 \pm \sqrt{2}/4 \qquad \omega = \sqrt{2\gamma_1+3} = \begin{cases} 2.39 \\ 2.07 \end{cases}$$

The corresponding points in parameter space are designated by X, Y in Figure 4. The root set corresponding to all allowed γ_1,γ_2 is sketched in Figure 5, and it will be observed that the values for ω computed above define those boundary parts of the root set which lie on the imaginary axis.

In this example, it is also possible to exactly determine the root boundary. Candidates for this boundary are besides the edge polynomials also points in the interior of the parameter region ABCE with

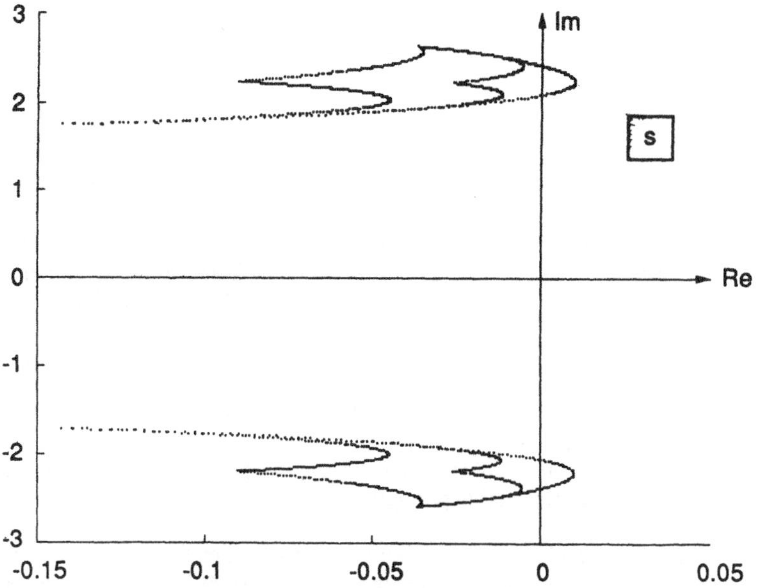

Fig. 5. Roots boundary

$$f(\sigma + j\omega; \gamma_1, \gamma_2) = 0$$

$$\frac{\partial(\mathrm{Ref}, \mathrm{Imf})}{\partial(\gamma_1, \gamma_2)} = 0$$

The relevant equations are

$$2\gamma_1\gamma_2 + (\gamma_1+\gamma_2)(6+\sigma+\sigma^2-\omega^2) + (1.25+3\sigma+\sigma^2+\sigma^3-\omega^2-3\sigma\omega^2) = 0$$
$$(\gamma_1+\gamma_2)(1+2\sigma) + (3+2\sigma+3\sigma^2 - \omega^2) = 0$$
$$2\omega(1+2\sigma)(\gamma_1-\gamma_2) = 0$$

For the complex root boundary, two different cases are distinguished:

$\sigma = -.5$

Then $\quad \omega_0^2 = 2.75$

$$\gamma_2 = -(3\gamma_1+1.25)/(2\gamma_1+3)$$

This is an isolated singular point. For variations along the given γ_1,γ_2 hyperbola the root pair $-.5\pm j\omega_0$ does not change.

$\gamma_1 = \gamma_2$

Because of the symmetry of $f(\cdot)$ with respect to γ_1,γ_2 it is obvious that for γ_1,γ_2 from the triangle DEF the same roots result as from the triangle DE'F. Therefore, the root boundaries for γ_1,γ_2 from ABCE and from ABCDF are the same. For γ_1,γ_2 from DF a part of the root boundary is built. This is for γ_1,γ_2 between X and Y unstable.

4. STABILITY TESTING IN PARAMETER REGION INTERIOR

We have already described how testing of edges and faces may proceed. In an m-dimensional parameter space (m>2) it is necessary to look successively at 3-dimensional boundaries (all but three of the γ_i take extreme values), 4-dimensional boundaries, ... the interior of the entire m-dimensional region. In each case, we seek to identify frequencies ω such that $j\omega$ is on the boundary of the root set of all polynomials. When looking at say 4-dimensional regions, this is done by setting up 5 simultaneous equations in 5 unknowns, viz. ω and the four variable γ_i, and seeking solutions which are real in ω and the γ_i, with each γ_i in the prescribed interval $[\underline{\gamma}_i,\overline{\gamma}_i]$. In the absence of such solutions, it is known that the entire 4-dimensional region defines stable polynomials if the 3-dimensional regions bounding it are known to define stable polynomials.

We shall explain the idea in more detail for the case when three parameters vary. It is a generalization of the two variable parameter case considered in the previous section; the generalization to more than three variable parameters is straightforward.

Let $\sigma+j\omega$ be a complex root of $f(s;\gamma_1,\gamma_2,\gamma_3)$ for $\gamma_i \in (\underline{\gamma}_i,\overline{\gamma}_i)$. Consider the effect of changing the γ_i on the root. In particular, let $\Delta\gamma_i$, i=1,2,3 denote very small changes in the γ_i, and let $\Delta\sigma$, $\Delta\omega$ denote the corresponding changes in the root. Then, neglecting second order terms,

$$\begin{bmatrix}\Delta\sigma\\ \Delta\omega\end{bmatrix} = \begin{bmatrix}\frac{\partial\sigma}{\partial\gamma_1} & \frac{\partial\sigma}{\partial\gamma_2} & \frac{\partial\sigma}{\partial\gamma_3}\\ \frac{\partial\omega}{\partial\gamma_1} & \frac{\partial\omega}{\partial\gamma_2} & \frac{\partial\omega}{\partial\gamma_3}\end{bmatrix}\begin{bmatrix}\Delta\gamma_1\\ \Delta\gamma_2\\ \Delta\gamma_3\end{bmatrix}$$

$$= \begin{bmatrix}\frac{\partial\sigma}{\partial\mathrm{Re}\,f} & \frac{\partial\sigma}{\partial\mathrm{Im}\,f}\\ \frac{\partial\omega}{\partial\mathrm{Re}\,f} & \frac{\partial\omega}{\partial\mathrm{Im}\,f}\end{bmatrix}\begin{bmatrix}\frac{\partial\mathrm{Re}\,f}{\partial\gamma_1} & \frac{\partial\mathrm{Re}\,f}{\partial\gamma_2} & \frac{\partial\mathrm{Re}\,f}{\partial\gamma_3}\\ \frac{\partial\mathrm{Im}\,f}{\partial\gamma_1} & \frac{\partial\mathrm{Im}\,f}{\partial\gamma_2} & \frac{\partial\mathrm{Im}\,f}{\partial\gamma_3}\end{bmatrix}\begin{bmatrix}\Delta\gamma_1\\ \Delta\gamma_2\\ \Delta\gamma_3\end{bmatrix}$$

$$= \begin{bmatrix}\frac{\partial\mathrm{Re}\,f}{\partial\sigma} & \frac{\partial\mathrm{Re}\,f}{\partial\omega}\\ \frac{\partial\mathrm{Im}\,f}{\partial\sigma} & \frac{\partial\mathrm{Im}\,f}{\partial\omega}\end{bmatrix}^{-1}\begin{bmatrix}\frac{\partial\mathrm{Re}\,f}{\partial\gamma_1} & \frac{\partial\mathrm{Re}\,f}{\partial\gamma_2} & \frac{\partial\mathrm{Re}\,f}{\partial\gamma_3}\\ \frac{\partial\mathrm{Im}\,f}{\partial\gamma_1} & \frac{\partial\mathrm{Im}\,f}{\partial\gamma_2} & \frac{\partial\mathrm{Im}\,f}{\partial\gamma_3}\end{bmatrix}\begin{bmatrix}\Delta\gamma_1\\ \Delta\gamma_2\\ \Delta\gamma_3\end{bmatrix} \tag{4.1}$$

Now we if we are on the boundary of the root set, there cannot exist perturbations $\Delta\gamma_i$ which can give arbitrary $\Delta\sigma$, $\Delta\omega$. So candidates for values of σ, ω and γ_i yielding a point on the boundary of the root set are given by

$$\mathrm{rank}\begin{bmatrix}\frac{\partial\mathrm{Re}\,f}{\partial\gamma_1} & \frac{\partial\mathrm{Re}\,f}{\partial\gamma_2} & \frac{\partial\mathrm{Re}\,f}{\partial\gamma_3}\\ \frac{\partial\mathrm{Im}\,f}{\partial\gamma_1} & \frac{\partial\mathrm{Im}\,f}{\partial\gamma_2} & \frac{\partial\mathrm{Im}\,f}{\partial\gamma_3}\end{bmatrix} \le 1 \tag{4.2}$$

Equivalently

$$\frac{\partial(\text{Re } f, \text{Im } f)}{\partial(\gamma_1,\gamma_2)} = 0 \tag{4.3a}$$

and

$$\frac{\partial(\text{Re } f, \text{Im } f)}{\partial(\gamma_1,\gamma_3)} = 0 \tag{4.3b}$$

as well as

$$\text{Re } f = 0 \qquad \text{Im } f = 0 \tag{4.3c}$$

It is enough to look for purely imaginary points on the boundary of the root set, i.e. to set $\sigma=0$. Then (4.3) represent four simultaneous equations in the four unknowns $\gamma_1,\gamma_2,\gamma_3,\omega$. In general there are a finite number of solutions. If and only if one of these solutions is real, with $\gamma_i \in [\underline{\gamma}_i,\overline{\gamma}_i]$, can there be a purely imaginary point on the boundary set.

The computation of solutions of simultaneous polynomial equations is a problem which has been studied. Older methods have depended on successive elimination of variables using resultants until a single equation in a single variable is obtained. This is solved, and then through successive back substitution, values of the other variables are obtained, see e.g. Bose (1982), and Hodge and Pedoe (1968).

Note that if ω is the variable eliminated from Re f = 0, Im f = 0 and all other equations are neglected, there results a single equation which corresponds to setting a Hurwitz determinant equal to zero. The terms in this equation depend on the γ_i. The question is then whether this determinant can be made zero for some choice of γ_i in the parameter region of interest or not. This is of course a natural question, and is roughly the approach exposed in Bose (1982).

Example:
Consider

$$f(s) = s^3 + 1 + (s^2+s)\gamma_2 + s\gamma_1\gamma_2 + \gamma_1\gamma_2\gamma_3$$

with $\gamma_i \in [\underline{\gamma}_i,\overline{\gamma}_i]$, i = 1,2,3.

For investigation of the root boundary, it is necessary to check all sides of the γ-cube, i.e. $\gamma_i \in \{\underline{\gamma}_i,\overline{\gamma}_i\}$, i = 1,2,3, and all points of the interior of the parameter region with

$$\text{Rank } \mathbf{J} \leqq 1 \qquad \text{Re } f = 0 \qquad \text{Im } f = 0$$

where $\mathbf{J}$ is the Jacobi matrix:

$$\mathbf{J} = \begin{bmatrix} \sigma\gamma_2+\gamma_2\gamma_3 & \sigma^2-\omega^2+\sigma+\sigma\gamma_1+\gamma_1\gamma_3 & \gamma_1\gamma_2 \\ \gamma_2 & 2\sigma+1+\gamma_1 & 0 \end{bmatrix}$$

the relevant equations are

$$\begin{aligned}
\mathrm{Re}\, f &= \sigma^3 - 3\sigma\omega^2 + 1 + \gamma_2(\sigma^2-\omega^2+\sigma) + \gamma_1\gamma_2\sigma + \gamma_1\gamma_2\gamma_3 \\
\mathrm{Im}\, f &= (3\sigma^2 - \omega^2 + \gamma_2(2\sigma+1) + \gamma_1\gamma_2)\omega \\
\gamma_1\gamma_2^2 &= 0 \\
\gamma_1\gamma_2(2\sigma+1+\gamma_1) &= 0 \\
(2\sigma+1+\gamma_1)(\sigma+\gamma_3) - \sigma^2 + \omega^2 - \sigma - \sigma\gamma_1 - \gamma_1\gamma_3 &= 0
\end{aligned}$$

These equations must be simultaneously fulfilled.

For $\gamma_2 = 0$ the polynomial family degenerates to

$$f(s) = s^3 + 1$$

a simple polynomial. Rank $\mathbb{J}$ is zero. No special investigation is necessary.

For $\gamma_1 = 0$ we obtain

$$f(s) = s^3 + 1 + (s^2+s)\gamma_2$$

and from rank $\mathbb{J} = 1$ the condition

$$(\gamma_2-2)\gamma_3 = 1$$

results, which is a hyperbola in the $\gamma_2\gamma_3$ plane. Along this hyperbola, there are pairs $\gamma_1=0$, γ_2,γ_3 which give possible boundary polynomials. But from the degeneration of the polynomial family f(s) it is obvious that rank $\mathbb{J} = 1$ follows from the degeneration of the parameter space to a straight line. Therefore, there exist internal points of the parameter space, which fulfill the necessary conditions for the root boundary. However, these points do not yield this boundary.

Next, the six sides of the parameter box must be checked. In general, this can be done by testing all boundaries of such a side and all candidates for the root boundary from the side inners. These are exactly the same steps as we have done before but on a lower dimensional space. In this way, we proceed for every side until the 2-dimensional faces are reached.

In our special case, the box sides are directly the 2-dimensional faces. The procedure of the last section can be used.

For γ_1 = constant we have Re f = 0 and Im f = 0, and

$$(2\sigma+1+\gamma_1)\gamma_1\gamma_2 = 0$$

With $\gamma_1 \neq 0 \neq \gamma_2$, and Im f = 0, we obtain

$$\begin{aligned}
2\sigma + 1 + \gamma_1 &= 0 \\
\omega^2 &= 3\sigma^2 + \gamma_2(2\sigma+1) + \gamma_1\gamma_2
\end{aligned}$$

and then

$$\begin{aligned}
\sigma &= -\frac{1}{2}(1+\gamma_1) \\
\omega^2 &= 3\sigma^2
\end{aligned}$$

The critical points of the γ_1-sides yield only a point in the s-space and because of the continuity conditions not a significant part of the root boundary.

In the same way one may proceed for γ_2- and γ_3-sides.

Recently, methods for solving simultaneous polynomial equations based on homotopy theory have been suggested, see Watson et al. (1987).

A number of further points should be noted. First, in this section, no special use has been made of the multilinearity, i.e. the same ideas will apply even if the dependence of the coefficients on the parameters is a general polynomial dependence.

Second, it is easy to recover various special cases. Suppose following Panier, Fan and Tits (1987) that the coefficients of even powers of f(·) depend on $\gamma_1,\ldots,\gamma_r$ and the coefficients of odd powers of f(·) depend on $\gamma_{r+1},\ldots,\gamma_m$. The condition (4.2) then becomes

$$\text{rank}\begin{bmatrix} \frac{\partial \text{Re}\, f}{\partial \gamma_1} & \cdots & \frac{\partial \text{Re}\, f}{\partial \gamma_r} & 0 & \cdots & 0 \\ 0 & \cdots & 0 & \frac{\partial \text{Im}\, f}{\partial \gamma_{r+1}} & \cdots & \frac{\partial \text{Im}\, f}{\partial \gamma_m} \end{bmatrix} \leq 1$$

Suppose for example that $\frac{\partial \text{Re}\, f}{\partial \gamma_i} = 0$, $i = 1\ldots r$ and $\frac{\partial \text{Im}\, f}{\partial \gamma_j} = 0$, $j = r+1,\ldots,m-1$. Now Re f is multilinear in $\gamma_1,\ldots,\gamma_r$, and accordingly can take no extreme value inside the region $\gamma_i \in [\underline{\gamma}_i, \overline{\gamma}_i]$ unless that value is also assumed on the boundary. Thus if for some ω, $\frac{\partial \text{Re}\, f}{\partial \gamma_i} = 0$ this continues to hold when the γ_i take extreme values. Similarly, if $\frac{\partial \text{Im}\, f}{\partial \gamma_j} = 0$, $j = r+1,\ldots, m-1$ for some ω, these equations continue to hold when the γ_j take extreme values. Hence the rank condition if fulfilled anywhere is necessarily fulfilled when all but one γ_i, say γ_m, take extreme values, i.e. it is fulfilled on the edge defined by variable γ_m. Consequently, it is only necessary to check edges for stability.

Another special case is provided by the shaping conditions of Djaferis and Hollot (1988). To fix ideas, suppose that f depends on four parameters, with

$$f(s;\gamma_1,\gamma_2,\gamma_3,\gamma_4) = \varphi_1(s)f_1(\gamma_1,\gamma_2) + \varphi_2(s)f_2(\gamma_1,\gamma_2) + \varphi_3(s)f_3(\gamma_1,\gamma_4) + \varphi_4(s)f_4(\gamma_3,\gamma_4)$$

The $\varphi_i(s)$ are of course independent of the γ_i. Moreover, $\varphi_i(j\omega) = E_{\varphi_i}(j\omega) + j\omega O_{\varphi_i}(j\omega)$ where $E_{\varphi_i}(j\omega) = \frac{1}{2}[\varphi_i(j\omega)+\varphi_i(-j\omega)]$, $O_{\varphi_i}(j\omega) = \frac{1}{2\omega}[\varphi_i(j\omega) - \varphi_i(-j\omega)]$, and the side conditions (shaping conditions)

$$E_{\varphi_1}O_{\varphi_2} - E_{\varphi_2}O_{\varphi_1} = 0 \qquad\qquad E_{\varphi_3}O_{\varphi_4} - E_{\varphi_4}O_{\varphi_3} = 0$$

hold identically in ω. The 2×4 Jacobian matrix condition becomes

$$\text{rank}\begin{bmatrix} E_{\varphi_1}\frac{\partial f_1}{\partial \gamma_1} + E_{\varphi_2}\frac{\partial f_2}{\partial \gamma_1} & E_{\varphi_1}\frac{\partial f_1}{\partial \gamma_2} + E_{\varphi_2}\frac{\partial f_2}{\partial \gamma_2} & E_{\varphi_3}\frac{\partial f_3}{\partial \gamma_3} + E_{\varphi_4}\frac{\partial f_4}{\partial \gamma_3} & E_{\varphi_3}\frac{\partial f_3}{\partial \gamma_4} + E_{\varphi_4}\frac{\partial f_4}{\partial \gamma_4} \\ O_{\varphi_1}\frac{\partial f_1}{\partial \gamma_1} + O_{\varphi_2}\frac{\partial f_2}{\partial \gamma_1} & O_{\varphi_1}\frac{\partial f_1}{\partial \gamma_2} + O_{\varphi_2}\frac{\partial f_2}{\partial \gamma_2} & O_{\varphi_3}\frac{\partial f_3}{\partial \gamma_3} + O_{\varphi_4}\frac{\partial f_4}{\partial \gamma_3} & O_{\varphi_3}\frac{\partial f_3}{\partial \gamma_4} + O_{\varphi_4}\frac{\partial f_4}{\partial \gamma_4} \end{bmatrix} \leq 1$$

Now the shaping conditions ensure that the minors formed from columns 1 and 2 and from columns 3 and 4 are zero automatically. Suppose the minor formed from columns 1 and 3 is zero. By the multilinearity, column 1 is independent of γ_1 and column 3 is independent of γ_3. The special form of f ensures that column 1 is independent of γ_3 and column 3 is independent of γ_1. Hence, if the minor formed from columns 1 and 3 is zero, it must remain so if γ_1 and γ_3 are varied to extreme values. The shaping condition ensures that the minors formed from columns 1 and 2 and columns 3 and 4 remain zero with this variation of γ_1 and γ_3. Similarly, one can argue that γ_2 and γ_4 could be varied to their extreme values. Hence if the Jacobian matrix has reduced rank somewhere, it has this property for all γ_i. A consequence of this is that the image of $f(j\omega;\gamma_1,\ldots,\gamma_m)$ as ω varies, $\gamma_i \in [\underline{\gamma}_i,\overline{\gamma}_i]$ is a set bounded by the images of the edges. In general, this is a polytope. But with the Jacobian matrix of rank 1, the image will be a line segment, and when of rank 0, it will be a point.

A third special case can be obtained by limiting the way in which the nonlinear parameter dependence arises. Specifically, assume that any one γ_i can occur bilinearly with at most one other parameter γ_j, and that in the polynomial $f(s;\gamma_1,\ldots,\gamma_m)$ the s-polynomial multiplying $\gamma_i\gamma_j$ is either even or odd. An easy calculation shows that this ensures that all 2x2 minors of the generalized Jacobian matrix are linear in the parameters. The solution of the associated simultaneous equations is made much easier in these circumstances.

5. DIFFERING AND CONVERGING NECESSARY AND SUFFICIENT CONDITIONS

We have referred earlier to the work of de Gaston and Safonov (1988), who exploited the observations of Zadeh and Desoer (1963) that the image of $f(j\omega;\gamma_1,\ldots,\gamma_m)$ for fixed ω and $\gamma_i \in [\underline{\gamma}_i,\overline{\gamma}_i]$ lies in the convex hull of $f(j\omega;\gamma_1,\ldots,\gamma_m)$ for $\gamma_i \in \{\underline{\gamma}_i,\overline{\gamma}_i\}$ to develop a test for stability based on Nyquist ideas.

It is possible to exploit the observation of Zadeh and Desoer (1963) in another way. Denote the corners of the allowed parameter space region by $A_1,\ldots,A_k$ where $k = 2^n$. Denote the corresponding points in the n-dimensional coefficient space by $B_1,\ldots,B_k$. Now a perusal of the argument of Zadeh and Desoer (which involves scalar functions dependent multilinearly on m parameters) shows that it extends very straightforwardly to vector functions. As a result, the image in coefficient space of any point in the allowed parameter region, i.e. in the convex hull of $A_1,\ldots,A_k$ necessarily lies in the convex hull of $B_1,\ldots,B_k$.

Figure 6 depicts a rectangular region in parameter space and certain straight lines in its image in coefficient space. These straight lines are the images of the edges in parameter space. It is possible to construct the convex hull of $B_1,\ldots,B_8$ by going with straight lines all possible so far unjoined pairs of points and then "filling in" the enclosed region. Thus straight lines such as B_4B_7, B_1B_6 etc. must be joined. Note that B_4B_7 is *not* the image of the straight line A_4A_7 (on a certain face) in parameter space. The image of A_4A_7 will in general be curved, and be within the convex hull determined by B_1 through B_8.

A necessary condition for robust stability is clearly that the edges in parameter space (or their images in coefficient space) are all stable. A sufficient condition is that the straight lines joining all possible pairs of corner points in coefficient space (i.e. those which are images of parameter space edges and those which are not) must be stable; for the Edge Theorem of Bartlett, Hollot and Lin (1988) ensures that all points in coefficient space in the convex hull of $B_1,\ldots,B_k$ will be stable, and so in particular those which are images of points in the defined region of parameter space.

Now if the necessary conditions for stability are fulfilled and the sufficiency ones are not, one can proceed in a similar fashion to de Gaston and Safonov (1988). That is, one partitions the original rectangular box in parameter space in two, and develops separate necessity and sufficiency conditions. More precisely, if in the example B_2B_7 proves to contain an unstable polynomial one could make a slice in parameter space parallel to

$A_1A_2A_3A_4$ or parallel to $A_1A_2A_6A_5$ thus ensuring that A_2,A_7 go into different rectangular boxes. Then the line B_2B_7 will no longer enter into a sufficiency condition.

To the original necessity conditions are added four more, while a number of the original sufficiency conditions fall away to be replaced by a greater number of collectively less demanding conditions.

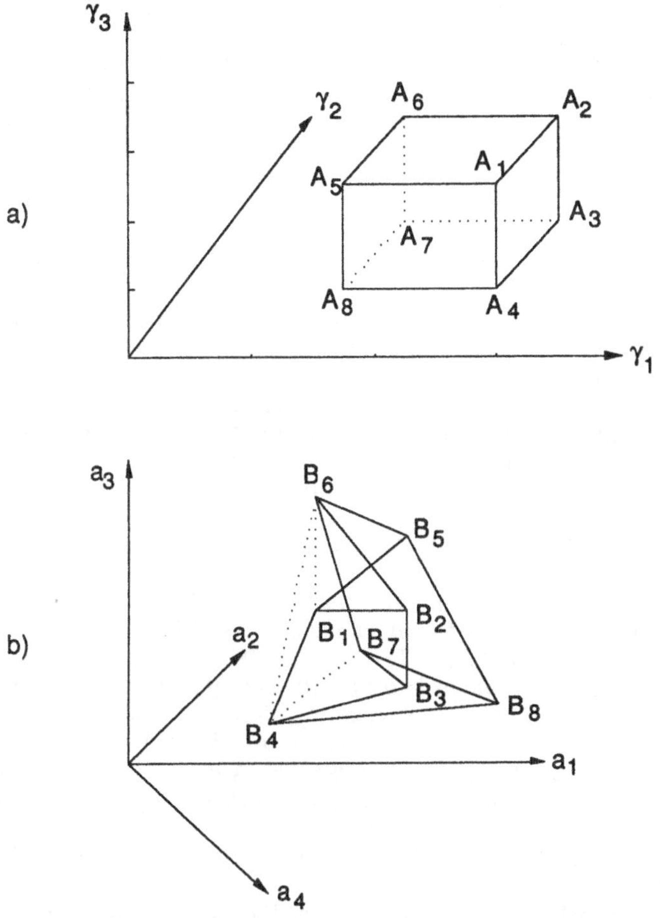

Fig. 6. Parameter and coefficient space convex hull covering. a) Parameter space 3-dimensional; b) coefficient space 4-dimensional

6. CONCLUDING REMARKS

This paper has extended consideration of the robust polynomial stability problem by allowing mild forms of nonlinear dependence of the polynomial coefficients on variable parameters. It is seen very rapidly that even this mild form of dependence introduceds substantial complications, so that for example the Edge Theorem applicable with affine dependence is probably no longer a valid tool. The key to examining interior points in parameter space is to consider a generalized Jacobian matrix and study the points where its rank is 1 or 0. Various special cases can be identified which allow a conclusion like that of the Edge Theorem to be applied. It would be interesting to expand this range of special cases.

REFERENCES

ACKERMANN, BARMISH, 1987, Internal Report, Deutsche Forschungs- und Versuchsanstalt für Luft- und Raumfahrt, DFVLR, Oberpfaffenhofen, FRG, to appear in *IEEE Trans. Autom. Control.*

ACKERMANN, J., HU, H.Z., KAESBAUER, D., 1988, *Robustness Analysis: A Case Study.* To appear in Proceedings of IEEE-CDC 1988.

ANDERSON, B.D.O., BOSE, N.K., and JURY, E.I., 1975, *IEEE Trans. Autom. Control,* Vol. **AC-20**, 53-66.

ANDERSON, B.D.O., and Scott, R.W., 1977, *Proc. IEEE,* **66**, 849-861.

BARTLETT, A.C., HOLLOT, C.V., and LIN Huang, 1988, *Root locations of an entire polytope of polynomials: it suffices to check the edges,* J. of Mathematics of Control, Signals and Systems, **1**, No. 1, pp. 61-71; see also Proc. ACC, 1987.

BOSE, N.K., 1982, *Applied Multidimensional System Theory.* Van Nostrand Reinhold Co., New York.

DASGUPTA, S., and ANDERSON, B.D.O., 1987, *Automatica,* **23**, 469-477.

DE GASTON, R.R.E., and SAFONOV, M.E., 1988, *IEEE Trans. Autom. Control,* **AC-33**, 156-171.

DJAFERIS, T.E., 1988, *Shaping Conditions for the Robust Stability of Polynomials with Multilinear Parameter Uncertainty.* Internal Report, Electrical and Computer Engineering Department, University of Massachusetts.

DJAFERIS, T.E., and HOLLOT, C.V., 1988, *Parameter Partitioning via Shaping Conditions for the Stability of Families of Polynomials.* Internal Report, Electrical and Computer Engineering Department, University of Massachusetts.

HODGE, W.V.D., and PEDOE, D., 1968, *Methods of Algebraic Geometry,* Vol. 1, Cambridge University Press, Cambridge.

HOLLOT, C.V., and BARTLETT, A.C., 1986, *IEEE Trans. Autom. Control,* **AC-31**, 355-356.

JACOBSON, N., 1964, *Lectures in Abstract Algebra,* Vol. III, Van Nostrand, Princeton.

KHARITONOV, V.L., 1979, *Differential Equations* , **14** 1483-1485.

PANIER, E.R., FAN, M.K.H., and TITS, A.L., 1987, *On the Stability of Polynomials with Uncoupled Perturbations in the Coefficients of Even and Odd Powers.* Internal Report, Department of Electrical Engineering, University of Maryland.

SAEKI, M., 1986, *IEEE Trans. Autom. Control,* **AC-31**, 935-940.

WATSON, L.T., BILLUPS, S.C., and MORGAN, A.P., 1987, *HOMPACK: A Suite of Codes for Globally Convergent Homotopy Algorithms.* ACM Transactions on Mathematical Software, **13**, No. 3, 281-310.

ZADEH, L., and DESOER, C.A., 1963, *Linear System Theory.* McGraw Hill Book Co., New York.

ZEHEB, 1987, Internal Report, Dept. of Electrical Engineering, Technion, Israel Institute of Technology, Haifa.

STABILITY CONDITIONS FOR POLYNOMIALS VIA QUADRATIC INEQUALITIES IN THEIR COEFFICIENTS

Adly T. Fam

Department of Electrical and Computer Engineering
State University of New York
Buffalo, New York 14260

INTRODUCTION

Stability conditions for monic polynomials of degree n and zeros in the unit circle involve the computation of determinants of rank of up to 2n. These determinants could be represented either explicitly, or iteratively.[1] In either case, each determinant requires the addition of up to 2n terms, each of which is the product of up to 2n coefficients or their complex conjugate.

In computing such determinants, finite wordlength effects are unavoidable. Even with floating point arithmetic and a large number of bits, the determinants of the highest ranks are sensitive to the finite computational accuracy. This is particularly the case for polynomials with zeros near the unit circle, and for large n. A determinant of rank near 2n which happens to be sufficiently near zero, could experience a change in sign as a result of finite wordlength effects. It is therefore desirable to develop stability criteria which incorporate the finite wordlength effects in some way.

In the sequel, conditions for the zeros to be in domains which approximate the unit circle from inside or outside are obtained. These conditions are quadratic in the coefficients of the polynomial tested, and therefore allow for exact evaluation even with fixed point arithmetic. Any desired degree of accuracy of approaching the unit circle from inside or outside is achieved simply by evaluating more quadratic expressions. The error is shifted from the computations to the domains being tested, with a complete characterization of their shape and how close they are to the unit circle.

The quadratic criteria are developed first for polynomials with real coefficients, and then easily extended to the complex coefficients case. Following a review of some proporties of polynomials in their coefficient space, the complex plane map of the convex hull of the coefficient space stability domain is obtained. This map is the basis of the quadratic test developed in either a sufficient or necessary form. Finally, the complexity of the proposed test is evaluated in terms of the required number of operations.

COEFFICIENT SPACE GEOMETRY

Following the notation in Fam,[2] each monic polynomial

$$P(z) = z^n + \alpha_1 z^{n-1} + \alpha_2 z^{n-2} + \dots + \alpha_n \tag{1}$$

with real coefficients is represented in the n-dimensional Euclidean space E^n by a point with coordinates $(\alpha_1, \alpha_2, \dots, \alpha_n)$. The domain of points in E^n corresponding to polynomials with zeros in the unit circle is denoted by D_n. The only two convex domains are D_1 and D_2, which are the straight line segment (-1,+1) in the α_1 space for D_1, and the interior of the triangle with vertices (-2,1), (0,-1), and (2,1) in the (α_1,α_2) space for D_2.

The convex hull of D_n, denoted by KD_n, is a simplex[2] with each of its n+1 vertices corresponding to one of the polynomials

$$\phi_{nr}(z) = (z+1)^{n-r}(z-1)^r, \quad r = 0, 1, \dots, n \tag{2}$$

Changing the basis over which P(z) is expanded from $\{1, z, z^2, \dots, z^n\}$ to the polynomials of (2), results in

$$P(z) = \sum_{r=0}^{n} \beta_r \phi_{nr}(z), \quad \sum_{r=0}^{n} \beta_r = 1 \tag{3}$$

where the β's are also the barycentric coordinates of the point representing P(z) in the α's coefficient space with respect to the vertices of KD_n. A polynomial is contained in KD_n if and only if

$$\beta_i \geqq 0, \quad i = 0, 1, \dots, n$$

and a necessary condition for stability is represented by

$$\beta_i > 0, \quad i = 0, 1, \dots, n$$

The α's and the β's are related by

$$[\beta_0\ \beta_1\ \dots\ \beta_n]^T = \Phi_n^{-1}[1\ \alpha_1\ \dots\ \alpha_n]^T \tag{4}$$

where the rth column of the matrix Φ_n is composed of the coefficients of ϕ_{nr} with the coefficient of z^n at the top.

The change of basis according to (2) also represents the bilinear transformation s = (z+1)/(z-1), which connects continuous-time systems stability to that of discrete-time systems. Matrices identical to, or closely related to Φ_n are well examined in the literature on bilinear transformations and have been introduced as early as in Unbenhauen.[3]

The bilinear transformation maps the point representing a polynomial in E^n to its barycentric coordinates with respect to the vertices of KD_n. This duality has been used to develop[4] continuous and discrete-time systems stability in a unified geometric setup, where it is found that

$$\Phi_n^{-1} = 2^{-n}\,\Phi_n \tag{5}$$

which is a matrix form of the observation that

$$s = \frac{z+1}{z-1}, \quad z = \frac{s+1}{s-1}$$

are equivalent.

MAPPING KD_n INTO THE COMPLEX PLANE

Let $F(z)$ be a convex linear combination of the monic polynomials $f_i(z)$, $i = 1, 2, \dots, m$

$$F(z) = \sum_{i=1}^{m} m_i f_i(z), \quad \sum_{i=1}^{m} m_i = 1, \; m_i \geq 0, \; i = 1, 2, \dots, m \tag{6}$$

each of which is of degree p and with zeros in a convex region K. A direct Corollary of Theorem (8,1) of Marden[1] is stated as follows.

Corollary. If K is a convex region which encloses all the zeros of each $f_i(z)$ of (6), then $F(z)$ has no zeros at any point at which K subtends an angle less than $\Psi = \pi/p$.

The zeros of $F(z)$ lie in a region $S(K,\Psi)$ of all points at which K subtends an angle of at least Ψ. Any $F(z)$ satisfying (6) has its zeros in $S(K,\Psi)$, and any point in $S(K,\Psi)$ is the zero of some $F(z)$ satisfying (6). However, it is important to notice that every polynomial of degree p with zeros in $S(K,\Psi)$ is not necessarily expressible as a convex combination as in (6).

Each polynomial in KD_n is a convex linear combination of the polynomials $\phi_{nr}^{n}(z)$ of (2), each of which has zeros at ±1. therefore, K is the line segment [-1,+1] in the complex plane, and $\Psi = \pi/n$. The domain which subtends angles $\geq \pi/n$ at the line segment [-1,+1] is bounded by the two circular arcs which pass by the points -1 and +1. The centers c_n and radius r_n of the two circles defining these arcs are

$$c_n = \pm j \tan (n-2)\pi/2n, \quad r_n = 1/\cos (n-2)\pi/2n \tag{7}$$

as depicted in Figure 1.

A polynomial in KD_n has its zeros in $S([-1,+1],\pi/n)$. A polynomial with all its zeros in the unit circle is represented by a point in D_n, which is contained in KD_n. It is possible however to construct polynomials with zeros in $S([-1,+1],\pi/n)$, but not all in the unit circle, which is not in KD_n. For example, the polynomial $P(z) = z^4 + 8z^2 + 16$ has two zeros at +2j and two at -2j, all in $S([-1,+1],\pi/4)$, but not all its β's are positive. The reason for this apparent anomaly is peculiar to mappings from the coefficient space to the complex plane. A point P that is moving in a domain D in E^n, produces a domain in the complex plane, C(D), traced by the zeros, which do not move independently as P changes. On the other hand, if we allow n zeros to move freely in C(D) they might map into a domain larger than D in the coefficient space. This is the case even if there movement is restricted to be in real or conjugate pair form. The mapping is one-to-one only in particular cases as for D_n.

CRITERION QUADRATIC IN THE COEFFICIENTS

The zeros of $P(z)$ are rotated by an angle of $-\theta$ by replacing z by $ze^{j\theta}$. Every zero of $P(ze^{j\theta})$ becomes real for some $\theta \epsilon [0,\pi/2]$ for polynomials with real coefficients, and $\theta \epsilon [0,\pi)$ for polynomials with complex coefficients. Since the positivity of the β's is a sufficient and necessary condition for the stability of all real zeros, and since every zero is rotated sufficiently to cross the real axis for some θ, then the positivity of the the β's of $Q(z)$, where

$$Q(z) = P(ze^{j\theta})\, P(ze^{-j\theta}) \tag{8}$$

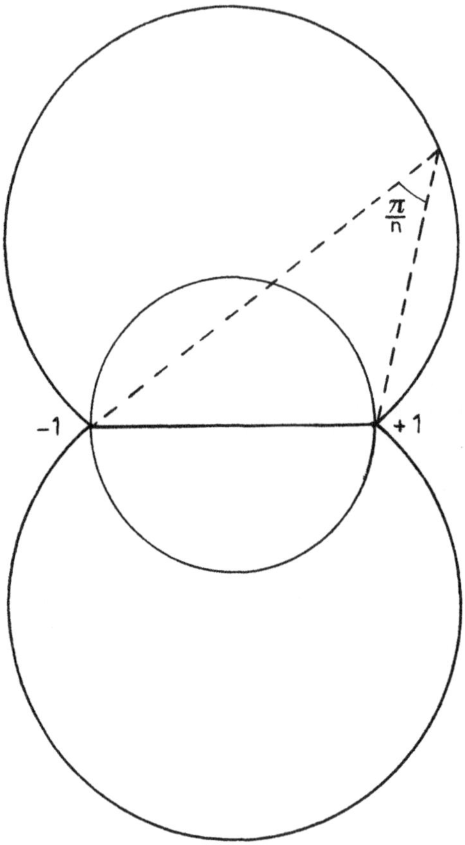

Fig. 1. The complex plane map of KD_n

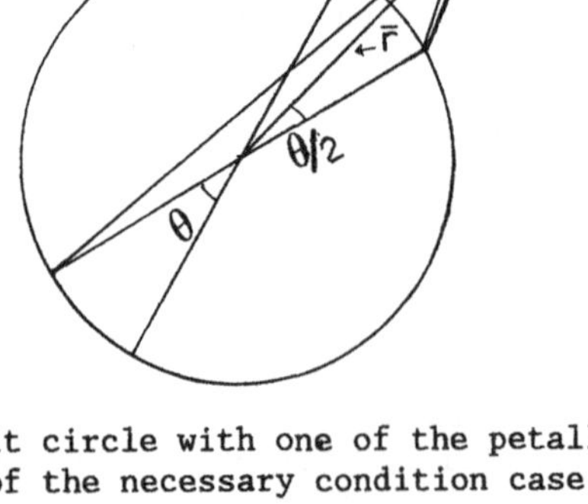

Fig. 2. The unit circle with one of the petallike extensions of the necessary condition case.

for all $\theta\varepsilon[0,\pi/2]$ is a sufficient and necessary for the zeros of $P(z)$ to be in the unit circle. For the case of polynomials with complex coefficients, $Q(z)$ is defined by

$$Q(z) = P(ze^{j\theta})\ \bar{P}(ze^{j\theta})$$

where $\bar{P}$ indicates a polynomial with the conjugate coefficients of P.

Necessary Conditions

By evaluating the β's of Q only for a finite number of rotations at angels $i\theta$, $i = 0, 1, 2, \ldots, R$, where θ is selected such that $R = \pi/4\theta$ is an integer, then their positivity defines a domain of zeros that is the intersection of the domain $S(K,\Psi)$ with rotated versions of itself for the given values of i. The line segment $[-1,+1]$ represents K here, and $\Psi = \pi/2n$ for all i, with the exception of $i = 0$ for polynomials with real coefficients, for which $\Psi = \pi/n$. Thus, the test is for a domain that contains the unit circle, but has petallike extensions, one of which is depicted in Figure 2. The number of "petals" increases and their size decreases as a larger R is used. The test is necessary for the zeros to be in the unit circle, and sufficient for the zeros not to be outside a circle of radius

$$\bar{r} = a + (a^2 + 1)^{1/2}, \quad a = \frac{\sin \theta/2}{\tan \pi/2n} \tag{9}$$

The annular region between the concentric circles of radii unity and $\bar{r}$, of width

$$\bar{\varepsilon} = \bar{r} - 1$$

could contain zeros of a polynomial that passes the above test. The number of rotations required to achieve the upper bound on the error $\bar{\varepsilon}$ is $R = \pi/4\theta$. Each rotation results in $2n+1$ quadratic inequalities. The total number of inequalities is therefore $I = (2n+1)\ \pi/4\theta$, in addition to $n+1$ linear inequalities for the computations of the β's in the real coefficients case. From the above, θ, n, and $\bar{\varepsilon}$ are related by

$$a = \frac{\sin \theta/2}{\tan \pi/2n} = \bar{\varepsilon}\ (\bar{\varepsilon} + 2)/2(\bar{\varepsilon} + 1) \tag{10}$$

For every rotation, the product of the form (8) could be evaluated by a fast convolution algorithm, requiring $O(n \log n)$ operations, where the logarithm is to the base 2, and the operations are complex multiplications and additions. For sufficiently small $\bar{\varepsilon}$, $\theta \cong 2\bar{\varepsilon} \tan \pi/2n$, and for large n

$$R \cong n/4\bar{\varepsilon}, \quad I \cong n^2/2\bar{\varepsilon} \tag{11}$$

Every rotation requires $O(n \log n)$ operations, and every inequality requires $O(n)$ operations, for a total computational cost of

$$C = O(n^3/\bar{\varepsilon}) \tag{12}$$

The inequalities result from multiplication by Φ_{2n}, and could be computed by any efficient algorithm for the bilinear transformation, with possible further reduction in the computational cost. In the complex coefficient case, $I = (2n+1)\ (\pi/2\theta + 1)$, with identical "order of" results as in the real case.

Sufficient Conditions

The conditions obtained above are necessary for the zeros to be in the unit circle, and sufficient for the zeros to be in a circle of radius

$$\bar{r} = \bar{\varepsilon} + 1$$

A polynomial with zeros in the unit circle could be mapped into one with zeros in a circle of radius r via the map

$$\alpha_i \rightarrow r^i \alpha_i$$

which could be used to convert the above conditions to necessary or sufficient conditions for the the zeros to be in a circle of any desired radius. In particular, sufficient conditions for the zeros to be in the unit circle result by mapping the coefficients by

$$\alpha_i \rightarrow \alpha_i (1+\bar{\varepsilon})^i \qquad (13)$$

followed by applying the above test for $\bar{\varepsilon}$. This is equivalent to a test for a circle of radius

$$\underline{r} = 1 - \underline{\varepsilon}, \ \underline{\varepsilon} = \bar{\varepsilon} \ /(1 + \bar{\varepsilon}) \qquad (14)$$

and petals inside the unite circle.

CONCLUSION

Criteria for the zeros of polynomials to be in a domain within ε from the unit circle, and expressed in terms of $O(n^2/\varepsilon)$ quadratic inequalities in their coefficients are introduced. The conditions could be made to be either sufficient or necessary, and within ε of being both.

In applications in which the characteristic polynomial coefficients of a control systems are complicated functions of some design parameters, stability conditions that are only quadratic in these functions could be particularly desirable.

REFERENCES

1. M. Marden, "Geometry of Polynomials," Mathematical Surveys No. 3, American Math. Society, Province, Rhode Island (1966).

2. A. T. Fam and J. S. Meditch, A canonical parameter space for linear systems design, IEEE Trans. Automat. Contr., AC-23:454 (1978).

3. R. Unbehauen, Ein beitrag zur stabilitätsuntersuchung linearer abtastsysteme, Regelungstechnik, 1:12 (1964).

4. A. T. Fam, On the geometry of stable polynomials of one and two variables, in: "Information Linkage Between Applied Mathematics and Industry," P. C. C. Wang, ed., Academic Press, New York (1979).

BOUNDARY IMPLICATIONS FOR INTERVAL POSITIVE RATIONAL FUNCTIONS:

PRELIMINARIES

N. K. Bose and J. F. Delansky

Department of Electrical Engineering
The Pennsylvania State University
University Park, PA 16802
United States of America

INTRODUCTION

The purpose of this documentation is to state the generalizations obtained on the topic of boundary implications in parameter space upon the properties of systems which are characterized by interval rational functions. These boundary implications in order that the positive real (complex) property holds for an interval rational function are formulated. The source for details pertaining to the proofs of the stated results is referred to and this source should be widely accessible.

INTERVAL STRICT POSITIVE REAL RATIONAL FUNCTIONS

Recently, Dasgupta (1987) considered interval rational functions,

$$F(s) = \frac{\sum_{k=0}^{n} [\underline{b}_k, \overline{b}_k] \, s^{n-k}}{s^m + \sum_{k=1}^{m} [\underline{a}_k, \overline{a}_k] s^{m-k}}, \tag{1}$$

where the generic coefficients b_k and a_k in the numerator and denominator are real with lower and upper bounds explicitly indicated in (2a) and (2b).

$$0 < \underline{b}_k \leq b_k \leq \overline{b}_k \, , \; k=0,1,\ldots,n \tag{2a}$$

$$0 < \underline{a}_k \leq a_k \leq \overline{a}_k \, , \; k=1,2,\ldots,m \tag{2b}$$

The numerator and denominator polynomials, $b(s)$ and $a(s)$, respectively, of a typical element $f(s) \varepsilon F(s)$ are subjected to the even-odd decomposition, exhibited in (3).

$$f(s) = \frac{b(s)}{a(s)} = \frac{p(s^2) + sq(s^2)}{u(s^2) + sv(s^2)} \tag{3}$$

The Kharitonov polynomials associated with b(s) and a(s), respectively, are

$$p_i(s^2) + sq_j(s^2) \ , \ i,j=1,2 \tag{4a}$$

and

$$u_k(s^2) + sv_\ell(s^2) \ , \ k,\ell=1,2 \tag{4b}$$

where

$$u_1(s^2) = \underline{a}_m + \bar{a}_{m-2}s^2 + \underline{a}_{m-4}s^4 + \bar{a}_{m-6}s^6 + \ldots \tag{5a}$$

$$u_2(s^2) = \bar{a}_m + \underline{a}_{m-2}s^2 + \bar{a}_{m-4}s^4 + \underline{a}_{m-6}s^6 + \ldots \tag{5b}$$

$$v_1(s^2) = \underline{a}_{m-1} + \bar{a}_{m-3}s^2 + \underline{a}_{m-5}s^4 + \bar{a}_{m-7}s^6 + \ldots \tag{5c}$$

$$v_2(s^2) = \bar{a}_{m-1} + \underline{a}_{m-3}s^2 + \bar{a}_{m-5}s^4 + \underline{a}_{m-7}s^6 + \ldots \ . \tag{5d}$$

Define $p_i(s^2)$ and $q_j(s^2)$, i,j=1,2 as above with m, $\underline{a}_k$ and $\bar{a}_k$ replaced, respectively, by n, $\underline{b}_k$ and $\bar{b}_k$. We introduce the definition for a strictly positive real (SPR) function, before stating Dasgupta's result (1987) in Theorem 1.

Definition 1: The rational function f(s) in (3) is SPR provided,

(a) f(s) is real for real s
(b) $a(s) \neq 0$, Re $s \geq 0$ and $b(s) \neq 0$, Re $s \geq 0$, i.e. a(s) and b(s) are Hurwitz
(c) Re $f(j\omega) > 0$, $-\infty \leq \omega \leq \infty$.

Theorem 1: All members of the set F(s) in (1) are SPR if and only if each of the sixteen members of the set

$$G(s) = \frac{p_i(s^2) + s\ q_j(s^2)}{u_k(s^2) + s\ v_\ell(s^2)} \ ; \ i,j,k,\ell=1,2 \tag{6}$$

is SPR.

The proof of Theorem 1 has been advanced by the authors of this paper via use of a standard result in interval analysis given, for example, by Moore (1966) and quoted below.

Lemma 1: Given $a_1 \leq a \leq a_2$, $b_1 \leq b \leq b_2$, then
$\min(a_1b_1, a_1b_2, a_2b_1, a_2b_2) \leq ab \leq \max(a_1b_1, a_1b_2, a_2b_1, a_2b_2)$.

INTERVAL POSITIVE REAL RATIONAL FUNCTIONS

Consider the interval rational functions

$$R(s) = \frac{\sum_{i=0}^{n} [\underline{n}_i, \overline{n}_i]\, s^{n-i}}{\sum_{i=0}^{m} [\underline{d}_i, \overline{d}_i]\, s^{m-i}} \tag{7}$$

where the generic coefficients n_i and d_i in the numerator and denominator are real with lower and upper bounds explicitly indicated in (8a) and (8b).

$$0 \le \underline{n}_i \le n_i \le \overline{n}_i\ , \quad i=0,1,\ldots,n \tag{8a}$$

$$0 \le \underline{d}_i \le d_i \le \overline{d}_i\ , \quad i=0,1,\ldots,m \tag{8b}$$

A typical element $r(s) \varepsilon R(s)$ will be denoted as

$$r(s) = \frac{n(s)}{d(s)}\ . \tag{9}$$

Define the augmented function $r_a(s)$ as

$$r_a(s) = r(s) + 1 = \frac{n(s)}{d(s)} + 1 = \frac{n(s) + d(s)}{d(s)} = \frac{a(s)}{d(s)}\ . \tag{10}$$

Definition 2 is standard and is available, for instance, in Temes and Lapatra (1977).

Definition 2: The rational function $r(s)$ in (9) is positive real (PR) provided $r_a(s)$ in (10) satisfies

(a) $r_a(s)$ is real for real s
(b) $a(s)$ is Hurwitz
(c) $\mathrm{Re}\, r_a(j\omega) - 1 = \mathrm{Re}\, r(j\omega) \ge 0,\ -\infty \le \omega \le \infty$.

Denote the Kharitonov polynomials associated with $n(s)$ and $d(s)$ by, respectively,

$$p_i(s^2) + sq_j(s^2),\ i,j = 1,2 \tag{11a}$$

and

$$u_k(s^2) + sv_\ell(s^2),\ k,\ell = 1,2. \tag{11b}$$

Each of the forms in (11a) and (11b) is the even-odd polynomial decomposition form, popular in circuit synthesis. The next theorem has been proved by the authors via the use of Lemma 1.

Theorem 2: All members of the set $R(s)$ in (7) are PR if and only if each of the sixteen members of the set

$$G_a(s) = \frac{p_i(s^2) + sq_j(s^2)}{u_k(s^2) + sv_\ell(s^2)} + 1,\ i,j,k,\ell=1,2 \tag{12}$$

satisfy conditions (a), (b), (c) of Definition 2.

INTERVAL POSITIVE RATIONAL FUNCTIONS

Consider the interval rational functions in (13a)

$$C(s) = \frac{P(s)}{Q(s)} , \tag{13a}$$

where the interval polynomials P(s) and Q(s) are

$$P(s) = \sum_{k=0}^{n} (\alpha_k + j\beta_k)s^k \; ; \; \alpha_k \varepsilon [\underline{\alpha}_k, \overline{\alpha}_k] \; , \; \beta_k \varepsilon [\underline{\beta}_k, \overline{\beta}_k] \; , \; k=0,1,\ldots,n \tag{13b}$$

$$Q(s) = \sum_{k=0}^{m} (\gamma_k + j\delta_k) \; s^k \; ; \; \gamma_k \varepsilon [\underline{\gamma}_k, \overline{\gamma}_k] \; , \; \delta_k \varepsilon [\underline{\delta}_k, \overline{\delta}_k] \; , \; k=0,1,\ldots,m \; . \tag{13c}$$

Obviously in (13b) and (13c) above, the α_k's, β_k's, γ_k's and δ_k's are all real. A typical element $c(s)\varepsilon C(s)$ will be denoted by

$$c(s) = \frac{p(s)}{q(s)} \; . \tag{14}$$

Define the augmented function $c_a(s)$ as

$$c_a(s) = c(s) + 1 = \frac{p(s) + q(s)}{q(s)} = \frac{a(s)}{q(s)} \; . \tag{15}$$

The function c(s) in (14) (Belevitch, 1968) is called positive (positive complex (PC)) provided

$$\text{Re } c(s) \geq 0 \text{ for Re } s \geq 0 \; . \tag{16}$$

Definition 3: The rational function c(s) in (14) is positive (PC) provided $c_a(s)$ in (15) satisfies

(a) a(s) is Hurwitz
(b) $\text{Re } c_a(j\omega) - 1 = \text{Re } c(j\omega) \geq 0, \; -\infty \leq \omega \leq \infty$.

The eight Kharitonov polynomials associated with each of the complex interval polynomials P(s) and Q(s) may be defined. Denote by C(s) the set of sixty-four extreme rational functions generated from the quotients of each of the elements in the Kharitonov polynomial set associated with P(s) after pairing with each of the elements in the corresponding set associated with Q(s). Let $C_a(s)$ be the augmented set obtained by adding 1 to each of the elements in the set C(s).

Theorem 3: All members of the set of rational functions in (13a) are PC if and only if all members of the set $C_a(s)$ satisfy conditions (a) and (b) in Definition 3.

The preceding theorem may be proved via use of a generalization to the complex number case the result stated in Lemma 1. This generalization, which is trivial to prove by applying Lemma 1 twice is stated in Lemma 2 below.

Lemma 2: Let (a+jb) and (c+jd) be two complex numbers where, obviously, a, b, c, and d are real and each is arbitrary but fixed in specified intervals given by $a_1 \leq a \leq a_2$, $b_1 \leq b \leq b_2$, $c_1 \leq c \leq c_2$ and $d_1 \leq d \leq d_2$. Suppose that the following sixteen inequalities,

$$a_i \; c_j + b_k \; d_\ell \geq 0$$

hold for $i,j,k,\ell=1,2$. Then it also follows that

$$ab + cd \geq 0$$

for each value of a, b, c, and d in their respective interval of variation.

The counterpart of the result in Theorem 3 is easy to give for the case of strict positive functions.

CONCLUSIONS

Recent results concerning boundary implications in parameter space for the strict positive real (complex) as well as positive real (complex) properties of interval rational functions are summarized. Details concerning proofs of the results are available in the publication of Bose and Delansky (1989).

ACKNOWLEDGEMENT

This research was partly supported by NSF Grant ECS 87-03215 and partly by IBM Grant PO 174688B-WF.

REFERENCES

Belevitch, V., 1968, "Classical Network Theory", Holden-Day, Inc., San Francisco.

Bose, N. K. and Delansky, J. F., 1989, Boundary implications for interval positive rational functions, IEEE Trans. Circuits and Systems, 36.

Dasgupta, S., 1987, A Kharitonov like theorem for systems under nonlinear passive feedback, Proc. IEEE Conf. Dec. and Cont., Los Angeles: 2062-2063.

Moore, R. E., 1966, "Interval Analysis", Prentice Hall, Inc., Englewood Cliffs.

Temes, G. C. and Lapatra, J. W., 1977, "Introduction to Circuit Synthesis and Design", McGraw-Hill Book Co., New York.

GUARANTEEING ULTIMATE BOUNDEDNESS AND EXPONENTIAL RATE OF CONVERGENCE FOR A CLASS OF UNCERTAIN SYSTEMS[1]

M. Corless
School of Aeronautics and Astronautics
Purdue University
West Lafayette
Indiana

F. Garofalo
Dipartimento di Informatica e Sistemistica
Universita' di Napoli
Naples
Italy

G. Leitmann
College of Engineering
University of California
Berkeley
California

ABSTRACT

For systems described by ordinary differential equations, we introduce the notion of exponential convergence to a ball containing the origin of the state space. For two specific classes of uncertain systems, controllers are presented which assure this behavior. For one of the system classes, the rate of exponential convergence can be made arbitrary large.

Key Words. Uncertain systems, exponential convergence, exponential stability, robust control, Lyapunov theory.

1. INTRODUCTION

A fundamental feedback control problem is that of obtaining a certain desired behavior from a system about which there is uncertain or incomplete information. In recent years much effort has focussed on utilizing Lyapunov theory to obtain controllers which yield desirable behavior from systems whose uncertainties are characterized deterministically (rather than stochastically); see, e.g., Refs. 3, 4, and the references therein.

In most of this literature, the desired behavior is asymptotic stability about the origin of the state space or a close approximation to this, e.g., all state trajectories are bounded and approach a sufficiently small neighborhood of the origin. Quite often one also desires that the state approaches the origin (or some sufficiently small neighborhood of it) in a sufficiently fast manner. To this end, Ref. 5 introduces a concept of exponential rate of convergence and for a specific class of uncertain systems presents controllers which guarantee this behavior; see also Refs. 1, 6.

[1] This paper is based on research supported by NSF and AFOSR under Grants MSM-87-06927 and ECS-86-02524, and by FORMEZ, Italy.

Here we introduce a notion which is slightly different from that of Ref. 5, the notion of exponential convergence to a ball, and for classes of systems more general than those considered in Ref. 5, we present controllers which guarantee this behavior; see also Ref. 2.

In Section 2, the concept of exponential convergence to a ball is introduced and a Lyapunov-type condition is given which assures this behavior.

In Section 3, a specific class of uncertain systems is considered and controllers are presented which assure convergence at a rate which is independent of the uncertainty and is the same as that of a "nominal" system.

In Section 4, another class of uncertain systems is considered and, for any given desired rate, exponential convergence is guaranteed by the controllers proposed there.

2. EXPONENTIAL CONVERGENCE TO A BALL

Consider a system described by

$$\dot{x}(t) = f(t, x(t)), \tag{1}$$

where $t \in \mathbb{R}$ is the "time" and $x(t) \in \mathbb{R}^n$ is the state. Suppose r is a non-negative real number. We have the following definition of desirable behavior with respect to

$$B(r) \triangleq \{x \in \mathbb{R}^n : \|x\| \leq r\} \ , \tag{2}$$

i.e., the closed ball with center at the origin and radius r.

Definition 2.1. System (1) is *(globally, uniformly) exponentially convergent to* B(r) iff there exists $\alpha > 0$ with the property that, for any initial conditions $t_0 \in \mathbb{R}$ and $x_0 \in \mathbb{R}^n$, there exists $c(x_0) \geq 0$ such that if $x(\cdot):[t_0, t_1) \to \mathbb{R}^n$ is any solution of (1) with $x(t_0) = x_0$ then

$$\|x(t)\| \leq r + c(x_0)\exp[-\alpha(t-t_0)] \quad \forall\, t \geq t_0 \,. \tag{3}$$

In the above definition α is called an *exponential rate of convergence.* Note that (3) implies,

$$\|x(t)\| \leq r + c(x_0) \quad \forall\, t \geq t_0 \,;$$

hence the solutions of (1) are *bounded* and can be extended indefinitely. Note also that (3) implies, given any $\varepsilon > 0$, there exists $T(x_0,\varepsilon) \geq 0$ such that

$$\|x(t)\| \leq r + \varepsilon \quad \forall\, t \geq t_0 + T(x_0,\varepsilon) \ ;$$

hence, using the terminology of Refs. 4 and 5, the solutions of (1) are *ultimately bounded* and

$$\limsup_{t \to \infty} \|x(t)\| \leq r \tag{4}$$

where

$$\limsup_{t \to \infty} \|x(t)\| \triangleq \lim_{t \to \infty} \sup\{\|x(s)\| : s \geq t\} \ .$$

The number r is called an *asymptotic (norm) bound* on the solutions of (1).

If system (1) satisfies the conditions of the above definition with

$$\lim_{x_0 \to 0} c(x_0) = 0, \tag{5}$$

then the system is said to be *(globally, uniformly) exponentially stable to within* B(r). If, in addition, r = 0, then the system is *exponentially stable about zero.*

As stated in Theorem 2.1, the following condition is sufficient to assure exponential convergence.

Condition 2.1. There exist a continuously differentiable function $V:\mathbb{R}^n \rightarrow \mathbb{R}$ and scalars $\gamma_1, \gamma_2 > 0$ which satisfy

$$\gamma_1 \|x\|^2 \le V(x) \le \gamma_2 \|x\|^2 \tag{6}$$

for all $x \in \mathbb{R}^n$ such that, for some scalars $\alpha > 0$ and[2] $\underline{V} \ge 0$,

$$V(x) > \underline{V} \;\Rightarrow\; DV(x)f(t, x) \le -2\alpha[V(x) - \underline{V}] \tag{7}$$

for all $t \in \mathbb{R}$ and $x \in \mathbb{R}^n$.

Theorem 2.1. Suppose Condition 2.1 is satisfied for system (1), and let

$$r \triangleq (\underline{V}/\gamma_1)^{1/2} . \tag{8}$$

Then system (1) is exponentially convergent to B(r) with rate α, where

$$c(x_o) \triangleq \begin{cases} 0, & \text{if } V(x_o) \le \underline{V}, \\ [(V(x_o) - \underline{V})/\gamma_1]^{1/2}, & \text{if } V(x_o) > \underline{V} . \end{cases} \tag{9}$$

Also, system (1) is exponentially stable to within B(r).

Proof. Ref. 2 contains a proof. □

Example 2.1. Linear Systems. Consider a linear time-invariant system described by

$$\dot{x}(t) = Ax(t) \tag{10}$$

with A Hurwitz, i.e.,

$$\mathrm{Re}(\lambda) < 0 \quad \forall \lambda \in \sigma(A), \tag{11}$$

where $\sigma(A)$ is the set of eigenvalues of A. Let $\alpha > 0$ be any number satisfying

$$\mathrm{Re}\,(\lambda) < -\alpha \quad \forall \lambda \in \sigma(A) . \tag{12}$$

Utilizing Theorem 2.1, we now show that (10) is exponentially stable about zero with rate α.

Choose any positive-definite symmetric matrix $Q \in \mathbb{R}^{n \times n}$. Since $A + \alpha I$ is Hurwitz, the equation

$$P(A + \alpha I) + (A + \alpha I)^T P + 2Q = 0 \tag{13}$$

has a unique solution $P \in \mathbb{R}^{n \times n}$, and this solution is symmetric and positive-definite; see

---

[2] Note that $DV(x) \triangleq [\frac{\partial V}{\partial x_1}(x) \; \frac{\partial V}{\partial x_2}(x) \; \cdots \; \frac{\partial V}{\partial x_n}(x)]$.

Ref. 7. Defining

$$V(x) \triangleq \tfrac{1}{2}x^T Px, \tag{14}$$

one has[3]

$$\tfrac{1}{2}\lambda_{min}(P)\|x\|^2 \leq V(x) \leq \tfrac{1}{2}\lambda_{max}(P)\|x\|^2 , \tag{15}$$

and in view of (13) it follows that

$$\begin{aligned} DV(x)Ax &= x^T PAx \\ &= \tfrac{1}{2}x^T[PA + A^T P]x \\ &= -\alpha x^T Px - x^T Qx \\ &\leq -2\alpha V(x) \ ; \end{aligned}$$

hence Condition 2.1 is satisfied with $\underline{V} = 0$. It now follows from Theorem 2.1 that (10) is exponentially stable about zero with rate α.

It should be clear from the above calculations that satisfaction of (13) for any $\alpha > 0$, any positive-definite $P \in \mathbb{R}^{n \times n}$, and any *semi positive-definite* $Q \in \mathbb{R}^{n \times n}$ assures exponential stability with rate α.

3. GUARANTEED EXPONENTIAL CONVERGENCE FOR A CLASS OF UNCERTAIN SYSTEMS

In this section we consider a specific class of uncertain systems and present controllers which assure that the feedback-controlled system is exponentially convergent with rate α to a ball of radius r_ε, where α and r_ε are independent of the uncertainty.

3.1. Systems under Consideration. Consider an uncertain system described by

$$\dot{x}(t) = f^o(t, x(t), \omega) + B(t, x(t))g(t, x(t), u(t), \omega) \tag{16}$$

where $t \in \mathbb{R}$ is the "time", $x(t) \in \mathbb{R}^n$ is the state, and $u(t) \in \mathbb{R}^m$ is the control. All the uncertainty in the system is characterized by the uncertain element ω. The only information assumed available on ω is a known set Ω to which ω belongs. It is assumed that for each $\omega \in \Omega$, B, $f(\cdot, \omega)$, and $g(\cdot, \omega)$ are continuous functions.

Assumption 3.1. There exists a continuously differentiable function $V:\mathbb{R}^n \to \mathbb{R}$ and scalars $\underline{V} \geq 0$ and $\gamma_1, \gamma_2, \alpha > 0$, which assure that, for all $\omega \in \Omega$, Condition 2.1 is satisfied for the system described by

$$\dot{x}(t) = f^o(t, x(t), \omega) \ . \tag{17}$$

Recalling Theorem 2.1, the above assumption implies that, for all $\omega \in \Omega$, system (17) is exponentially convergent with rate α to a ball of radius $r = (\underline{V}/\gamma_1)^{1/2}$.

Assumption 3.2. There exist continuous functions $\kappa, \rho:\mathbb{R}\times\mathbb{R}^n \to \mathbb{R}_+$ such that, for all $\omega \in \Omega$,

---

[3] If all the eigenvalues of $M \in \mathbb{R}^{nxn}$ are real, $\lambda_{min(max)}(M)$ denotes the smallest (largest) eigenvalue of M.

$$u^T g(t, x, u, \omega) \geq -\beta_1(t, x, \omega)\|u\| + \beta_2(t, x, \omega)\|u\|^2 \quad (18a)$$

where $\beta_1(t, x, \omega)$, $\beta_2(t, x, \omega) \geq 0$, and

$$\beta_1(t, x, \omega) \leq \kappa(t, x), \quad (18b)$$
$$\beta_1(t, x, \omega) \leq \beta_2(t, x, \omega)\rho(t, x) \quad (18c)$$

for all $t \in \mathbb{R}$, $x \in \mathbb{R}^n$, and $u \in \mathbb{R}^m$.

Remark 3.1. As an example of a function satisfying the above assumption consider

$$g(t, x, u, \omega) = u + a(t, x, u, \omega)$$

where

$$\|a(t, x, u, \omega)\| \leq k_1\|x\| + k_2\|u\| + k_3$$

for all $t \in \mathbb{R}$, $x \in \mathbb{R}^n$, $u \in \mathbb{R}^m$, $\omega \in \Omega$, and

$$k_2 < 1 .$$

A short calculation yields

$$u^T g(t, x, u, \omega) \geq -(k_1\|x\| + k_3)\|u\| + (1-k_2)\|u\|^2 ;$$

hence Assumption 3.2 is assured with

$$\kappa(t, x) = k_1\|x\| + k_3 ,$$
$$\rho(t, x) = (1-k_2)^{-1}(k_1\|x\| + k_3) .$$

3.2. Proposed Controllers. Consider any functions V, κ, ρ, which assure Assumptions 3.1 and 3.2. Choose any scalar $\varepsilon > 0$ and any continuous functions $\kappa^c, \rho^c : \mathbb{R}\times\mathbb{R}^n \rightarrow \mathbb{R}_+$ which satisfy

$$\kappa^c(t, x) \geq \kappa(t, x), \quad (19a)$$
$$\rho^c(t, x) \geq \rho(t, x) \quad (19b)$$

for all $t \in \mathbb{R}$, $x \in \mathbb{R}^n$, and let

$$\eta(t, x) \triangleq \kappa^c(t, x)B(t, x)^T DV(x)^T . \quad (19c)$$

Let $s: \mathbb{R}^m \rightarrow \mathbb{R}^m$ be any continuous function which satisfies

$$\|z\|s(z) = \|s(z)\|z \quad (19d)$$

(i.e., s(z) has the same direction as z) and

$$\|z\| > 1 \Rightarrow \|s(z)\| \geq 1 - 1/\|z\| \quad (19e)$$

for all $z \in \mathbb{R}^m$. Defining

$$p^\varepsilon(t, x) \triangleq -\rho^c(t, x)s(\eta(t, x)/\varepsilon) , \quad (19f)$$

a proposed controller is given by

$$u(t) = p^\varepsilon(t, x(t)) . \quad (20)$$

As an example of a function satisfying the above requirements on s consider

$$s(z) = \begin{cases} z & \text{if} \quad \|z\| \leq 1 \\ \|z\|^{-1} z & \text{if} \quad \|z\| > 1 \end{cases} ,$$

or

$$s(z) = (1 + \|z\|)^{-1} z .$$

3.3. Systems with Proposed Controllers. Consider a system described by (16) and subject to one of the controllers proposed in Section 3.2. The resulting closed-loop system can be described by

$$\dot{x}(t) = f^o(t, x(t), \omega) + B(t, x(t))g(t, x(t), p^\varepsilon(t, x(t)), \omega) , \tag{21}$$

and its properties are given by the following theorem.

Theorem 3.1. Consider an uncertain system described by (16), satisfying Assumptions 3.1 and 3.2, subject to control given by (19)-(20), and let

$$r_\varepsilon \triangleq [(\underline{V} + \varepsilon/2\alpha)/\gamma_1]^{1/2} . \tag{22}$$

For each $\omega \in \Omega$, the closed-loop system (21) has the following properties.

(i) Existence of solutions.[4]

(ii) Indefinite extension of solutions.[4]

(iii) Exponential convergence with rate α to $B(r_\varepsilon)$, where

$$c(x_o) \triangleq \begin{cases} 0 & \text{if} \quad V(x_o) \leq \underline{V}_\varepsilon \\ \\ [(V(x_o) - \underline{V}_\varepsilon)/\gamma_1]^{1/2} & \text{if} \quad V(x_o) > \underline{V}_\varepsilon \end{cases} , \tag{23a}$$

$$\underline{V}_\varepsilon \triangleq \underline{V} + \varepsilon/2\alpha . \tag{23b}$$

(iv) Exponential stability to within $B(r_\varepsilon)$.

Proof. Ref. 2 contains a proof. □

Remark 3.2. The feedback-controlled system (21) has a convergence rate which is the same as that of system (17). Also, it is clear from (22) that the asymptotic bound r_ε for (21) can be made arbitrarily close to that of (17) by choosing ε sufficiently small.

4. GUARANTEED EXPONENTIAL CONVERGENCE WITH AN ARBITRARY RATE

In this section, we treat a class of uncertain systems which is a generalization of the class treated in Ref. 5. For any given $\alpha > 0$ we present controllers which assure that, for

---

[4] A precise definition of this property is given in Ref. 4.

any allowable uncertainty, the feedback-controlled system is exponentially convergent with rate α to a ball of radius r_ε. Also, by choice of a controller parameter ε, $r_\varepsilon > 0$ can be made arbitrarily small.

4.1. Systems under Consideration. Consider an uncertain system described by

$$\dot{x}(t) = Ax(t) + Bg(t, x(t), u(t), \omega) \tag{24}$$

where $t \in \mathbb{R}$, $x(t) \in \mathbb{R}^n$, $u(t) \in \mathbb{R}^m$, and $\omega \in \Omega$ are as previously described.

Assumption 4.1. (A, B) is controllable.

Assumption 4.2. There exist continuous functions $\kappa, \underline{\lambda} : \mathbb{R} \times \mathbb{R}^n \to \mathbb{R}_+$ such that, for all $\omega \in \Omega$,

$$u^T g(t, x, u, \omega) \geq -\beta_1 (t, x, \omega)\|u\| + \beta_2(t, x, \omega)\|u\|^2 \tag{25a}$$

where $\beta_1 (t, x, \omega) \geq 0$ and

$$\beta_1 (t, x, \omega) \leq \kappa(t, x) \tag{25b}$$

$$\beta_2(t, x, \omega) \geq \underline{\lambda}(t, x) > 0 \tag{25c}$$

for all $t \in \mathbb{R}$, $x \in \mathbb{R}^n$, and $u \in \mathbb{R}^m$.

Assumption 4.2 is a stronger version of Assumption 3.2; if 4.2 is satisfied then 3.2 is assured, for example, with

$$\rho(t, x) = \underline{\lambda}(t, x)^{-1} \kappa(t, x) .$$

The functions discussed in Remark 3.1 satisfy 4.2.

For the systems treated in Ref. 5, the function g has the special form considered in Remark 3.1. The systems treated in Ref. 6 are similar to those considered here. There, the matrices A and B need not be constant, but, $\kappa(\cdot)$ should satisfy $\kappa(t, x) \leq \kappa_1 \|x\|$ for some constant $\kappa_1 \geq 0$.

4.2. Proposed Controllers. For a given $\alpha > 0$, a proposed controller is given by

$$u(t) = p(t, x(t)) , \tag{26}$$

where

$$p(t, x) = p^\alpha(t, x) + p^\varepsilon(t, x) \tag{27a}$$

and p^α, p^ε are constructed as follows.

To construct p^α choose any scalar $\sigma > 0$ and any positive-definite symmetric matrix $Q \in \mathbb{R}^{n \times n}$, and consider the positive-definite solution $P \in \mathbb{R}^{n \times n}$ of

$$PA + A^T P + 2\alpha P - 2\sigma PBB^T P + 2Q = 0 . \tag{27b}$$

The existence of a unique positive-definite solution to (27b) is guaranteed by the controllability of (A, B). Choose any continuous function $\gamma: \mathbb{R} \times \mathbb{R}^n \to \mathbb{R}_+$ which satisfies

$$\gamma(t, x) \geq \underline{\lambda}(t, x)^{-1} \sigma . \tag{27c}$$

Then let

$$p^\alpha(t, x) \triangleq - \gamma(t, x) B^T P x . \tag{27d}$$

Defining

$$V(x) \triangleq \tfrac{1}{2}x^T Px \quad , \tag{27e}$$

the controller p^ε is given by (19). Hence,

$$p^\varepsilon(t, x) = -\rho^c(t, x)s(\eta(t, x)/\varepsilon) \quad ,$$

where

$$\eta(t, x) = \kappa^c(t, x)B^T Px \quad .$$

4.3. Systems with Proposed Controllers. Consider a system described by (24) and subject to one of the controllers proposed in the previous section. The resulting feedback-controlled system can be described by

$$\dot{x}(t) = Ax(t) + Bg(t, x(t), p(t, x(t)), \omega) \quad , \tag{28}$$

and its properties are given by the following theorem.

Theorem 4.1. Consider an uncertain system described by (24) and satisfying Assumptions 4.1, 4.2. Consider any $\alpha > 0$ and suppose (24) is subject to control given by (26), (27), (19).

With

$$r_\varepsilon \triangleq (\varepsilon/2\alpha\gamma_1)^{1/2} \quad , \tag{29}$$

the feedback-controlled system (28) has the following properties for all $\omega \in \Omega$.

(i) Existence of solutions.[4]

(ii) Indefinite extension of solutions.[4]

(iii) Exponential convergence with rate α to $B(r_\varepsilon)$, where

$$c(x_o) \triangleq \begin{cases} 0, & \text{if } V(x_o) \le \underline{V}_\varepsilon, \\ [(V(x_o) - \underline{V}_\varepsilon)/\gamma_1]^{1/2}, & \text{if } V(x_o) > \underline{V}_\varepsilon, \end{cases}$$

$$\underline{V}_\varepsilon \triangleq \varepsilon/2\alpha \quad .$$

(iv) Exponential stability to within $B(r_\varepsilon)$.

Proof. Ref. 2 contains a proof. □

REFERENCES

1. ANDERSON, B.D.O., and MOORE, J.B., *Linear System Optimization with Prescribed Degree of Stability,* Proceedings of IEE, Vol. 116, pp. 2083-2087, 1969.
2. CORLESS, M., *Guaranteed Rates of Exponential Convergence for Uncertain Systems,* Journal of Optimization Theory and Applications (to appear).
3. CORLESS, M., and LEITMANN, G., *Controller Design for Uncertain Systems via Lyapunov Functions,* Proceedings of the 1988 American Control Conference, Atlanta, Georgia, 1988.

4. CORLESS, M., and LEITMANN, G., *Deterministic Control of Uncertain Systems: A Lyapunov Theory Approach,* Deterministic Nonlinear Control of Uncertain Systems: Variable Structure and Lyapunov Control, Edited by A. Zinober, IEE Publishers, London, England (to appear).

5. GAROFALO, F., and LEITMANN, G., *Guaranteeing Ultimate Boundedness and Exponential Rate of Convergence for a Class of Nominally Linear Uncertain Systems,* Journal of Dynamic Systems, Measurement, and Control (to appear).

6. HAMANO, F., BOYKIN, W.H., JR., and WARREN, M.E., *Global Stabilization of a System with Linearly Bounded Uncertainties,* International Symposium on Design and Systems, Tokyo, 1984.

7. KALMAN, R. E., and BERTRAM, J. E., *Control System Analysis and Design via the "Second Method" of Lyapunov, I: Continuous-Time Systems,* Journal of Basic Engineering, Vol. 82, pp. 371-393, 1960.

ON MEASURES OF STABILITY ROBUSTNESS

FOR LINEAR UNCERTAIN SYSTEMS

Rama K. Yedavalli

Department of Aeronautical and Astronautical Engineering
The Ohio State University
Columbus, Ohio 43210

ABSTRACT

This paper addresses the aspect of developing "measures of stability robustness" for linear uncertain systems with state space description. A brief overview of the current research as well as a new result on this topic are presented.

INTRODUCTION

Recently, the aspect of developing 'measures of stability robustness' for linear uncertain systems with state space description has received much attention [1]-[19]. For a discussion on this topic for nonlinear systems, one may refer to [20]. The several results available in the literature for the linear system case can be categorized according to the characterization of the uncertainty, such as 'structured' and 'unstructured;' 'time varying' and 'time invariant;' 'complex' and 'real' parameters. Also, the stability robustness bounds developed do depend on the type of parameter space region specified (such as hyper rectangle, sphere etc.) In the next section, we attempt to summarize the results available in the recent literature based on the above considerations.

A BRIEF PERSPECTIVE

The starting point for the problem at hand is to consider a linear state space system described by

$$\dot{x}(t) = [A_0 + E]\, x(t) \tag{1}$$

where x is an n dimensional state vector, asymptotically stable matrix and E is the 'perturbation' matrix. The issue of 'stability robustness measures' involves the determination of bounds on E which guarantee the preservation of stability of (1). Evidently, the characterization of the perturbation matrix E has considerable influence on the derived result. In what follows, we summarize a few of the available results, based on the characterization of E.

I. Time Varying (Real) Unstructured Perturbation with Spectral Norm: Sufficient Bound

For this case, the perturbation matrix E is allowed to be time varying, i.e. E(t) and a bound on the spectral norm (σ_{max} E(t) where $\sigma(\cdot)$ is the singular value of ($\cdot$)) is derived. When a bound on the norm of E is given, we refer to it as 'unstructured' perturbation. This norm produces a spherical region in parameter space. The following result is available for this case [3]-[4]:

$$\sigma_{max}(E(t)) < \frac{1}{\sigma_{max}(P)} \tag{2}$$

where P is the solution to the Lyapunov matrix

$$PA_0 + A_0^T P + 2I = 0 \tag{3}$$

See Refs [10], [13] and [16] for results related to this case.

II. Time Varying (Real) Structured Variation

Case 1: Independent Variations (Sufficient Bound) [11]-[12]

$$E_{ij}(t) \leq \forall_t |E_{ij}(t)|_{max} = \epsilon_{ij} \tag{4}$$

$$\epsilon = \mathrm{Max}_{ij}\, \epsilon_{ij}$$

$$\epsilon_{ij} < \frac{1}{\sigma_{max}(P_m U_e)_s} U_{eij} \tag{5}$$

where P satisfies equation (3) and $U_{eij} = \epsilon_{ij}/\epsilon$. For cases when ϵ_{ij} are not known, one can take $U_{eij} = |A_{0ij}|/|A_{0ij}|_{max}$. $(\cdot)_m$ denotes the matrix with all modulus elements and $(\cdot)_s$ denotes the symmetric part of ($\cdot$).

Case 2: Linear Dependent Variation (Sufficient Bounds [17]

$$E(t) = \sum_{i=1}^{r} \beta_i(t) E_i \tag{6}$$

where E_i are constant, given matrices and β_i are the uncertain parameters. For this case, we have

$$\text{i)} \qquad |\beta_j| < 1/\sigma_{max} \left(\sum_{i=1}^{r} |P_i|\right) \qquad j=1,2,\ldots r \tag{7}$$

This is a hyper rectangle region in parameter (β) space.

$$\text{ii)} \qquad \sum_{i=1}^{r} |\beta_i|\ \sigma_{max}(P_i) < 1 \tag{8}$$

This is a diamond shaped region in β space.

$$\text{iii)} \qquad \sum_{i=1}^{r} \beta_i^2 < 1/\sigma_{max}^2 (P_e) \tag{9}$$

This is a spherical region in β space. In these expressions, $P_i = (PE_i + E_i^T P)/2 = (PE_i)s$ $i=1,2,\ldots r$ and $P_e = [P_1\ P_2 \ldots P_r]$. It may be noted that the bound in (7) can be simplified to

$$|\beta_1| < 1/\sigma_{max}(P_1) \tag{10}$$

when r=1. This was not explicitly stated in [17].

III. Complex (Real), Unstructured Perturbation [6], [9] and [19]: For this case, the bound is given by

$$||E|| < \frac{1}{\sup_{\omega \geq 0} ||(j\omega I - A_0)^{-1}||} = \underline{r}_k \tag{11}$$

Here $||(\cdot)||$ can be any operator norm. Hinrichsen and Pritchard label r_k as the "stability radius." When E is real, it is called the "Real Stability Radius" and is denoted by r_R. Note that when E is complex $r_k = r_c$ is a necessary and sufficient bound whereas when E is real, r_R becomes a sufficient bound. However, with A_0 being a 2 x 2 matrix and E being real, r_R becomes a necessary and sufficient bound and is given by

$$r_R(A_{0_{2x2}}) = \text{Min}[\text{Trace}(A_0), \sigma_{min}(A_0)] \tag{12}$$

The following case is in a way a hybrid situation. Hinrichsen and Pritchard [7] considered the perturbation matrix to be of the form

$$E = BDC$$

where D is the 'uncertain' matrix and B and C are known scaling matrices defining the 'structure' of the perturbation. With this characterization of E which can be complex, they give a bound on the norm of D, $||D||$. They call this bound "structured stability radius." Notice that E as above does not capture the entire class of structured perturbation, which would be covered by

$$E = \sum_{i=1}^{r} B_i D_i C_i \tag{13}$$

But, Hinrichsen and Pritchard do not consider the case of (13). Hence, we label the result of [7] as belonging to norm bounded complex, semi-structured variation.

IV. Norm Bounded, Complex (Real) Semi-Structured Variation $E = BDC$. The result is

$$||D|| < \frac{1}{\sup_{\omega \geq 0} ||C(j\omega I - A_0)^{-1}B||} \tag{14}$$

Again, when E is complex, the bound above is a necessary and sufficient bound whereas for real E, it is only a sufficient bound.

V. Time Invariant, (Real) Structured Perturbation E_{ij} = Constant

Case i: Independent Variations [18]-[19]: (Sufficient Bounds). For this case, E can be characterized as

$$E = S_1 D S_2 \tag{15}$$

where S_1 and S_2 are constant, known matrices and $|D_{ij}| \leq d_{ij}d$ with $d_{ij} \geq 0$ are given and $d > 0$ is the unknown. Let U be the matrix with elements $U_{ij} = d_{ij}$. Then the bound on d is given by [19]

$$d < \frac{1}{\sup_{\omega \geq 0} \rho([S_2(j\omega I - A_0)^{-1}S_1]_m U)} = \mu_J = \mu_Q \tag{16}$$

Notice that the characterization of E (with time invariant) in (4) is accommodated by the characterization in (15). $\rho(\cdot)$ is the spectral radius of $(\cdot)$.

<u>Case ii: Linear, Dependent Variation</u>: For this case, E is characterized (as in (6) before), by

$$E = \sum_{i=1}^{r} \beta_i E_i \tag{17}$$

and bounds on $|\beta_i|$ are sought.

This type of representation represents a 'polytope of matrices' as discussed in [14]. In this notation, the interval matrix case (i.e. the independent variation case) is a special case of the above representation where E_i contains a single nonzero element, at a different place in the matrix for different i.

For the time invariant, real structured perturbation case, there are no computationally tractable necessary and sufficient bounds either for polytope of matrices or for interval matrices (even for a 2 x 2 case). Even though some derivable necessary and sufficient conditions are presented in [21] for any general variation in E (not necessarily linear dependent and independent case), there are no easily computable methods available to determine the necessary and sufficient bounds at this stage of research. So most of the research, at this point of time, seems to aim at getting better (less conservative) sufficient bounds. In the next section, we extend the method of [18]-[19] to give sufficient bounds for the linear dependent variation case.

SUFFICIENT BOUNDS FOR LINEAR DEPENDENT CASE

<u>Linear Dependent Uncertainty</u>: In what follows, we consider the case where the uncertain parameters in E are assumed to enter linearly, as in (17). Our intention is to give a bound on $|\beta_i|$.

We now present a bound on $|\beta_i|$ and show that the resulting bound specializes to (16) for the independent variation case. The proposed bound is less conservative than (16) when applied to the situation in which E is given by (17) and yields the same bound as in (16) when applied to the independent variation case (when E is given by (4)). This is exactly the type of situation that arises in Zhou and Khargonekar, [17], where they consider the liner dependency case and specialize it to the independent variation case of Yedavalli, [11].

<u>Remark</u>: It should be mentioned at the outset that it is very important to distinguish between the independent variation case and the dependent variation case at the problem formulation stage. In the independent variation case one gives bounds on ϵ_{ij} (and consequently on ϵ), whereas in the dependent variation case, one gives bounds on $|\beta_i|$. This is particularly crucial in the comparison of different techniques. Proper comparison is possible only when the basis, namely whether one is considering the dependent case or the independent case, is established beforehand. It may

be noted that the techniques aimed at the independent variation case can accommodate the dependent variation situation, but at the expense of some conservatism; whereas the technique aimed at the dependent case, while it gives a less conservative bound for that case, cannot accommodate the independent variation case (unless it is established, additionally, to handle that situation, as is done in [17] and also later in this paper for the new proposed bound).

Main Theorem: Consider the system (1) with E as in (17). Then (1) is stable if

$$|\beta_i| < \frac{1}{\sup_{\omega\geq 0} \rho(\sum_{i=1}^{r} |(j\omega I - A_0)^{-1}E_i|)} = \mu_d \text{ for } r > 1 \tag{18a}$$

and

$$|\beta_1| < \frac{1}{\sup_{\omega\geq 0} \rho[(j\omega I - A_0)^{-1}E_1]} = \mu_d \text{ for } r = 1 \tag{18b}$$

Proof: Given in Appendix

It can be shown that the bound (16) becomes a special case of (18) when one notes that in the independent variation case each E_i will contain a single element and is given by

$$E_{i(n-1)+j} = U_{eij} e_i e_j^T \tag{19}$$

where e_i is an n-dimensional column matrix with 1 in the i-th entry and 0 elsewhere. Note that U_{eij} is a scalar and $e_i e_j^T$ is a matrix.

Remark: The bound of (18), when specialized to the independent variation case (i.e., when each E_i contains a single element, at a different place for different i), will be denoted by μ_{ind}. Thus, $\mu_{ind} = \mu_J = \mu_Q$.

Example 1: Consider

$$A_0 = \begin{bmatrix} -3 & -2 \\ 1 & 0 \end{bmatrix}$$

and let

$E = \beta\begin{bmatrix} 1 & 1 \\ 1 & 1 \end{bmatrix}$ (i.e., dependent case)

μ_Q	μ_J	μ_d (proposed)	ZK[17]	[12]
0.329	0.329	1.0	1.0	0.236

If, instead, all the elements in E are assumed to vary independently, then we use

$$E_1 = \begin{bmatrix} 1 & 0 \\ 0 & 0 \end{bmatrix}, \quad E_2 = \begin{bmatrix} 0 & 1 \\ 0 & 0 \end{bmatrix}, \quad E_3 = \begin{bmatrix} 0 & 0 \\ 1 & 0 \end{bmatrix}, \quad E_4 = \begin{bmatrix} 0 & 0 \\ 0 & 1 \end{bmatrix}$$

in the expression (17) and get

$$|E_{ij}| < \mu_{ind} = 0.329$$

which is, of course, the same bound as μ_J and μ_Q.

It may be noted that the bound $\mu_d = 1.0$ is also a necessary and sufficient bound.

Example 2: Consider the same A_0 as in Example 1 and let

$$E = \beta\begin{bmatrix} -1 & 1 \\ 0 & 0 \end{bmatrix}$$

μ_Q	μ_J	μ_d (proposed)	ZK[17]	[12]
1.52	1.52	2.0	2.0	1.0

Example 3: Let us consider the example given in [17] in which the perturbed system matrix is given by

$$(A_0 + BKC) = \begin{bmatrix} -2+k_1 & 0 & -1+k_1 \\ 0 & -3+k_2 & 0 \\ -1+k_1 & -1+k_2 & -4+k_1 \end{bmatrix}$$

Taking the nominally stable matrix to be

$$A_0 = \begin{bmatrix} -2 & 0 & -1 \\ 0 & -3 & 0 \\ -1 & -1 & -4 \end{bmatrix}$$

the error matrix with k_1 and k_2 as the uncertain parameters is given by

$$E = k_1E_1 + k_2E_2$$

where

$$E_1 = \begin{bmatrix} 1 & 0 & 1 \\ 0 & 0 & 0 \\ 1 & 0 & 1 \end{bmatrix} \quad \text{and} \quad E_2 = \begin{bmatrix} 0 & 0 & 0 \\ 0 & 1 & 0 \\ 0 & 1 & 0 \end{bmatrix}$$

The following are the bounds on $|k_1|$ and $|k_2|$ obtained by [17] and the proposed method (corresponding to the bound given by expression (7))

μ_y	$\mu_J = \mu_Q$	ZK[17]	proposed bound
0.815	0.875	1.55	1.75

It may be noted that, in this paper, we do not have counterparts to the bounds given by expressions (8) and (9) in Zhou and Khargonekar's paper [17].

CONCLUSIONS

This paper presents some new results on the stability robustness measures for linear state space models with structured, dependent uncertainty. These are less conservative compared to the existing bounds, and are obtained by using a frequency domain approach.

REFERENCES

1. Zheng, D.Z., "A Method for Determining the Parameter Stability Regions of Linear Control Systems," IEEE Transactions, Vol. AC-29, No. 2, pp. 183-185. February 1984.
2. Eslami, M. and Russell, D.L., "On Stability with Large Parameter Variations Stemming from the Direct Method of Lyapunov," IEEE Transactions, Vol. AC-25, No. 6, pp. 1231-1234, December 1980.
3. Chang, S.S.L. and Peng, T.K.C., "Adaptive Guaranteed Cost Control of Systems with Uncertain Parameters," IEEE Transactions, Vol. AC-17, pp. 474-483, August 1972.
4. Patel, R.V. and Toda, M., "Quantitative Measures of Robustness for Multivariable Systems," Proceedings of Joint Automatic Control Conference, TP8-A, 1980.
5. Patel.R.V., Toda, M., and Sridhar, B., "Robustness of Linear Quadratic State Feedback Designs in the Presence of System Uncertainty," IEEE Transactions, Vol. AC-22, pp. 945-949, December 1977.
6. Hinrichsen, D. and Pritchard, A.J., "Stability Radius of Linear Systems," Systems and Control Letters, Vol. 7, pp. 1-10, 1986.
7. Hinrichsen, D. and Pritchard, A.J., "Stability Radius for Structured Perturbations and the Algebraic Riccati Equation," Systems and Control Letters, Vol. 8, pp. 105-113, 1986.
8. Barmish, B.R. and Leitmann, G., "On Ultimate Boundedness Control of Uncertain Systems in the Absence of Matching Assumptions," IEEE Transactions, Vol. AC-27, pp. 153-158, February 1982.
9. Martin, J.M., "State Space Measures for Stability Robustness," IEEE Transactions on Automatic Control, Vol. AC-32, pp. 509-512, June 1987.
10. Yedavalli, R.K., Banda, S.S., and Ridgely, D.B., "Time Domain Stability Robustness Measures for Linear Regulators," AIAA Journal of Guidance, Control and Dynamics, pp. 520-525, July-August 1985.
11. Yedavalli, R.K., "Improved Measures of Stability-Robustness for Linear State Space Models," IEEE Transactions on Automatic Control, Vol. AC-30, pp 577-579, June 1985.
12. Yedavalli, R.K., "Perturbation Bounds for Robust Stability in Linear State Space Models," International Journal of Control, Vol. 42, No. 6, pp. 1507-1517, 1985.
13. Yedavalli, R.K. and Liang, Z., "Reduced Conservation in Stability Robustness Bounds by State Transformation," IEEE Transactions on Automatic Control, Vol. AC-31, pp. 863-866, September 1986.
14. Barmish, B.R., Fu, M. and Saleh, S. "Stability of a Polytope of Matrices: Counterexamples," IEEE Transactions on Automatic Control, Vol. AC-33, pp. 569-572, June 1987.
15. Keel, L.H., Bhattacharyya, S.P., and Howze, J.W., "Robust Control with Structured Perturbations," IEEE Transactions on Automatic Control, Vol. AC-33, pp. 68-79, January 1988.
16. Hyland, D.C. and Bernstein, D.S., "The Majorant Lyapunov Equations: A Nonnegative Matrix Equation for Robust Stability and Performance of Large Scale Systems," IEEE Transactions on Automatic Control, Vol. AC-32,pp. 1005-1013, November 1987.
17. Zhou, K. and Khargonekar, P., "Stability Robustness Bounds for Linear State Space Models with Structured Uncertainty," IEEE Transactions on Automatic Control, Vol. AC-32, pp. 621-623, July 1987.
18. Juang, Y.T., Kuo, T.S., and Hsu, C.F., "New Approach to Time Domain Analysis for Stability Robustness of Dynamic Systems," International Journal of Systems Science, Vol. 18, No. 7, pp. 1363-1376, 1987.
19. Qiu, L. and Davison, E.J., "New Perturbation Bounds for the Robust Stability of Linear State Space Models," Proceedings of the 25th Conference on Decision and Control, Athens, Greece, pp. 751-755, 1986.

20. Corless, M. and Da, D., "New Criteria for Robust Stability," Proceedings of the International Workshop on 'Robustness in Identification and Control,' Torino, Italy, June 1988.

21. Tesi, A. and Vicino, A., "Robustness Analysis for Uncertain Dynamical Systems with Structured Perturbations," Proceedings of the International Workshop on 'Robustness in Identification and Control,' Torino, Italy, June 1988.

APPENDIX

Proof of Main Theorem

It is known that the perturbed system

$$\dot{x}(t) = (A_0 + E)\, x(t) \tag{A-1}$$

(where A_0 is an asymptotically stable matrix) is asymptotically stable if

$$\sup_{\omega\geq 0} \rho[(j\omega\, I - A_0)^{-1}E] < 1 \tag{A-2}$$

(For a proof see [18] or [19]). Let $(j\omega I - A_0)^{-1} = M(\omega)$. Now with E given by

$$E = \sum_{i=1}^{r} \beta_i E_i \tag{A-3}$$

the perturbed system (A-1) is asymptotically stable if

$$\sup_{\omega\geq 0} \rho[M(\omega)\, (\sum_{i=1}^{r} \beta_i E_i)] < 1 \tag{A-4}$$

$$\text{But } \max_j|\beta_j| \sup_{\omega\geq 0} \rho[\sum_{i=1}^{r} |M(\omega)E|] \geq \sup_{\omega\geq 0} \rho(\sum_{i=1}^{r} |\beta_i M(\omega) E_i|)$$

$$\geq \sup_{\omega\geq 0} \rho(\sum_{i=1}^{r} |\beta_i M(\omega) E_i|)$$

$$\geq \sup_{\omega\geq 0} \rho[M(\omega)(\sum_{i=1}^{r} \beta_i E_i)]$$

The satisfaction of condition (18a) implies the satisfaction of (A-4) and hence the perturbed system is asymptotically stable. For r=1, we see that

$$|\beta_1| \sup_{\omega\geq 0} \rho[(M(\omega)E_1)] = \sup_{\omega\geq 0} \rho[M(\omega)(\beta_1 E_1)]$$

Hence (18b) implies (A-4) and hence the result.

ROBUST STABILIZATION OF LINEAR TIME-INVARIANT SYSTEMS VIA LINEAR CONTROL

Kehui Wei

DFVLR - INSTITUT FUR DYNAMIK DER FLUGSYSTEME
D-8031 Oberpfaffenhofen, FRG

Abstract--This paper investigates the problem of designing a single linear static feedback control to simultaneously stabilize a family of multi-input linear dynamical systems. The family of systems $\Sigma(A(q), B(q))$; $q \in Q$, represented by their state space matrices, may be uncountable thus allowing for the possibility of a continuum of variations in system parameters. Sufficient conditions related to the given state space matrices $A(q)$ and $B(q)$ are given under which there does exist a single robust controller stabilizing the family of systems. A recursive algorithm is also provided to compute a desired constant feedback gain matrix K.

I. INTRODUCTION

In recent years, the problem of designing a feedback control law to simultaneously stabilize a family of systems, or an uncertain system, has received considerable attention. A main motivation for this study comes from the following multi-model problem of robust control, proposed by J. Ackermann in Ackermann (1980 and 1985): Given a finite number of linear systems described by state equations, determine whether there exists a single linear constant feedback control which can stabilize all the systems. This problem arises if a nonlinear plant is linearized at different operating points and a constant feedback law is sought to stabilize the system at all the operating points. The problem is of particular interest in aircraft control, e. g., see Kreisselmeier and Steinhauser (1980) and Franklin and Ackermann (1981). To allow further for a continuum of variations in the system parameters, a more general formulation of the multi-model problem is as follows: Given an uncertain dynamical systems whose parameters are only known within a predescribed compact (either discrete or continuum) set, provide conditions under which it is possible to design a constant feedback controller which guarantees uniform asymptotic stability of the origion for all admissible variations of uncertainties. Such a controller might be appropriately called a robust stabilizer.

One of considerable methods to tackle this problem is to treat the uncertain system as a nominal system with uncertain perturbations. By using the knowledge of the nominal system, one can construct a feedback control to stabilize the nominal system. Then, the admissible perturbation bound for the closed nominal system may be determined, e.g., see Patel, Toda and Sridhar (1977) and Yedavalli (1985). When desired pertubation bounds are given, one may directly check the robust stability of the closed loop uncertain system by using recently developed methods, e.g., see Karitonov (1978), Bartlett, Hollot and Huang (1988) and Barmish (1988). However, those methods are analysis in nature, the stabilizability of a given uncertain system is not known beforehand. In addition, with those methods, usually only small "size" of perturbations is allowable. When the perturbations of a given system excceed the allowable bound, there is no guiding line which leads to finding a desired robust control.

In Ackermann (1980, 1985), parameter space technique has been used to solve the multi-model problem. When a pole assignment region is prespecified, for each system one may map the region to the parameter space and then use computer graphic methods to find out if there is an intersection for all systems. This method is specially useful for low order single input systems.

Given the preceding literature, the main aim of this paper is to study the stabilizability of uncertain linear time-invariant systems and the related robust control design procedure. In this paper, sufficient conditions are provided under which an uncertain system will be stabilizable by a single constant static feedback control. Once the stabilizability of a given uncertain system is determined through our criteria, a concrete design method to synthesize a desired robust controller is also provided.

II. SYSTEMS AND DEFINITIONS

We consider a linear time-invariant uncertain system $\Sigma(A(q), B(q))$ (or uncertain system for short) described by the state equation

$$\dot{x}(t) = A(q)x(t) + B(q)u(t) \; ; \; t \geq 0$$

where $x(t) \in R^n$ is the state; $u(t) \in R^m$ is the control; $q \in Q \subset R^k$ is the model uncertainty which is restricted to a prescribed compact bounding set Q. Within this framework, $A(\cdot)$ and $B(\cdot)$ must be $n \times n$ and $n \times m$ dimensional matrix functions on the set Q, respectively. Hence for fixed $q \in Q$, A(q) and B(q) are the model matrices which result.

Definition 2.1: An uncertain system $\Sigma(A(q), B(q))$ is said to be stabilizable (with respect to Q) via linear control if there exists an $m \times n$ constant matrix K such that the characteristic polynomial

$$P(s,q) \triangleq \det (sI - A(q) - B(q)K)$$

is Hurwitz invariant, i. e., for every $q \in Q$, all the zeroes of P(s,q) are in the strict left half of the complex plane.

In this paper, we will provide conditions under which an uncertain system $\Sigma(A(q), B(q))$ is stabilizable via linear control. To describe the conditions we introduce some definitions.

Definition 2.2: A square matrix function $\Phi : Q \rightarrow R^{t \times t}$ with entries $\phi_{ij}(q)$ is said to be antisymmetric if the following conditions hold:

i) Each diagonal term $\phi_{ii}(q)$ is a sign invariant uncertain function of q, represented by θ (a nonzero constant is considered to be a special case of θ).

ii) If $i > j$ and $\phi_{ij}(q) \not\equiv 0$, then $\phi_{jl}(q) \equiv 0$ for all l satisfying $i \geq l > j$ and if $i < j$ and $\phi_{ij}(q) \not\equiv 0$, then $\phi_{jl}(q) \equiv 0$ for all l satisfying $j > l \geq i$.

It is convenient to describe antisymmetric matrix functions by using "0" and "d" for nondiagonal entries of a matrix Φ. An entry of "d" in the matrix is viewed as a "don't-care" term. This notation is illustrated below.

Example 2.3: Some antisymmetric uncertain matrix functions are described by

$$\begin{bmatrix} \theta & 0 & 0 & 0 \\ d & \theta & 0 & 0 \\ d & d & \theta & 0 \\ d & d & d & \theta \end{bmatrix}; \quad \begin{bmatrix} \theta & 0 & 0 & 0 \\ d & \theta & 0 & d \\ d & d & \theta & d \\ d & 0 & 0 & \theta \end{bmatrix};$$

$$\begin{bmatrix} \theta & 0 & 0 & d \\ d & \theta & d & d \\ d & 0 & \theta & d \\ 0 & 0 & 0 & \theta \end{bmatrix}; \quad \begin{bmatrix} \theta & 0 & 0 & 0 \\ d & \theta & d & d \\ d & 0 & \theta & d \\ d & 0 & 0 & \theta \end{bmatrix}.$$

The motivation for defining antisymmetry in the case when $\Phi(q)$ is a nonsquare matrix is derived from a characterization of antisymmetry which is available in the square case. The next definition enables us to develop this characterization.

Definition 2.4: Suppose $\Phi : Q \rightarrow R^{t \times l}$ is a rectangular matrix function. Then the matrix function

$\Phi^+ : Q \to R^{(t+1)\times(l+1)}$ is said to be an up-augmentation of $\Phi(q)$ if it has the form

$$\Phi^+(q) \triangleq \left[\begin{array}{c:ccc} \theta & 0 & 0 & \cdots\ 0 \\ \hdashline d & & & \\ \vdots & & & \\ d & & \Phi(q) & \\ \vdots & & & \\ d & & & \end{array}\right]; \tag{2.4.1}$$

and is said to be a down-augmentation of $\Phi(q)$ if it has the form

$$\Phi^+(q) \triangleq \left[\begin{array}{ccc:c} & & & d \\ & \Phi(q) & & d \\ & & & \vdots \\ & & & d \\ \hdashline 0 & 0 & \cdots\ 0 & \theta \end{array}\right] \tag{2.4.2}$$

where θ is a sign invariant uncertain function of q.

The following observation is an easy consequence of the definition of antisymmetry.

Observation 2.5: A square matrix function $\Phi(q)$ is antisymmetric if and only if it can be generated from a sign invariant scaler function θ via a sequence of augmentations (either up or down).

We are now prepared to define antisymmetry in the nonsquare case.

Definition 2.6: A rectangular matrix function $\Phi : Q \to R^{t\times l}$ is said to be antisymmetric if it can be generated from some vector function c(q) via a sequence of augmentations (either up or down). The vector function $c(q) \triangleq (c_0(q)\ \ c_1(q) \ldots\ c_v(q))' \in R^{v+1}$ is called the core of $\Phi(q)$. A core c(q) is called a Hurwitz core if the correspondent uncertain polynomial $c(s,q) \triangleq c_0(q)s^v + c_1(q)s^{v-1} + \cdots + c_v(q)$ is a Hurwitz invariant polynomial with a sign invariant leading coefficient $c_0(q)$ for all $q \in Q$. The matrix function $\Phi(q)$ is said to be Hurwitz antisymmetric if it is antisymmetric and is generated from a Hurwitz core.

Example 2.7: Two illustrations of antisymmetric matrix functions are shown below.

$$\begin{bmatrix} c_0 & d & d \\ c_1 & d & d \\ 0 & \theta & d \\ 0 & 0 & \theta \end{bmatrix}; \quad \begin{bmatrix} \theta & 0 & d \\ d & 2 & d \\ d & 3 & d \\ 0 & 0 & \theta \end{bmatrix}.$$

Notice that the first matrix is generated by two down-augmentations; the second matrix is generated by an up-augmentation followed by a down-augmentation. The second matrix is Hurwitz antisymmetric because the core (2 3)' is a Hurwitz core.

Definition 2.8: Consider an n×(n+1) uncertain matrix pencil $M(s,q) \triangleq sT(q) + N(q) \triangleq \{m_1, m_2, \ldots, m_{n+1}\}$ where m_i are column vectors of M(s,q). Let $S \triangleq (s^n\ \ s^{n-1} \ldots\ s\ 1)$ and $M_i \triangleq \det\{m_1, m_2, \ldots, m_{i-1}, m_{i+1}, \ldots, m_{n+1}\} \triangleq S\,\phi_i(q)$ where $\phi_i(q)$ are column vectors. Then, the coefficient matrix $\Phi(q)$ of M(s,q) is defined as follows:

$$\Phi(q) \triangleq \{\ \phi_1(q), \phi_2(q), \ldots, \phi_n(q)\ \}.$$

Definition 2.9: An n×(n+1) uncertain matrix pencil M(s,q) as in Definition 2.8 is said to have Hurwitz antisymmetry property if its coefficient matrix $\Phi(q)$ satisfies the following condition: Some columns of $\Phi(q)$ can be permuted to a Hurwitz antisymmetric matrix $\Phi^*(q)$ as in Definition 2.6.

III. MAIN RESULTS

We now state our main results. First, we consider a special uncertain system $\Sigma(A(q), B_0(q))$ with $B_0(q)=(0\ 0\ \ldots\ 0\ I(q))'$ where I(q) is an m×m lower triangle matrix and each diagonal term of I(q) is sign invariant, i.e.,

$$B_0(q) = \begin{bmatrix} 0 & 0 & \cdots & 0 \\ \vdots & \vdots & & \vdots \\ 0 & 0 & & \\ \theta_1 & 0 & & \\ b_{21} & \theta_2 & & \\ & & \cdots & 0 \\ b_{m1} & b_{m2} & & \theta_m \end{bmatrix} \qquad (3.0.1)$$

where $\theta_1, \theta_2, \ldots, \theta_m$ are sign invariant uncertain functions of q.

Theorem 3.1: (See Section V for proof.) An uncertain system $\Sigma(A(q), B_0(q))$ is stabilizable via linear control if in the first (n-m) rows of the matrix (sI-A(q)) there is an (n-m)×(n-m+1) submatrix M(s,q) having Hurwitz antisymmetry property.

We now consider more general cases.

Definition 3.2: we define elementary matrices as follows:

$$T = \begin{bmatrix} 1 & & & & \\ & \ddots & & & \\ & & 1 \cdots & a(q) & \\ & & \ddots & \vdots & \\ & & & 1 & \\ & & & & \ddots \\ & & & & & 1 \end{bmatrix}; \qquad T = \begin{bmatrix} 1 & & & & \\ & \ddots & & & \\ & & 0 & 1 & \\ & & & \cdots & \\ & & 1 & 0 & \\ & & & & \ddots \\ & & & & & 1 \end{bmatrix};$$

$$T = \begin{bmatrix} 1 & & & & \\ & \ddots & & & \\ & & 1 & & \\ & & & \theta & \\ & & & & 1 \\ & & & & & \ddots \\ & & & & & & 1 \end{bmatrix}$$

where θ is a sign invariant uncertain function of q and a(q) is an arbitrary function of q.

Definition 3.3: An uncertain system $\Sigma(A(q), B(q))$ is said to be admissible if B(q) satisfies the following condition: There exists a nonsinguler uncertain matirx $T(q)=T_1\, T_2 \ldots T_p$ such that

$$T(q)B(q) = B_0(q)$$

where $B_0(q)$ is as in (3.0.1), T_i : i=1,2,...,p are all elementary matrices as in Definition 2.10 and T(q) is called a transformation matrix.

Theorem 3.4: (See Section V for proof.) An admissible uncertain system $\Sigma(A(q), B(q))$ is stabilizable via linear control if in the first (n-m) rows of the matrix (sT(q) - T(q)A(q)) there is an (n-m)× (n-m+1) submatrix M(s,q) having Hurwitz antisymmetry property.

IV. PRELIMINARY LEMMAS FOR PROOF OF THEOREM 3.1 AND 3.4

To prove our main results, we need some key lemmas.

Definition 4.1: An (nth-order, continuous coefficient) gain controlled uncertain polynomial is a family of polynomials $\{f(s,k,q) : k \in R^m, q \in Q\}$ all having degree n with real coefficients which depend continuously on $(k,q) \in R^m \times Q$. For notational convenience, let $S \triangleq (s^n \; s^{n-1} \; \ldots \; s \; 1)$ and $\alpha(k,q) \triangleq [\alpha_0(k,q) \;\; \alpha_1(k,q) \;\; \ldots \;\; \alpha_n(k,q)]'$, then

$$f(s,k,q) \triangleq S\alpha(k,q). \tag{4.1.1}$$

We often refer to $k \in R^m$ as the control gain vector.

Definition 4.2: A gain controlled uncertain polynomial f(s,k,q) is said to be Hurwitz invarilizable (over Q) if there exists a gain vector $k^* \in R^m$ such that the uncertain polynomial $f(s,k^*,q)$ is Hurwitz invariant (over Q), that is, for every $q \in Q$, all the zeros of $f(s,k^*,q)$ lie in the strict left half of the complex plane.

Definition 4.3: Let $G=(1 \; k_1 \; k_2 \; \ldots \; k_m)'$. A gain controlled uncertain polynomial f(s,k,q) as in (4.1.1) is said to have affine coefficients to control gain k if there exists a continous matrix function $\Phi : Q \rightarrow R^{(n+1)\times(m+1)}$ such that

$$\alpha(k,q) = \Phi(q)G \tag{4.3.1}$$

or consequently,

$$f(s,k,q) = S\Phi(q)G. \tag{4.3.2}$$

The following lemma is the main result of Wei and Barmish (1985).

Lemma 4.4: (See Wei and Barmish (1985) for proof.) Suppose f(s,k,q) ; $q \in Q$ as in (4.1.1) is a gain controlled uncertain polynomial with affine coefficient to control gain k, i. e., $f(s,k,q) = S\Phi(q)G$. Then f(s,k,q) is Hurwitz invarilizable if the following condition holds: $\Phi(q)$ contains an (n+1) row submatrix $\Phi^*(q)$ which is Hurwitz antisymmetric.

The following lemma is a direct consequece of Lemma 2.7 of Wei and Barmish (1985).

Lemma 4.5: (See Wei and Barmish (1985) for proof.) Suppose f(s,q) is an nth-order Hurwitz invariant uncertain polynomial with a sign invariant leading coefficient and f'(s,q) is an (n+1)th-order uncertain polynomial with a sign invariant leading coefficient. Then there exists a constant k such that

$$f^*(s,q) = kf(s,q) + f'(s,q)$$

is also a Hurwitz invariant polynomial with a sign invariant leading coefficient.

V. PROOF OF THEOREM 3.1 AND 3.4

Proof of Theorem3.1: Without lost of generality, we assume that the submatrix $M_{i\,i-1}$ containing the entries in the first i=n-m+1 columns and the first i-1=n-m rows of the matrix (sI-A(q)) has Hurwitz antisymmetry property. Let A_1 be the submatrix containing the entries in the first i columns and the first i rows of A(q), A_2 be the submatrix containing the entries in the first i+1 columns and the first i+1 rows of A(q) and so on. Let

$$K = \begin{bmatrix} -k_1 & -k_2 \cdots & -k_i & & 0 \\ & & & -k_{i+1} & \\ & & & & \cdots \\ 0 & & & & -k_n \end{bmatrix}$$

where $k_1, k_2, \cdots, k_n$ are design parameters. In the sequel, we will compute $k_1, k_2, \cdots, k_n$ through an iterative procedure.

Step 1: Consider the system $\Sigma(A_1(q), B_1(q))$ where $B_1(q) \triangleq (0\,0 \ldots \theta_1)'$. Let

$K_1 \triangleq (-k_1\ -k_2 \cdots -k_i)$, $G_1 \triangleq (1\ -k_1\ -k_2 \cdots -k_i)$, $S_1 \triangleq (s^i\ s^{i-1} \ldots s\ 1)$ and

$$P_1(s,K_1,q) \triangleq \det(sI - A_1(q) - B_1(q)K_1).$$

Expanding the determinant through the last row yields

$$P_1(s, K_1,q) = S_1\Phi_1(q)G_1.$$

By the hypothesis of the theorem, $\Phi_1(q)$ has Hurwitz antisymmetry property. It follows from lemma 4.4 that one can find $k_1\ k_2 \cdots k_i$ so that $P_1(s, K_1,q)$ is a Hurwitz invariant polynomial with a sign invariant leading coefficient.

Step 2: Now consider the system $\Sigma(A_2(q), B_2(q))$ where

$$B_2(q) = \begin{bmatrix} 0 & 0 \\ \vdots & \vdots \\ 0 & 0 \\ \theta_1 & 0 \\ b_{21} & \theta_2 \end{bmatrix}.$$

Let

$$K_2 = \begin{bmatrix} -k_1 & -k_2 & \cdots & -k_i & 0 \\ 0 & 0 & \cdots & 0 & -k_{i+1} \end{bmatrix}.$$

A straightforward computation yields

$$\begin{aligned} P_2(s,K_2,q) &= \det(sI - A_2(q) - B_2(q)K_2) \\ &= k_{i+1}\theta_2(q)P_1(s,K_1,q) + f_1(s,q,K_1) \end{aligned}$$

where $f_1(s,q,K_1)$ is an (i+1)th-order uncertain polynomial with a sign invariant leading coefficient and $\theta_2(q)$ is a sign invariant uncertain function. It follows from Lemma 4.5 that there exists a k_{i+1} such that $P_2(s,K_2,q)$ is again a Hurwitz invariant polynomial with a sign invariant leading coefficient.

Step 3: Continue the above iterative procedure. One can find $k_{i+2}, k_{i+3}, \cdots, k_n$ to guarantee that

$$P(s,K,q) \triangleq \det(sI - A(q) - B_0(q)K)$$

is Hurwitz invariant for all $q \in Q$. []

Proof of Theorem 3.4: Consider

$$\begin{aligned} P'(s,K,q) &= \det(T(q)(sI-A(q)-B(q)K)) \\ &= \det(T(q)) \det(sI-A(q)-B(q)K) \\ &= \det(T(q)P(s,K,q)). \end{aligned}$$

Since $\det(T(q)) \neq 0$ for all $q \in Q$, the characteristic polynomial $P(s,K,q) \triangleq \det(sI-A(q)-B(q)K)$ is Hurwitz invariant if and only if $P'(s,K,q)$ is Hurwitz invariant. However,

$$\begin{aligned} P'(s,K,q) &= \det(T(q)(sI-A(q)) - T(q)B(q)K) \\ &= \det(T(q)(sI-A(q)) - B_0(q)K) \\ &= \det(sT(q) - T(q)A(q) - B_0(q)K). \end{aligned}$$

Now one can follow the similar procedure as in Proof of Theorem 3.1 to construct control gain K guaranteeing that $P'(s,K,q)$ is Hurwitz invariant. []

VI. ILLUSTRATIVE EXAMPLE

To illustrate our main results, we take a practical problem on Boeing 929 Jetfoil from Clark (1978). The system under consideration is described by $\Sigma(A(q), B(q))$:

$$\dot{x}(t) = A(q)x(t) + B(q)u(t)\ ;\ t \geq 0$$

where $q \in Q = \{1,2,3\}$ and

$$A(1) = \begin{bmatrix} -11.8 & -0.63 & -4.25 & 29.6 \\ 1 & 0 & 0 & 0 \\ -0.9 & 0.036 & -4.1 & 3.1 \\ 0.97 & 0.56 & -0.8 & 3.4 \end{bmatrix}; \quad B(1) = \begin{bmatrix} 10 & -8.5 \\ 0 & 0 \\ -0.06 & 3.73 \\ 0 & 0.98 \end{bmatrix};$$

$$A(2) = \begin{bmatrix} -12.98 & -0.693 & -4.675 & 32.56 \\ 1 & 0 & 0 & 0 \\ -0.99 & 0.0396 & -4.51 & 3.41 \\ 1.067 & 0.616 & -0.88 & -3.74 \end{bmatrix}; \quad B(2) = \begin{bmatrix} 11 & -9.35 \\ 0 & 0 \\ -0.066 & 4.103 \\ 0 & 1.078 \end{bmatrix};$$

$$A(3) = \begin{bmatrix} -10.9 & -0.63 & -3.92 & 27.3 \\ 1 & 0 & 0 & 0 \\ -0.82 & 0.036 & -3.7 & 2.7 \\ 0.87 & 0.56 & -0.73 & -3.1 \end{bmatrix}; \quad B(3) = \begin{bmatrix} 10 & -7.83 \\ 0 & 0 \\ -0.06 & 3.36 \\ 0 & 0.88 \end{bmatrix}.$$

Our objective is to determine if there exists a single constant static feedback control which can stabilize all the three systems. If so, we then design a desired control. To apply our method, let

$$T(1) = \begin{bmatrix} 1 & 0 & 500/3 & -625.6803 \\ 0 & 1 & 0 & 0 \\ 0 & 0 & 1 & -3.8061 \\ 0 & 0 & 0 & 1 \end{bmatrix};$$

$$T(2) = \begin{bmatrix} 1 & 0 & 500/3 & -625.6803 \\ 0 & 1 & 0 & 0 \\ 0 & 0 & 1 & -3.8061 \\ 0 & 0 & 0 & 1 \end{bmatrix};$$

$$T(3) = \begin{bmatrix} 1 & 0 & 500/3 & -627.4659 \\ 0 & 1 & 0 & 0 \\ 0 & 0 & 1 & -3.8182 \\ 0 & 0 & 0 & 1 \end{bmatrix}.$$

We obtain

$$T(1)A(1) = \begin{bmatrix} -768.71 & -345.01 & -187.04 & -1581.05 \\ 1 & 0 & 0 & 0 \\ -4.59 & -2.10 & -1.06 & -9.84 \\ 0.97 & 0.56 & -0.8 & 3.4 \end{bmatrix}; \quad T(1)B(1) = \begin{bmatrix} 0 & 0 \\ 0 & 0 \\ -0.06 & 0 \\ 0 & 0.98 \end{bmatrix};$$

$$T(2)A(2) = \begin{bmatrix} -845.58 & -379.51 & -205.74 & 2940.94 \\ 1 & 0 & 0 & 0 \\ -5.05 & -2.30 & -1.16 & 17.64 \\ 1.067 & 0.616 & -0.88 & -3.74 \end{bmatrix}; \quad T(2)B(2) = \begin{bmatrix} 0 & 0 \\ 0 & 0 \\ -0.066 & 0 \\ 0 & 1.078 \end{bmatrix};$$

$$T(3)A(3) = \begin{bmatrix} -693.46 & -346.01 & -162.54 & 2422.44 \\ 1 & 0 & 0 & 0 \\ -4.142 & -2.102 & -0.913 & 14.536 \\ 0.87 & 0.56 & -0.73 & -3.1 \end{bmatrix}; \quad T(3)B(3) = \begin{bmatrix} 0 & 0 \\ 0 & 0 \\ -0.06 & 0 \\ 0 & 0.88 \end{bmatrix}.$$

By Theorem 3.4 we only need check the first two rows of sT(q)-T(q)A(q). It is easy to see that the submatrix M(s,q) containing the entries in the column 1, 2, 3 have Hurwitz property. In fact, the coefficient matrix $\Phi(q)$ of M(s,q) is

$$\Phi(1) = \begin{bmatrix} 1 & 166.67 & 0 \\ 768.71 & 187.04 & -166.67 \\ 345.01 & 0 & -187.04 \end{bmatrix};$$

$$\Phi(2) = \begin{bmatrix} 1 & 166.67 & 0 \\ 845.58 & 205.74 & -166.67 \\ 379.51 & 0 & -205.74 \end{bmatrix};$$

$$\Phi(3) = \begin{bmatrix} 1 & 166.67 & 0 \\ 693.46 & 162.54 & -166.67 \\ 346.01 & 0 & -162.54 \end{bmatrix}$$

and the last two columns of $\Phi(q)$ can be permuted to an antisymmetric matrix with a Hurwitz core. Hence, we conclude that the system is robust stabilizable.

To design a robust controller, let

$$K = \begin{bmatrix} 0 & k_1 & k_2 & 0 \\ 0 & 0 & 0 & k_3 \end{bmatrix}.$$

Following the computation procedure given in Section V, we obtain a robust stabilizer as follows:

$$K = \begin{bmatrix} 0 & -8 & 4 & 0 \\ 0 & 0 & 0 & -9 \end{bmatrix}.$$

The eigenvalues of the three closed loop systems are -18.8940, -1.2511± 8.4768 i, -0.1638; -25.1524, -2.4591± 10.5177 i, -1.1254 and -20.4995, -2.1652± 9.6176, -1.0301, respectively. Hence, the closed loop systems are stable.

VII. CONCLUSION

In the paper, we provided sufficient conditions under which a family of multi-input dynamic systems are simultaneously stabilizable by a single constant feedback controller. A concreat synthesis method is also given to design a desired robust controller.

With regard to further research, it may be possible to provide some degree of relaxation on the antisymmetry requirement. Also, it is possible to generate the result to the cases where the eigenvalues of the closed loop system are required in some special regions of the complex plane.

REFERENCES

Ackermann, J. (1980). Parameter space design of robust control systems. IEEE Trans. Aut. Control, **AC-25**, 1058.

Ackermann, J. (1985). Design of robust controllers by multi-model method. Proc. 7th Symp. on Math. Theory of Networks and Systems, Stockholm.

Barmish, B. R. (1988). A generalization of Kharitonov's four polynomial concept for robust stability problems with linearly dependent coefficient perturbations. Proc. of the American Control Conference, Atlanta.

Bartlett, A. C., C. V. Hollot and Huang Lin (1988).Root locations of an entire polytope of polynomials: It suffices to check the edges. Math. of Control, Signal and Systems, **1**, 61.

Clark, R. N. (1978). Instrument fault detection. IEEE Trans. Aerosp. Electron. Syst. **AES-14**, 456.

Franklin, S. N. and J. Ackermann (1981). Robust fight control: A design example. J. Guidance Control, **4**, 597.

Kharitonov, C. L. (1978). Asymptotic stability of an equilibrium position of a family of linear differetial equations. Differensialnye Uravneniya, **14**, 2086.

Kreisselmeier, G. and R. Steinhauser (1983). Application of vector performance optimization to robust control loop design for a fighter aircraft. Int. J. Control, **37**, 251.

Patel, R. V., M. Toda and B. Sridhar (1977). Robustness of linear quadratic state feedback designs in the presence of system uncertainty. IEEE Trans. Aut. Control, **AC-22**, 290.

Wei, K. H. and B. R. Barmish (1985). On making a polynomial Hurwitz invariant by choice of feedback gains. Proc. of 24th IEEE Conference on Decision and Control, Fort Lauderdale.

Yedavalli, R. K., (1985). Perturbation bounds for robust stability in linear state space model. Int. J. Control, **42**, 1507.

U–PARAMETER DESIGN: FEEDBACK SYSTEM DESIGN WITH GUARANTEED ROBUST STABILITY

Peter Dorato, Yunzhi Li and Hong Bae Park

Department of Electrical and Computer Engineering
University of New Mexico
Albuquerque, NM 87131, U.S.A.

INTRODUCTION

We propose here an extension of the Q–parameter design technique developed by Youla, Jabr and Bongiorno [1], and Desoer, Liu, Murray, and Saeks [2] for the design of nominally stable closed-loop systems. The basic idea behind the Q–parameter approach is the characterization of all compensators, which guarantee closed-loop stability for a nominal plant, in terms of a compensator parameter Q(s), where Q(s) is an arbitrary stable function. Here stable is taken to be BIBO stable, i.e., Q(s) is proper and all its poles have negative real parts. This free parameter function, Q(s), is then used to design a nominally optimal system, or to meet other design objectives. Boyd et al. [3] exploit this parameterization to develop computer-aided design software which permits the minimization of a performance measure, while simultaneously meeting a set of additional deisgn specifications. The key point is that with Q–parameterization many design specifications reduce to convex constraints on the Q(s) function space, and by further parameterization of Q(s), the optimal design problem can be reduced to a convex programming in a finite dimensional space. However, the Q–parameterization approach only guarantees stability of a fixed "nominal" plant. No robustness of the solution is assured for plant uncertainties. To provide for the design of closed-loop systems which are guaranteed to be robustly stable, we propose a "U–parameterization" of the compensator in terms of an arbitrary strongly bounded real (SBR) function, U(s). We define an SBR function as a function U(s) with the usual properties:

(i) U(s) is real for s real
(ii) U(s) is analytic for $\text{Re}\, s \geq 0$
(iii) $|U(j\omega)| < 1$, all real ω.

It is well known, see for example Kimura [4], that for additive unstructured plant perturbations the compensator which guarantees robust stabilization can be expressed in the "fractional" form

$$C(s) = \frac{A(s)\,U(s) + B(s)}{C(s)\,U(s) + D(s)} \tag{1}$$

where U(s) is an arbitrary SBR function. It is also known, see for example Dorato, Park and Li [5], that compensators which guarantee simultaneous stabilization of two plants can also be written in the form (1), where U(s) is an arbitrary SBR function. We propose then that this free SBR parameter-function U(s) be used to minimize a performance measure for the nominal system, or be used to meet other specifications for the nominal system. This then guarantees a closed-loop system which is optimal when the plant is at its nominal value, and is at least stable as the plant is perturbed from its nominal value.

The development here is limited to linear, single-input-single-output systems characterized by plants with rational transfer functions.

REVIEW OF Q–PARAMETER DESIGN

There are two major approaches to Q–parameterization. One is the Bezout-identity approach as developed in references [1] and [2]. The other is the interpolation approach used in Zames and Francis [6] for the H^∞ sensitivity minimization problem. We review here the latter approach to Q–parameterization. It is shown in [6] that if the compensator C(s) is parameterized by the stable function Q(s), via the equation

$$C(s) = \frac{Q(s)}{1 - P(s)\,Q(s)}\,, \tag{2}$$

where

$$Q(s) = B_p(s)\,\tilde{Q}(s) + B_p^2(s)\,Q_1(s)\,, \tag{3}$$

with $B_p(s)$ given by the Blaschke product

$$B_p(s) = \prod_i \left[\frac{\alpha_i - s}{\bar{\alpha}_i + s}\right], \tag{4}$$

where α_i are the poles of the plant P(s) in Res > 0, then the closed-loop system will be nominally internally stable for <u>any</u> stable $Q_1(s)$, if $\tilde{Q}(s)$ is a stable function which interpolates to $\tilde{Q}(\alpha_i) = 1/\tilde{P}(\alpha_i)$ where $\tilde{P}(s) = B_p(s)\,P(s)$. Here the free design parameter is the arbitrary stable function $Q_1(s)$. A critical property of Q–parameterization is that key transfer functions for the closed-loop system are affine in the Q–parameter. For example, the sensitivity function is given by

$$S(s) = \frac{1}{1 + P(s)\,C(s)} = 1 - P(s)\,Q(s) \tag{5}$$

This fact is exploited in [6] to obtain a solution to the H^∞ weighted sensitivity problem where the Q–parameter is selected to minimize the H^∞ norm,

$$\| S(s)\, W(s) \|_\infty \tag{6}$$

and in [1] where it is used to minimize H^2 matrix norms for multiple-input-multiple-output systems.

Also, as noted in the introduction, many design specifications translate into convex constraints on the parameter Q.

To summarize, by introduction of the Q–parameter in the compensator one can guarantee stability of the nominal closed loop system and obtain closed-loop transfer functions which are affine in Q. Optimal design problems can then be reduced to a minimization problem of the form

$$\inf_{Q(s) \in K} \| T_1(s) + T_2(s)\, Q(s) \| \tag{7}$$

where $\| \bullet \|$ is a suitable norm and K is the class of stable transfer functions, or if additional specifications are to be met, as in reference [3], a convex set of stable transfer functions.

SIMULTANEOUS AND ROBUST STABILITY THEORY

It is shown in Vidyasagar and Viswanadham [7], that two plants $P_0(s)$ and $P_1(s)$ can be simultaneously stabilized by a fixed compensator if and only if the "difference" plant $P_1(s) - P_0(s)$ can be stabilized by a stable compensator. It is further shown in [7] that C(s) can be computed, when it exists, from

$$C(s) = R(s)\,(1 - R(s)\, P_0(s))^{-1} \tag{8}$$

where $R(s) = (U(s) - D_A(s))/N_A(s)$ and U(s) is a unit in H^∞ (a stable function whose inverse is also stable) which interpolates to $U(\alpha_i) = D_A(\alpha_i)$, where α_i are the zeros of $N_A(s)$ in Res > 0, and $N_A(s)$ and $D_A(s)$ are stable functions in the fractional representation of $P_1(s) - P_0(s)$, i.e., $P_1 - P_0 = N_A\, D_A^{-1}$. In reference [5] it is shown that all units which meet the above interpolation conditions can be parameterized by an arbitrary strongly bounded real function U(s). From the form of C(s) given by (8) it then follows that all compensators which guarantee the simultaneous stabilization of two plants can be written in the form (1) where U(s) is an arbitrary SBR function. In reference [5] an algorithm is generated for interpolation with units which leads to functions A(s), B(s), C(s), and D(s) with lowest possible degree. This is critical if the degree of the compensator is to be kept as low as possible.

In reference [4] it is shown that a compensator of the form (2) will yield a closed-loop system which is stable for all perturbed plants $P(s) = P_0(s) + \delta P(s)$ with perturbations bounded by

$$| \delta P(j\omega) | \leq | r(j\omega) | , \text{ all real } \omega \tag{9}$$

if Q(s) is given by

$$Q(s) = \frac{B_p(s)\, U(s)}{r(s)} \tag{10}$$

where U(s) is an SBR function which interpolates to the points $U(\alpha_i) = \beta_i$ where

$$\beta_i = \frac{r(\alpha_i)}{\widetilde{P}_0(\alpha_i)} \tag{11}$$

In the above formulas $B_p(s)$ is the Blaschke product given in (4), $\widetilde{P}_0(s) = B_p(s)\, P_0(s)$, and r(s) is a given stable function with all its zeros in Res < 0 which bounds the plant perturbation. From the classical Nevanlinna-Pick interpolation theory, see for example Delsarte et al. [8], it is known that all SBR functions which interpolate given points in Res > 0 can be parameterized in terms of an arbitrary SBR function and that U(s) can be written

$$U(s) = \frac{A_1(s)\, U_1(s) + B_1(s)}{C_1(s)\, U_1(s) + D_1(s)} \tag{12}$$

where $A_1(s)$, $B_1(s)$, $C_1(s)$, and $D_1(s)$ are fixed functions and $U_1(s)$ is an arbitrary SBR fuction. It is this function $U_1(s)$ that can be used for further design, i.e. nominal H^2 or H^∞ optimization. With U(s) given by (12) one once more obtains a compensator of the form given in (1), with U(s) replaced by $U_1(s)$. Algorithms for the computation of A_1, B_1, C_1, and D_1 in (12) are given in Krein and Nudelman [9] and Dorato and Li [10].

U–PARAMETER DESIGN

From the discussion in the previous section it follows that the compensator which guarantees either simultaneous stabilization of two-plants or robust stabilization for additive unstructured plant perturbations can always be parameterized as in (1), where U(s) is an arbitrary SBR function. The algorithms for the computation of the functions A(s), B(s), C(s), and D(s) given in references [5] and [10] represent the best available algorithms in the sense that the degree of the functions are lower than other existing algorithms for interpolation with units or SBR functions. As previously noted this is important in keeping down the complexity of the compensator C(s). If the sensitivity function; or some other transfer function of interest, is written in terms of U(s) it will in general be of the fractional form

$$\frac{T_1(s)\,U(s) + T_2(s)}{T_3(s)\,U(s) + T_4(s)} \tag{13}$$

where T_1, T_2, T_3, and T_4 are known functions and U(s) is an arbitrary SBR function. By suitable rationalization these known functions can always by expressed as polynomial functions. Thus U–parameterization leads to a fractional form for transfer functions; rather than the affine form generated by Q–parameterization. This will, of course, complicate any optimization problem defined on a transfer function, however by further parameterization of the U–parameter-function; for example by using polynomial coefficients as design parameters, the optimization problem can be reduced to a nonlinear programming problem. A general U–parameter optimization problem, in terms of a norm $\| \bullet \|$ may be expressed as

$$\inf_{U(s) \in B} \left\| \frac{T_1(s)\,U(s) + T_2(s)}{T_3(s)\,U(s) + T_4(s)} \right\| \tag{14}$$

where B is the set of SBR functions. The solution of the optimization problem in (14) then yields a closed-loop system which is nominally optimal <u>and</u> robustly stable. While general analytical solutions of this optimization problem are not currently available, specific problems can be solved by nonlinear programming techniques. A simple example illustrating the U–parameter design approach follows.

EXAMPLE

Consider the problem of designing a compensator which minimizes the H^2–norm of weighted sensitivty

$$\| S(s)\, W(s) \|_2 = \left(\int_{-\infty}^{\infty} | S(j\omega)\, W(j\omega) |^2 \, d\omega \right)^{1/2}$$

for the nominal plant $P_0(s) = (1-s)/(2-s)(1+s)$ with weighting function $W(s) = 1/(s+1)$, while guaranteeing that the closed-loop system is robustly stable for all plant perturbations which satisfy $| \delta P(j\omega) | \leq 1/20$, for all real ω.

In this case $B_p(s) = (2-s)/(2+s)$, $r(s) = 1/20$, and from robust stabilization theory, see for example [4] or [5], the required compensator is given by $C(s) = Q(s)/(1-P_0(s)\,Q(s))$ where

$$Q(s) = \frac{20(2-s)}{(2+s)} \bullet \frac{-0.6 + \left(\frac{2-s}{2+s}\right) U(s)}{1 - 0.6\left(\frac{2-s}{2+s}\right) U(s)}$$

where U(s) is an arbitrary SBR function. The compensator in this case is given by (1) with

$$A(s) = 20s^3 - 60s^2 + 80$$

$$B(s) = 12s^3 + 12s^2 - 48s - 48$$

$$C(s) = 0.6s^3 - 19.4s^2 + 57.6s - 42.4$$

$$D(s) = s^3 - 7s^2 - 4s + 28$$

and the weighted sensitivity is given by (14) with

$$T_1(s) = 0.6s^3 - 19.4s^2 + 57.6s - 42.4$$

$$T_2(s) = s^3 - 7s^2 - 4s + 28$$

$$T_3(s) = 0.6s^4 + 1.2s^3 - 1.8s^2 - 4.8s - 2.4$$

$$T_4(s) = s^4 + 6s^3 + 13s^2 + 12s + 4$$

The simplest choice for U(s) is $U(s) = \alpha$, where $|\alpha| < 1$. If the parameter-function U(s) is further parameterized this way, the following nonlinear programming problem results

$$\inf_{|\alpha| < 1} \phi(\alpha)$$

where $\phi(\alpha) = \| S(s)\, W(s) \|_2$ is evaluated from integral tables. The solution of this one-dimensional constrained optimization problem is given by $\alpha = 0.42$ with a performance value of $\phi = 8.1898$ (compared with $\phi = 12.5000$ for $\alpha = 0$).

CONCLUSIONS

We have outlined here a design approach which permits optimal design for nominal plant operation while guaranteeing robust stability of the closed-loop system for the perturbed plant operation. This is an extension to the control of uncertain systems of the Q-parameter design approach, which allows for optimization of a nominal plant while guaranteeing only nominal closed-loop stability. We refer to this new approach as the U-parameter approach. The interpolation algorithms developed for units in H^∞ in [5] and SBR functions in [10] are especially pertinent to this approach, since they result in compensators with low degrees of complexity. While all the analytical machinery available for the Q-parameter theory is not available in the U-parameter theory, specific problems can be reduced to standard nonlinear programming probelms. Further examples and details on the U-parameter design approach may be found in Li [11].

REFERENCES

[1] D.C. Youla, H.A. Jabr and J.J. Bongiorno, Jr., "Modern Wiener-Hopf Design of Optimal Controllers – Part II: The Multivariable Case," IEEE Trans. Automat. Contr., Vol. AC–21, No. 3, pp. 319–338, June 1976.

[2] C.A. Desoer, R–W. Liu, J. Murray, and R. Saeks, "Feedback System Design: The Fractional Representation Approach to Analysis and Synthesis," IEEE Trans. Automat. Contr., Vol. AC–25, No. 3, pp. 399–412, June 1980.

[3] S.P. Boyd, V. Balakrishnan, C.H. Barratt, N.M. Khraishi, X.M. Li, D.G. Meyer, and S.A. Norman, "A new CAD Method and Associated Architectures for Linear Controllers," IEEE Trans. Automat. Contr., Vol. AC–33, No. 3, pp. 268–283, March 1988.

[4] H. Kimura, "Robust Stabilization for a Class of Transfer Functions," IEEE Trans. Automat. Contr., Vol. AC–29, No. 9, pp. 788–793, September 1984.

[5] P. Dorato, H–B. Park, and Yunzhi Li, "An Algorithm for Interpolation with Units in H^∞, with Applications to Feedback Stabilization," to be published in Automatica, May 1989.

[6] G. Zames and B.A. Francis, "Feedback, Minimax Sensitivity, and Optimal Robustness," IEEE Trans. Automat. Contr., Vol. AC–28, No. 5, pp. 585–601, May 1983.

[7] M. Vidyasagar and N. Viswanadham, "Algebraic Design Techniques for Reliable Stabilization," IEEE Trans. Automat. Contr., Vol. AC–27, No. 5, pp. 1085–1095, October 1982.

[8] Ph. Delsarte, Y. Genin and Y. Kamp, "On the Role of the Nevanlinna-Pick Problem in Circuit and System Theory," Int. J. Circuit Theory Appl., Vol. 9, pp. 177–187, 1981.

[9] M.G. Krein and A.A. Nudelman, The Markov Moment Problem and External Problems, Translations of Mathematical Monographs, Vol. 50, American Mathematical Society, Providence, Rhode Island, 1977.

[10] P. Dorato and Yunzhi Li, "A Modification of the Classical Nevanlinna-Pick Interpolation Algorithm with Applications to Robust Stabilization," IEEE Trans. Automat. Contr., Vol. 31, No. 7, pp. 645–648, July 1986.

[11] Yunzhi Li, "U–Parameter Design: Feedback System Design with Guaranteed Robust Stability," Ph.D. Dissertation, Department of Electrical and Computer Engineering, University of New Mexico, 1989.

NEW CRITERIA FOR ROBUST STABILITY[1]

M. Corless and D. Da
School of Aeronautics and Astronautics
Purdue University
West Lafayette
Indiana

ABSTRACT

We consider a class of uncertain systems whose uncertainties are characterized by certain structural conditions and a known bound. Given that the "nominal system" has a "Lyapunov matrix" P we present conditions on the uncertainty bound which assure that P is also a Lyapunov matrix for the uncertain system.

1. INTRODUCTION AND PROBLEM STATEMENT

Consider a system described by

$$\dot{x}(t) = f^o(t, x(t)) \tag{1.1}$$

where $t \in \mathbb{R}$ is "time", $x(t) \in \mathbb{R}^n$ is the state, and $f^o : \mathbb{R} \times \mathbb{R}^n \to \mathbb{R}^n$. Suppose that P belongs to P^n, the set of positive-definite symmetric members of $\mathbb{R}^{n \times n}$. We say that P is a *Lyapunov Matrix (LM)* for (1.1) iff there exists a matrix $Q \in P^n$ such that

$$x^T P f^o(t, x) \le -\|x\|_Q^2 \qquad \forall t \in \mathbb{R},\ x \in \mathbb{R}^n, \tag{1.2}$$

where

$$\|x\|_Q \triangleq (x^T Q x)^{1/2} . \tag{1.3}$$

From a stability viewpoint, the existence of P as a LM for (1.1) has the following significance. If $x(\cdot) : [t_o, t_1) \to \mathbb{R}^n$ is any solution of (1.1), then

$$\|x(t)\| \le c(x_o) e^{-\alpha(t - t_0)} \tag{1.4}$$

for all $t \ge t_o$ where $x_o \triangleq x(t_0)$ and [2]

[1] This paper is based on research supported by NSF under Grant MSM-87-06927.

[2] If all the eigenvalues of $M \in \mathbb{R}^{n \times n}$ are real, $\lambda_m(M)$ and $\lambda_M(M)$ denote the minimum and maximum eigenvalues, respectively, of M.

$$c(x_o) \triangleq \|x_o\|_P / \lambda_m(P)^{1/2}\,, \qquad \alpha \triangleq \lambda_m(P^{-1}Q)\,, \tag{1.5}$$

i.e., (1.1) is *globally, uniformly, exponentially, stable* about zero with rate $\alpha > 0$; see Refs. 3, 5.

Consider now an *uncertain system* described by

$$\dot{x}(t) = f(t, x(t), \omega) \tag{1.6a}$$

$$\omega \in \Omega \tag{1.6b}$$

where Ω is some known, non-empty set and $f : \mathbb{R} \times \mathbb{R}^n \times \Omega \to \mathbb{R}^n$ is known. All the uncertainty in the system is represented by the lumped uncertain element ω. This uncertain element could be an element of $\mathbb{R}^q$ representing unknown constant parameters; it could be a function from $\mathbb{R}$ into $\mathbb{R}^q$ representing unknown time varying parameters; it could also be a function from $\mathbb{R} \times \mathbb{R}^n$ into $\mathbb{R}^q$ representing nonlinear elements which are difficult to characterize. Each $\omega \in \Omega$ specifies a function $f(\cdot, \omega) : \mathbb{R} \times \mathbb{R}^n \to \mathbb{R}^n$.

We say that $P \in \mathcal{P}^n$ is a *Common Lyapunov Matrix (CLM)* for (1.6) iff there exists a matrix $Q \in \mathcal{P}^n$ such that for every uncertainty $\omega \in \Omega$,

$$x^T P f(t, x, \omega) \le -\|x\|_Q^2 \tag{1.7}$$

for all $t \in \mathbb{R}$ and $x \in \mathbb{R}^n$.

Clearly, the existence of a CLM for (1.6) implies that (1.6a) is exponentially stable with a rate which is independent of ω.

In this paper, we consider uncertain systems described by (1.6) with

$$f(t, x, \omega) = f^o(t, x) + \beta \Delta f(t, x, \omega) \tag{1.8a}$$

where $\beta \in \mathbb{R}_+$,

$$\Delta f(t, x, \omega) = \sum_{j=1}^{L} D_j g_j(t, x, \omega)\,, \tag{1.8b}$$

$D_j \in \mathbb{R}^{n \times k_j}$, $j = 1, 2, \ldots, L$, and

$$\{(g_1(t, x, \omega), g_2(t, x, \omega), \ldots, g_L(t, x, \omega)) : \omega \in \Omega\}$$
$$= \{(v_1, v_2, \ldots, v_L) : v_j \in \mathbb{R}^{k_j}, \|v_j\| \le \|E_j x\|, j = 1, 2, \ldots, L\} \tag{1.8c}$$

for some $E_j \in \mathbb{R}^{l_j \times n}$, $j = 1, 2, \ldots, L$.

Thus, a system under consideration here can be described by

$$\dot{x} = f^o(t, x) + \beta \sum_{j=1}^{L} D_j g_j(t, x, \omega) \tag{1.9a}$$

where

$$\|g_j(t, x, \omega)\| \le \|E_j x\|\,, \qquad j = 1, 2, \ldots, L, \qquad \forall\, \omega \in \Omega\,. \tag{1.9b}$$

The known matrices D_j and E_j describe the structure of the uncertain terms.

As an example, consider a system with uncertain matrices $\omega_j \in \mathbb{R}^{k_j \times l_j}$, $j = 1, 2, \ldots, L$, described by (1.6) with

$$f(t, x, \omega) = Ax + \beta \sum_{j=1}^{L} D_j \omega_j E_j x \tag{1.10a}$$

where $A \in \mathbb{R}^{n \times n}$ and

$$\omega \in \Omega = \{(\omega_1, \omega_2, \ldots, \omega_L) : \omega_j \in \mathbb{R}^{k_j \times l_j}, \|\omega_j\| \le 1, j = 1, 2, \ldots, L\}\,. \tag{1.10b}$$

In this example,

$$f^o(t, x) = Ax \ , \tag{1.11}$$
$$g_j(t, x, \omega) = \omega_j E_j x \ .$$

Remark 1.1. Some of the literature on stability robustness of uncertain systems considers an uncertain term of the form

$$\Delta f(t, x, \omega) = \sum_{j=1}^{L} \omega_j(t, x) A_j x \tag{1.12a}$$

where $A_j \in \mathbb{R}^{n \times n}$, $\omega_j(t,x) \in \mathbb{R}$, $j = 1,2, ...,L$, and Ω is the set of continuous functions $\omega : \mathbb{R} \times \mathbb{R}^n \to \mathbb{R}^L$ which satisfy

$$|\omega_j(t, x)| \leq 1 \quad , \quad j = 1,2, ... L \tag{1.12b}$$

for all $t \in \mathbb{R}$ and $x \in \mathbb{R}^n$; e.g., see Refs. 1, 2, 6, 19-24.

If each matrix A_j has rank one then Δf can be described by (1.8) as follows. Since A_j has rank one, there exist matrices $D_j \in \mathbb{R}^{n \times 1}$ and $E_j \in \mathbb{R}^{1 \times n}$ such that

$$A_j = D_j E_j \qquad ;$$

hence

$$\Delta f(t, x, \omega) = \sum_{j=1}^{L} D_j \, g_j \, (t, x, \omega)$$

where

$$g_j(t, x, \omega) = \omega_j(t, x) E_j x$$

and (1.8b) holds.

We consider the following problem. Suppose the *nominal system,*

$$\dot{x} = f^o(t, x) \tag{1.13}$$

has P as a LM. Find a bound $\bar{\beta} > 0$ such that for each $\beta < \bar{\beta}$, P is a CLM for the uncertain system (1.6), (1.8). Such a bound can be regarded as a *measure* of *robustness* of the system's stability with respect to uncertainties whose structure is characterized by the matrices D_j, E_j, $j = 1, 2, ..., L$.

2. A NECESSARY AND SUFFICIENT CONDITION

For systems in which equality holds identically in (1.2), the following lemma provides a necessary and sufficient condition for P to be a CLM for the uncertain system (1.6), (1.8).

Lemma 2.1. Suppose P is a LM for the nominal system (1.13) and

$$x^T P f^o(t, x) = -\|x\|_Q^2 \qquad \forall t \in \mathbb{R} \, , x \in \mathbb{R}^n \tag{2.1}$$

with $Q \in \mathcal{P}^n$. Let

$$\beta^* \triangleq \delta^{-1} \ , \tag{2.2}$$
$$\delta \triangleq \max\left\{ \sum_{j=1}^{L} \|D_j^T P x\| \, \|E_j x\| : x \in \mathbb{R}^n \, , \, \|x\|_Q^2 = 1 \right\} .$$

Then P is a CLM for the uncertain system (1.6), (1.8) iff

$$\beta < \beta^* \ . \tag{2.3}$$

Proof. Ref. 4 contains a proof. □

For systems satisfying (1.2), it can readily be seen from the proof of Lemma 2.1 that, (2.3) is a *sufficient condition* for P to be a CLM for (1.6), (1.8).

For systems satisfying (2.1), β^* is the largest measure of robustness for the given LM. However, its computation involves solving a constrained optimization problem. For this reason, the next section presents robustness measures which can be more conservative than β^* but which are easier to compute.

3. SUFFICIENT CONDITIONS

For a prescribed LM for the nominal system, the following lemma yields a robustness measure which depends on the choice of an arbitrary matrix $R \in P^n$

Lemma 3.1. Suppose P is a LM for the nominal system (1.13); consider any $R \in P^n$ and let

$$\begin{aligned} \bar{\beta}(R) &\triangleq \gamma(R)^{-1} , \\ \gamma(R) &\triangleq \sum_{j=1}^{L} \gamma_j(R) , \\ \gamma_j(R) &\triangleq [\lambda_M(R^{-1}PD_jD_j^TP)\lambda_M(R^{-1}E_j^TE_j)]^{1/2}\lambda_M(Q^{-1}R) , \end{aligned} \tag{3.1}$$

where $Q \in P^n$ satisfies (1.2).

If

$$\beta < \bar{\beta}(R) \tag{3.2}$$

then P is a CLM for the uncertain system (1.6), (1.8).

Proof. The proof proceeds by showing that

$$x^T Pf(t, x, \omega) \leq -[1 - \beta / \bar{\beta}(R)]\lambda_m(R^{-1}Q)\|x\|_R^2 \tag{3.3}$$

for all $t \in \mathbb{R}$, $x \in \mathbb{R}^n$, $\omega \in \Omega$. The details are given in Ref. 4. □

The above lemma provides a robustness measure $\bar{\beta}(R)$ which depends on the choice of an arbitrary matrix $R \in P^n$. This suggests the question of the existence of a best R. This question is answered in the next lemma.

Lemma 3.2. Consider any $P, Q \in P^n$. Then

$$\bar{\beta}(R) \leq \bar{\beta}(Q) \qquad \forall R \in P^n$$

where $\bar{\beta}(R)$ is defined in (3.2).

Proof. Consider any $R \in P^n$. Clearly, it suffices to show that

$$\gamma_j(Q)^2 \leq \gamma_j(R)^2 \qquad j = 1, 2, \ldots, L, \tag{3.4}$$

where

$$\begin{aligned} \gamma_j(Q)^2 &= \lambda_M(Q^{-1}PD_jD_j^TP)\lambda_M(Q^{-1}E_j^TE_j) , \\ \gamma_j(R)^2 &= \lambda_M(R^{-1}PD_jD_j^TP)\lambda_M(R^{-1}E_j^TE_j)\lambda_M(Q^{-1}R)^2 . \end{aligned} \tag{3.5}$$

Utilizing Lemma 6.1 (see Appendix), one obtains

$$\begin{aligned} \lambda_M(Q^{-1}E_j^TE_j) &\leq \lambda_M(Q^{-1}R)\lambda_M(R^{-1}E_j^TE_j) , \\ \lambda_M(Q^{-1}PD_jD_j^TP) &\leq \lambda_M(Q^{-1}R)\lambda_M(R^{-1}PD_jD_j^TP) , \end{aligned}$$

hence, recalling (3.5), one can readily see that (3.4) holds. □

4. A NONLINEAR EXAMPLE

Consider an uncertain nonlinear system described by

$$\dot{x}_1 = -x_1 + x_1 x_2^2 \tag{4.1a}$$

$$\dot{x}_2 = -x_2 - x_1^2 x_2 + \beta\omega(t, x) \tag{4.1b}$$

$$\omega \in \Omega \tag{4.1c}$$

where $x_1, x_2 \in \mathbb{R}$ and $\beta \in \mathbb{R}_+$. The uncertainty set Ω is the set of continuous functions from $\mathbb{R} \times \mathbb{R}^2 \rightarrow \mathbb{R}$ which satisfy

$$|\omega(t, x)| \leq |x_1| \qquad \forall t \in \mathbb{R}, x \in \mathbb{R}^2 . \tag{4.2}$$

We wish to find a bound $\bar{\beta} \in \mathbb{R}_+$ which assures that (4.1) is exponentially stable for all $\beta < \bar{\beta}$.

Clearly, system (4.1) can be described by (1.6), (1.8) with L = 1,

$$f^o(t, x) \triangleq \begin{bmatrix} -x_1 & + & x_1 x_2^2 \\ -x_2 & - & x_1^2 x_2 \end{bmatrix}, \quad D_1 \triangleq \begin{bmatrix} 0 \\ 1 \end{bmatrix}, \quad E_1 \triangleq [1 \;\; 0] .$$

Also, letting

$$P \triangleq Q \triangleq \begin{bmatrix} 1 & 0 \\ 0 & 1 \end{bmatrix},$$

(2.1) is satisfied; hence P is a LM for the nominal system

$$\dot{x}_1 = -x_1 \;\; + x_1 x_2^2$$

$$\dot{x}_2 = -x_2 \;\; - x_1^2 x_2$$

and this system is exponentially stable with rate 1.

Recalling Lemma 2.1, P is a CLM for (4.1) iff $\beta < \beta^*$ where β^* is given by (2.2). For this example β^* is readily calculated to be 2. Hence (4.1) is exponentially stable if

$$\beta < 2 \quad .$$

Using the results of Section 3, one obtains the more conservative bound $\bar{\beta}(Q) = 1$.

5. LINEAR TIME-INVARIANT NOMINAL SYSTEMS

In this section we consider uncertain systems whose nominal parts are linear and time-invariant, i.e.,

$$\dot{x} = Ax + \sum_{j=1}^{L} D_j g_j(t, x, \omega) \tag{5.1a}$$

$$\omega \in \Omega \tag{5.1b}$$

where $A \in \mathbb{R}^{n \times n}$, all other quantities are as defined in Section 1, and the functions g_j, $j = 1, 2, \cdots, L$, satisfy (1.8c).

A necessary and sufficient condition for the existence of a LM for the nominal system

$$\dot{x} = Ax \tag{5.2}$$

is that A be Hurwitz, i.e., all the eigenvalues of A have negative real parts. In fact, one can show that A is Hurwitz iff for each $Q \in P^n$, there exists $P \in P^n$ which satisfies

$$PA + A^T P + 2Q = 0 \quad ; \tag{5.3}$$

see Ref. 10. Note that (5.3) is equivalent to

$$x^T PAx = -\|x\|_Q^2 \qquad \forall x \in \mathbb{R}^n \quad ; \tag{5.4}$$

i.e., P is an LM for (5.2).

In earlier literature, Refs. 15, 16 considered systems with a single, unstructured, uncertain term, i.e., $L = 1$, $D_1 = E_1 = I$, and the system is described by

$$\dot{x} = Ax + \beta\, g(t, x, \omega) \tag{5.5a}$$

where

$$\|g(t, x, \omega)\| \le \|x\| \qquad \forall \omega \in \Omega \ . \tag{5.5b}$$

These references demonstrate that if A is Hurwitz and $P, Q \in P^n$ are chosen to satisfy (5.3) then P is a CLM for (5.5) if

$$\beta < \mu(Q)$$

where

$$\mu(Q) \triangleq \lambda_m(Q)/\lambda_M(P) = \lambda_m(Q)\lambda_m(P^{-1}) \ . \tag{5.6}$$

For a system described by (5.5), the robustness measure $\bar{\beta}(R)$ defined in Lemma 3.1 is given by

$$\bar{\beta}(R) = [\lambda_m(P^{-2}R)\lambda_m(R)]^{1/2}\lambda_m(R^{-1}Q) \quad ; \tag{5.7}$$

hence

$$\mu(Q) = \bar{\beta}(I) \ .$$

Recalling Lemma 3.1, it follows that

$$\mu(Q) \le \bar{\beta}(Q) = [\lambda_m(P^{-2}Q)\lambda_m(Q)]^{1/2} \quad ; \tag{5.8}$$

i.e., $\bar{\beta}(Q)$ is less conservative than $\mu(Q)$.

Consider now a system with a single, structured, uncertain term, i.e.,

$$\dot{x} = Ax + \beta D g(t, x, \omega) \tag{5.9a}$$

where $D \in \mathbb{R}^{n \times k}$ and

$$\{g(t, x, \omega) : \omega \in \Omega\} = \{v \in \mathbb{R}^k : \|v\| \le \|Ex\|\} \tag{5.9b}$$

for some $E \in \mathbb{R}^{l \times n}$. Define a transfer function $G : C \to C^{l \times k}$ by

$$G(s) \triangleq E(sI - A)^{-1}D \tag{5.10}$$

and let

$$\|G\|_\infty \triangleq \sup_{\eta \in \mathbb{R}} \|G(j\eta)\| \ . \tag{5.11}$$

Refs. 12, 13 demonstrate that there exists a CLM for (5.9) iff

(i) A is Hurwitz and

(ii)

$$\|G\|_\infty \beta < 1 \ . \tag{5.12}$$

In addition to demonstrating that conditions (i), (ii) are sufficient for the existence of a CLM for (5.9), Refs. 8, 9 demonstrate that these conditions are necessary and sufficient for exponential stability of the following uncertain system which contains complex uncertainties

$$\dot{x} = Ax + \beta D\omega Ex \ ,$$
$$\omega \in \Omega = \{\omega \in C^{k\times l} : \|\omega\| \leq 1\} \ ;$$

see also Ref. 14.

For systems described by (5.1) and (1.8c) with $l_j = k_j$, $j = 1, 2, \cdots, L$, Ref. 6 contains a condition which is necessary and sufficient for an LM of (5.2) to be a CLM for (5.1) - (1.8c). This condition utilizes the notion of a structured singular value. See also Ref. 2.

6. APPENDIX

The following lemma is used in the proof of Lemma 3.2.

Lemma 6.1. Suppose A, B, C $\in \mathbb{R}^{n\times n}$ are symmetric with A, B positive semi-definite and C positive definite. Then

$$\lambda_M(AB) \leq \lambda_M(AC)\lambda_M(C^{-1}B) \ .$$

Proof. Since $C \in P^n$, there exists a nonsingular matrix $T \in \mathbb{R}^{n\times n}$ such that

$$C = T^T T \ .$$

Also, for any matrix $M \in \mathbb{R}^{n\times n}$ with real eigenvalues,

$$\lambda_M(M) = \lambda_M(TMT^{-1}) = \lambda_M(T^{-1}MT) \ .$$

Since A, B, and C are symmetric, the eigenvalues of AC and $C^{-1}B$ are real; hence,

$$\begin{aligned}\lambda_M(AC)\lambda_M(C^{-1}B) &= \lambda_M(AT^TT)\lambda_M(T^{-1}T^{-T}B)\\ &= \lambda_M(TAT^T)\lambda_M(T^{-T}BT^{-1})\\ &= \|TAT^T\|\,\|T^{-T}BT^{-1}\|\\ &\geq \|TABT^{-1}\|\\ &\geq \lambda_M(TABT^{-1})\\ &= \lambda_M(AB) \ ;\end{aligned}$$

i.e.,

$$\lambda_M(AB) \leq \lambda_M(AC)\lambda_M(C^{-1}B) \ .$$

□

ACKNOWLEDGEMENTS

Discussions with Dr. E. P. Ryan, University of Bath were very useful.

REFERENCES

1. BECKER, N., and GRIMM, W., *Comments on "Reduced Conservatism in Stability Robustness Bounds by State Transformation"*, IEEE Transactions on Automatic Control, Vol. 33, pp. 223-224, 1988.
2. BOYD, S., and YANG, Q., *Structured and Simultaneous Lyapunov Functions for System Stability Problems,* Technical Report No. L-104-88-1, Stanford University, 1988.
3. CORLESS, M., *Guaranteed Rates of Exponential Convergence for Uncertain Systems,* Journal of Optimization Theory and Applications (to appear).
4. CORLESS, M., and DA, D., *Some Robustness Measures in Lyapunov Stability Theory,* in preparation.
5. CORLESS, M., GAROFALO, F., and LEITMANN, G., *Guaranteeing Exponential Convergence for Uncertain Systems,* this proceedings.
6. DOYLE, J., and PACKARD, A., *Uncertain Multivariable Systems from a State Space Perspective,* Proceedings of the 1987 American Control Conference, Minneapolis, Minnesota, pp. 2147-2152, 1987.
7. ESLAMI, M., and RUSSEL, D.L., *On Stability with Large Parameter Variations: Stemming from the Direct Method of Lyapunov,* IEEE Transactions on Automatic Control, Vol. AC-25, pp. 1231-1234, 1980.
8. HINRICHSEN, D., and PRITCHARD, A.J., *Stability Radii of Linear Systems,* Systems & Control Letters, Vol. 7, pp. 1-10, 1986.
9. HINRICHSEN, D., and PRITCHARD, A.J., *Stability Radius for Structured Perturbations and the Algebraic Riccati Equation,* Systems & Control Letters, Vol. 8, pp. 105-113, 1986.
10. KALMAN, R.E., and BERTRAM, J.E., *Control System Analysis and Design Via the "Second Method" of Lyapunov, I: Continuous-Time Systems,* Journal of Basic Engineering, Vol. 32, pp. 317-393, 1960.
11. KANTOR, J.C., and KEENAN, M.R., *Stability Constraints for Nonlinear State Feedback,* Proceedings of the 1987 American Control Conference, Minneapolis, Minnesota, pp. 2126-2131, 1987.
12. KHARGONEKAR, P.P., PETERSEN, I.R., and ZHOU, K., *Feedback Stabilization of Uncertain Systems,* 25th Annual Allerton Conference on Communications, Control and Computing, Allerton Park, University of Illinois, 1987.
13. KHARGONEKAR, P.P., PETERSEN, I.R., and ZHOU, K., *Robust Stabilization of Uncertain Systems and H^{∞} Optimal Control,* in preparation.
14. MARTIN, J.M., and HEWER, G.A., *Smallest Destabilizing Perturbations for Linear Systems,* International Journal of Control, Vol. 45, pp. 1495-1504, 1987.
15. MICHAEL, G.J., and MERRIAM, C.W., III, *Stability of Parametrically Disturbed Linear Optimal Control Systems,* Journal of Mathematical Analysis and Applications, Vol 28, pp. 294-302, 1969.
16. PATEL, R.V., and TODA, M., *Quantitative Measures of Robustness for Uncertain Systems,* Proceedings of the 1986 Joint Automatic Control Council, 1986.
17. PATEL, R.V., TODA, M., and SRIDHAR, B., *Robustness of Linear Quadratic State Feedback Designs in the Presence of System Uncertainty,* IEEE Transactions on Automatic Control, Vol. AC-22, pp. 945-949, 1977.
18. QUI, L., and DAVIDSON, E.J., *New Perturbation Bounds for the Robust Stability of Linear State Space Models,* Proceedings of the 1986 Conference on Decision and Control, Athens, Greece, pp. 751-755, 1986.
19. YEDAVALLI, R.K., *Improved Measures of Stability Robustness for Linear State Space Models,* IEEE Transactions on Automatic Control, Vol. AC-30, pp. 557-579, 1985.

20. YEDAVALLI, R.K., *Perturbation Bounds for Robust Stability in Linear State Space Models,* International Journal of Control, Vol. 42, pp. 1507-1517, 1985.

21. YEDAVALLI, R.K., *Stability Analysis of Interval Matrices: Another Sufficient Condition,* International Journal of Control Vol. 43, pp. 767-772, 1986.

22. YEDAVALLI, R.K., BANDA, S.S., and RIDGELY, D.D, *Time-Domain Stability Robustness Measures for Linear Regulators,* Journal of Guidance, Vol. 8, pp. 520-524, 1985.

23. YEDAVALLI, R.K., and LIANG, L., *Reduced Conservatism in Stability Robustness Bounds by State Transformation,* IEEE Transactions on Automatic Control, Vol. AC-31, pp. 863-866, 1986.

24. ZHOU, K., and KHARGONEKAR, P.P., *Stability Robustness Bounds For Linear State-Space Models with Structured Uncertainty,* IEEE Transactions on Automatic Control, Vol. AC-32, pp. 621-623, 1987.

AUTHOR INDEX

SUBJECT INDEX